Handbook of Nephrology & Hypertension

Fifth Edition

D1584931

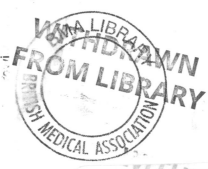

www.bma.org.uk/library

Handbook of Nephrology & Hypertension

Fifth Edition

Editors

Christopher S. Wilcox, M.D., Ph.D., F.R.C.P.(U.K.), F.A.C.P.

George E. Schreiner Professor of Nephrology
Director, Georgetown Cardiovascular-Kidney Institute
Chief, Division of Nephrology and Hypertension
Vice Chair for Academic Affairs, Department of Medicine
Georgetown University Medical Center
Washington, DC

C. Craig Tisher, M.D.

Professor of Medicine, Pathology and Anatomy & Cell Biology
Dean, College of Medicine
Folke H. Peterson/Dean's Distinguished Professor
Division of Nephrology, Hypertension, and Transplantation
University of Florida College of Medicine
Gainesville, Florida

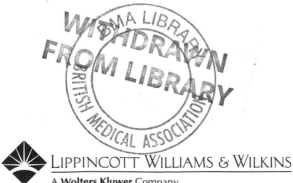

LIPPINCOTT WILLIAMS & WILKINS
A **Wolters Kluwer** Company
Philadelphia • Baltimore • New York • London
Buenos Aires • Hong Kong • Sydney • Tokyo

Acquisitions Editor: Lisa McAllister
Developmental Editor: Nicole T. Dernoski
Supervising Editor: Dave Murphy
Production Editor: Kate Sallwasser, Silverchair Science + Communications
Senior Manufacturing Manager: Ben Rivera
Compositor: Silverchair Science + Communications
Printer: RR Donnelley

© 2005 by LIPPINCOTT WILLIAMS & WILKINS
530 Walnut Street
Philadelphia, PA 19106 USA
LWW.com

Printed in the USA

Library of Congress Cataloging-in-Publication Data

Handbook of nephrology & hypertension / editors, Christopher S. Wilcox, C. Craig Tisher.-- 5th ed.
   p. ; cm.
   Rev. ed of: Nephrology and hypertension / editors, C. Craig Tisher, Christopher S. Wilcox. 1999.
   Includes bibliographical references and index.
   ISBN 0-7817-5076-8
   1. Nephrology--Handbooks, manuals, etc. 2. Kidneys--Diseases--Handbooks, manuals, etc. 3. Hypertension--Handbooks, manuals, etc. I. Title: Handbook of nephrology and hypertension. II. Wilcox, Christopher S. III. Tisher, C. Craig, 1936- IV. Nephrology and hypertension.
   [DNLM: 1. Kidney Diseases--Handbooks. 2. Hypertension, Renal--Handbooks. WJ 39
   H236 2004]
   RC903.H357 2004
   616.6'1--dc22

                                                                    2004011738

10 9 8 7 6 5 4 3 2 1

To Audrae A. Tisher and Linda Wilcox, and to the many Fellows in the Division of Nephrology and Hypertension at the University of Florida and at Georgetown University who have contributed to previous editions of this book.

Contents

Contributing Authors

From the Division of Nephrology, Hypertension, and Transplantation at the University of Florida College of Medicine, Gainesville, Florida:

Thomas G. Baumgartner, Pharm.D., M.Ed.
Clinical Professor of Pharmacy, Medicine, Nursing, and Dentistry
Division of Gastroenterology, Hepatology, and Nutrition

Geraldine Shaw Bichier, M.B.B.Ch., M.D.
Assistant Professor of Medicine
Center for Clinical Trials Research

Janet M. Caruso, M.D.
Assistant Professor of Medicine

Ronald M. Goldin, M.D.
Senior Clinical Fellow in Nephrology

Richard J. Johnson, M.D., F.A.C.P.
Professor and Chief, Division of Nephrology, Hypertension, and Transplantation
J. Robert Cade Professor of Nephrology

Kirsten M. Madsen, M.D., Ph.D.
Associate Professor of Medicine

Edward A. Ross, M.D.
Associate Professor of Medicine

C. Craig Tisher, M.D.
Professor of Medicine, Pathology and Anatomy & Cell Biology
Dean, College of Medicine
Folke H. Peterson/Dean's Distinguished Professor

Jill W. Verlander, D.V.M.
Associate Scientist
Department of Medicine and Anatomy & Cell Biology

I. David Weiner, M.D.
Associate Professor of Medicine and Physiology
Chief, Renal Section
Malcom Randall Veterans Affairs Medical Center

Charles S. Wingo, M.D.
Professor of Medicine and Physiology

From the Division of Nephrology at the University of Alabama, Birmingham, Alabama:

Anupam Agarwal, M.D.
Associate Professor of Medicine

Matthew Kapturczak, M.D.
Assistant Professor of Medicine

From the Division of Nephrology, Hennepin County Medical Center, University of Minnesota School of Medicine, Minneapolis, Minnesota:

John R. Silkensen, M.D.
Assistant Professor of Medicine

From the Division of Nephrology and Hypertension, Georgetown University Medical Center, Washington, DC:

Oscar Adler, M.D., Ph.D.
Senior Nephrology Fellow

Shakil Aslam, M.D.
Assistant Professor of Medicine

Awad A. El-Magbri, M.B.Ch.B., M.D., M.R.C.P.(U.K.)
Senior Nephrology Fellow

Joyce M. Gonin, M.B.Ch.B.
Associate Professor of Medicine

Aaron Francis Kulick, M.D.
Senior Nephrology Fellow

Francisco Llach, M.D.
Professor of Medicine
Director of Clinical Nephrology

Connie C. Mere, M.D.
Senior Nephrology Fellow

Paul S. Modlinger, M.D.
Senior Nephrology Fellow

Kinjal R. Patel, M.D.
Senior Nephrology Fellow

Adam M. Pearlman, M.D.
Senior Nephrology Fellow

Julie Raggio, M.D.
Senior Nephrology Fellow

Robert J. Rubin, M.D.
Distinguished Professor of Medicine

Brendan J. Smyth, Ph.D., M.D.
Clinical Pharmacology Research Fellow
Clinical Pharmacology Division

Jason G. Umans, M.D., Ph.D.
Associate Professor of Medicine and of Obstetrics and Gynecology

Christopher S. Wilcox, M.D., Ph.D., F.R.C.P.(U.K.), F.A.C.P.
George E. Schreiner Professor of Nephrology
Director, Georgetown Cardiovascular-Kidney Institute
Chief, Division of Nephrology and Hypertension
Vice Chair for Academic Affairs, Department of Medicine

From Division of Nephrology, Department of Medicine, University of Puerto Rico, San Juan, Puerto Rico:

Lillian J. Borrego Conde, M.D.
Assistant Professor of Nephrology

From Department of Medicine, Mahidol University and Ramathibodi Hospital, Bangkok, Thailand:

Chagriya Kitiyakara, M.D.
Assistant Professor of Medicine

From Carolina Hospital and McLeod Hospital, Florence, South Carolina:

Wen-Ting Ouyang, M.D., M.R.C.P.(U.K.), F.A.C.P.

Preface

The fifth edition of this clinical text has been extensively revised and rewritten. Many chapters have new authors. New chapters have been added to address growing points on the subject. There is now a chapter on hypertension and renal disease in pregnancy. Also, there are four new chapters that detail the use of specific classes of drugs in hypertension. Included is an up-to-date table of the outcomes of the major controlled clinical trials describing the use of these drugs to prevent cardiovascular complications of hypertension or the progression of chronic kidney disease. Another new chapter on the strategies for prevention of progressive renal failure synthesizes the information in the chapters on individual drug classes. Another new chapter describes the management of anemia in renal disease, detailing the use of erythropoietin and its analogs, iron, and other therapy for the patient with chronic renal failure or end-stage renal disease. The section on hypertension, diagnosis, and management has been extensively expanded. The section on the use of drugs in renal failure has undergone major revision to make the information more comprehensive and of practical use to the clinician. It is our aim to provide the physician with the information needed to make the best treatment choices.

The original structure of previous editions, in which many chapters are coauthored by a Fellow and a faculty physician, has been retained. We believe that this combination provides an ideal balance. On one hand, contributions from a Fellow ensure that the information is current and strictly relevant to the needs of the practicing clinician. On the other hand, contributions from our large and diverse faculty at the Universities of Florida and Georgetown ensure that there is an internationally recognized expert in the field as the senior author of each chapter. As the two editors, we have remained closely involved with the development of the chapters. Extensive editorial input gives the book balance and cohesion. The aim is to provide a concise, yet sufficiently detailed, text so that the reader can derive useful, accurate, quantitative, and current information to aid in the care of patients with nephrologic and hypertensive problems.

This book is designed to provide all the information in the fields of nephrology and hypertension required by a resident in training, by a general internist or family practitioner, or by a physician in another specialty. This text should be quite useful for those preparing for the board examinations in internal medicine.

This book is intended as a practical clinical manual. However, nephrology and hypertension encompass a wide variety of disciplines that include physiology, anatomy, pathology, biochemistry, immunology, molecular biology, pharmacology, and cell biology. Therefore, key findings from these diverse disciplines are included in the text to provide the practitioner with the information needed to make rational clinical judgments.

C.S.W.
C.C.T.

Approach to the Patient with Renal Disease

1

Renal Structure in Relation to Function

Kirsten M. Madsen and Jill W. Verlander

I. **Gross Anatomy.** The kidneys are located retroperitoneally from the T-12 to the L-3 vertebra. The right kidney is positioned slightly lower than the left. Each kidney is approximately 11–12 cm long, 5–7.5 cm wide, and 2.5–3 cm thick. Kidney weight in adult men is 125–170 g and in adult women is 115–155 g. On the medial margin is a cleft, the hilus, through which the renal pelvis, the renal artery and vein, lymphatics, and a nerve plexus pass into the sinus of the kidney (Fig. 1.1). The renal pelvis, an expansion of the upper end of the ureter, continues into funnel-shaped tubes called *the calyces* that connect with the renal papillae. The kidney is covered by a tough fibrous capsule that is normally smooth and easily removable.

The kidney can be divided into the cortex and medulla. In humans, the medulla forms 8–18 renal pyramids, the bases of which are located at the corticomedullary junction (Fig. 1.1). The apices of the pyramids extend toward the renal pelvis, each forming a papilla. From the base of the pyramids, medullary rays consisting of collecting ducts and the straight portions of proximal and distal tubules extend into the cortex. Based on segmentation of the nephron (Fig. 1.2), the medulla can be divided into an outer medulla, which in turn can be subdivided into an outer and inner stripe, and an inner medulla, which includes the renal papilla.

The functional unit of the kidney is the nephron, which consists of a renal corpuscle, or glomerulus, and its associated tubule (Fig. 1.2). The tubular portion of the nephron is composed of three major subdivisions: the proximal convoluted tubule (PCT), the loop of Henle, and the distal convoluted tubule (DCT). The latter continues into the collecting duct system, which is derived from the ureteric bud and, strictly speaking, is not part of the nephron. The loop of Henle includes the proximal straight tubule (pars recta of the proximal tubule), the thin limb segments, and the thick ascending limb (TAL) (pars recta of the distal tubule).

Each human kidney contains approximately 1.2 million nephrons. Those originating from outer and midcortical glomeruli have short loops of Henle that bend in the inner stripe of the outer medulla. Juxtamedullary nephrons originating from glomeruli located near the corticomedullary junction have long loops of Henle that reach into the inner medulla. In the human kidney, 10–15% of the glomeruli belong to long-looped nephrons.

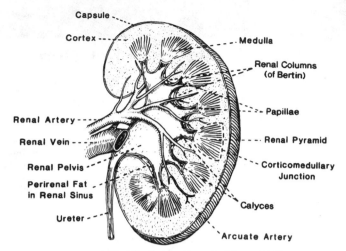

FIG. 1.1. Cut surface of a bisected kidney.

II. Microscopic Anatomy

A. Glomerulus. The glomeruli are located in the cortex. The human glomerulus measures approximately 200 µm in diameter and includes a capillary tuft and the surrounding parietal epithelium of Bowman's capsule. The glomerulus is responsible for the formation of an ultrafiltrate of plasma. It consists of a capillary network lined by a thin, fenestrated endothelium, a central mesangial region, and the visceral epithelium with its associated basement membrane (Fig. 1.3A). The filtration barrier between the blood and the urinary space is composed of the fenestrated endothelium, the peripheral glomerular basement membrane, and the slit pores between the foot processes of the visceral epithelial cells (Fig. 1.3B). The thin *endothelium* is perforated by pores, or fenestrae, measuring approximately 70–100 nm in diameter. It constitutes the initial barrier to the passage of blood constituents but is not believed to represent a significant barrier to the passage of macromolecules.

The *glomerular basement membrane* is located between the endothelium and the visceral epithelium and is approximately 300 nm thick. It is composed of three layers: a central dense layer, the lamina densa, and two electron-lucent layers—the lamina rara externa and lamina rara interna. The glomerular basement membrane is believed to constitute a size-selective as well as a charge-selective barrier to the passage of macromolecules. It is composed of various glycoproteins, including type IV and type V collagen, laminin, fibronectin, and negatively charged glycosaminoglycans rich in heparan sulfate. These anionic sites appear to be important in

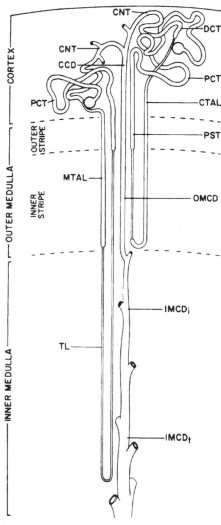

FIG. 1.2. Relationships between various segments of the nephron and zones of the kidney. CCD, cortical collecting duct; CNT, connecting segment; CTAL, cortical thick ascending limb; DCT, distal convoluted tubule; IMCD$_i$, initial inner medullary collecting duct; IMCD$_t$, terminal inner medullary collecting duct; MTAL, medullary thick ascending limb; OMCD, outer medullary collecting duct; PCT, proximal convoluted tubule; PST, proximal straight tubule; TL, thin limb of the loop of Henle.

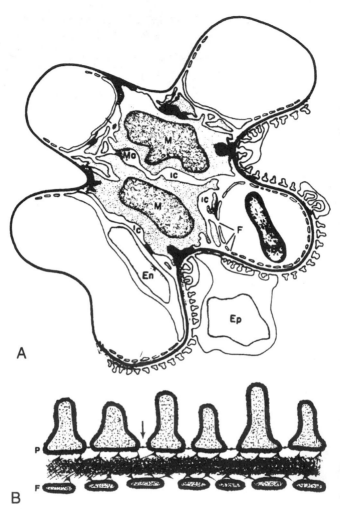

FIG. 1.3. A: Relationship among endothelial cells (En), epithelial cells (Ep), and mesangial cells (M) of the glomerulus. F, endothelial fenestrae; IC, intercellular channels; Ma, mesangial matrix. (From Latta H. Ultrastructure of the glomerulus and juxtaglomerular apparatus. In: Orloff J, Berliner RW, eds. *Handbook of physiology, Section 8: renal physiology.* Bethesda: American Physiological Society, 1973:1–29, with permission.) **B:** Glomerular basement membrane with adjoining endothelial fenestrae (F) and epithelial foot processes (P) with slit pores (*arrow*). (From Kanwar YS, Farquhar MG. Anionic sites in the glomerular basement membrane: in vivo and in vitro localization to the lamina rarae by cationic probes. *J Cell Biol* 1979;81:137–153, with permission.)

establishing the charge-selective properties of the filtration barrier.

The *visceral epithelial cells*, or *podocytes*, have long cytoplasmic processes that divide into foot processes, or pedicles, that are in close contact with the glomerular basement membrane. The space between adjacent foot processes is called the *filtration slit*, or *slit pore*, and it is closed by a thin membrane, the slit diaphragm. A recently identified protein, nephrin, which is located in the slit diaphragm, is believed to constitute a key component of the filtration barrier. The foot processes possess a negatively charged surface coat that is rich in sialic acid and is important for maintaining the normal structure and function of the filtration barrier. Removal of the anionic surface coat causes the foot processes to disappear and to be replaced by a continuous band of cytoplasm along the glomerular basement membrane. Similar changes called *foot process fusion* or *effacement* are observed in various proteinuric conditions.

The *mesangium* is separated from the capillary lumen by the endothelium and consists of mesangial cells and surrounding mesangial matrix. The mesangial cells provide structural support for the capillary loops. They contain numerous filaments and have contractile as well as phagocytic properties. Mesangial cells are stimulated to contract by angiotensin II, arginine vasopressin, and thromboxane, a response that is inhibited by prostaglandin E_2. Cell contraction is believed to limit filtration, perhaps by reducing the area of the glomerular filter. Mesangial cells are also phagocytic, and in certain forms of glomerulonephritis they appear to be involved in the sequestration of immune complexes from the glomerular tuft. Glomerular injury is often associated with mesangial cell proliferation and mesangial expansion.

The *parietal epithelium* of Bowman's capsule is continuous with the visceral epithelium at the vascular pole. At the urinary pole there is an abrupt transition from the parietal epithelium to the epithelium of the proximal tubule.

B. Juxtaglomerular Apparatus. The juxtaglomerular apparatus located at the vascular pole of the glomerulus has tubular and vascular components. The vascular components include the terminal portion of the afferent arteriole, the initial portion of the efferent arteriole, and the extraglomerular mesangium between the arterioles. The tubular component is a specialized part of the TAL called the *macula densa*. A population of cells in the vascular portion of the juxtaglomerular apparatus contains numerous granules. These granular cells secrete renin, which, via the generation of angiotensin, is involved in regulation of tubuloglomerular feedback and in control of aldosterone-stimulated sodium and potassium transport. The cells of the macula densa sense changes in the concentration of sodium chloride in the luminal fluid, which initiates the tubuloglomerular feedback response and regulates renin secretion. Therefore, the juxtaglomerular apparatus plays an important role in the control of renal hemodynamics and glomerular filtration as well as salt excretion.

C. Proximal Tubule. The proximal tubule includes an initial pars convoluta, or PCT, and a pars recta, or proximal straight tubule that is located in the medullary ray (Fig. 1.2). The PCT has numerous lateral cell processes that extend from the apical to the basal surface of the cell and interdigitate with similar cell processes from adjacent cells (Fig. 1.4). Mitochondria are located in these processes in close proximity to the cell membrane. The presence of these lateral cell processes and interdigitations gives rise to a complex extracellular compartment between the cells. This intercellular space is separated from the tubule lumen by the tight junction, or zonula occludens. A prominent endocytic–lysosomal system is present in the cells and is important in the reabsorption and catabolism of proteins from the tubule fluid. Based on morphologic differences, the proximal tubule can be subdivided into three distinct segments: The S_1 segment corresponds to the initial PCT; the S_2 segment corresponds to the terminal PCT and the initial proximal straight tubule; and the S_3 segment constitutes the remainder of the proximal straight tubule.

The main function of the proximal tubule is the reabsorption of sodium, chloride, bicarbonate, potassium, phosphate, water, and organic solutes, such as glucose and amino acids, and the secretion of organic acids and bases, including common drugs such as sali-

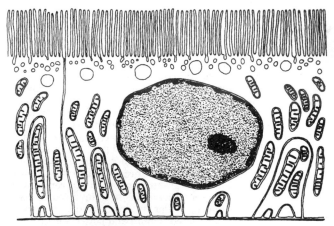

FIG. 1.4. Proximal tubule cell.

cylates, barbiturates, penicillin, and many diuretics. Much of the sodium reabsorption is an active process mediated by the Na^+/K^+-ATPase, or sodium pump, located in the basolateral plasma membrane. The transport of the various anions and organic solutes across the luminal membrane is coupled with the reabsorption of sodium down its concentration gradient. Fluid reabsorption is accomplished primarily by isosmotic water flow through the cells and the intercellular spaces via the water channel protein aquaporin-1, located in the apical and basolateral plasma membrane.

D. Thin Limb of the Loop of Henle. The thin limb of the loop of Henle extends from the proximal tubule to the TAL (Fig. 1.2). Short-looped nephrons have only a short descending thin limb segment that is located in the inner stripe of the outer medulla. Long-looped nephrons have both a long descending and a long ascending thin limb. Four morphologically distinct segments can be identified in the thin limb. All are lined by a flat epithelium containing few cell organelles.

The thin limb of the loop of Henle is important in the countercurrent multiplication mechanism. The descending limb is permeable to water but impermeable to sodium, whereas the ascending limb is almost impermeable to water but highly permeable to sodium and modestly permeable to urea. Accordingly, water diffuses out of the descending limb through aquaporin-1 water channels, and, subsequently, sodium exits the ascending limb through its concentration gradient. Thus, the countercurrent mechanism is involved in the maintenance of a hypertonic medullary interstitium and in the formation of a dilute tubule fluid.

E. Distal Tubule. The distal tubule includes the TAL, which can be subdivided into a medullary and a cortical segment, the macula densa, and the DCT (Fig. 1.2). The transition from the TAL to the DCT occurs shortly after the macula densa. Cells of the TAL and the DCT possess extensive invaginations of the basolateral plasma membrane and interdigitations of cell processes between adjacent cells. Numerous elongated mitochondria are located in the lateral cell processes in close proximity to the plasma membrane. In contrast to the proximal tubule, the luminal membrane of the distal tubule does not possess a brush border (Fig. 1.5). The ultrastructural composition of the distal tubule is characteristic of an epithelium involved in active transport. Both the TAL and the DCT are responsible for active reabsorption of sodium chloride, which is important in the countercurrent multiplication process and the urinary concentrating and diluting mechanisms. Because the TAL is relatively impermeable to water, the active reabsorption of sodium chloride creates a hypertonic interstitium and ensures the delivery of a hypotonic tubule fluid to the DCT. The TAL is the site of action for loop

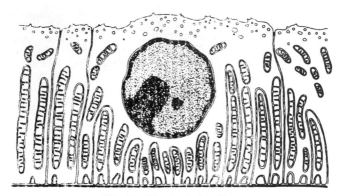

FIG. 1.5. Distal tubule cell.

diuretics (e.g., furosemide), whereas thiazide diuretics exert their effect mainly on the DCT.

The *connecting segment* is located between the distal tubule and the collecting duct (Fig. 1.2). It is a transition region where a mixture of cells from adjacent regions can be encountered, including DCT cells, connecting tubule cells, and collecting duct cells (intercalated and principal cells). The connecting segment is an important site of potassium secretion and calcium absorption.

F. Collecting Duct. The collecting duct system can be divided into the cortical, outer medullary, and inner medullary collecting duct (IMCD) (Fig. 1.2). The cortical collecting duct includes the initial collecting tubule and the segment located in the medullary ray. The epithelium of both the cortical collecting duct and the outer medullary collecting duct is composed of two distinct cell types, *principal cells* and *intercalated cells*, the latter constituting approximately one-third of the cells. Principal cells have a light cytoplasm with few cell organelles and a relatively smooth luminal surface (Fig. 1.6), whereas intercalated

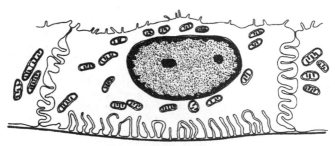

FIG. 1.6. Principal cell.

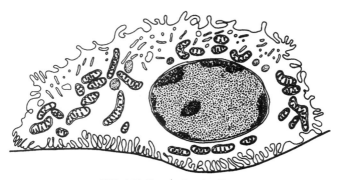

FIG. 1.7. Intercalated cell.

cells have a dark-staining cytoplasm with many mito-chondria and numerous small tubulovesicles (Fig. 1.7). The luminal surface of intercalated cells is covered with microprojections that are either microvilli or microplicae. Two different configurations of intercalated cells have been observed: type A cells, which are involved in hydro-gen ion secretion, and type B cells, which secrete bicar-bonate. A main function of principal cells in the cortical collecting duct is potassium secretion.

Intercalated cells gradually disappear in the early por-tion of the IMCD and are absent in the papillary portion. Cells in the terminal two-thirds of the IMCD are believed to constitute a distinct cell type that is called the *IMCD cell*. The IMCD cells have a very light cytoplasm and few organelles. They increase in height as the collecting duct descends toward the papillary tip. The IMCD cells are involved in the absorption of urea from the tubule lumen into the surrounding interstitium, which is important for the generation of a hypertonic renal medulla. The princi-pal cells and the IMCD cells are responsive to antidiuretic hormone. In the presence of antidiuretic hormone, water is reabsorbed from the collecting duct through the vaso-pressin-regulated water channel, aquaporin-2, located on the luminal cell surface. Other members of the water channel family, aquaporin-3 and aquaporin-4, are present within the basolateral membrane of the principal cells and IMCD cells. Reabsorbtion of water through these channels leads to the formation of a hypertonic urine. In the absence of antidiuretic hormone, the collecting duct is relatively impermeable to water, and a hypotonic urine is formed.

G. **Interstitium.** The interstitium is composed of intersti-tial cells and a loose, flocculent, extracellular material rich in glycosaminoglycans. Interstitial tissue is sparse in the cortex, where two types of interstitial cells have been described: one that resembles a fibroblast and another, less common mononuclear cell. In the medulla, there is a gradual increase in the amount of interstitial tissue from the outer medulla to the papillary tip. Three different types of interstitial cells have been described in the medulla: type I, the typical renomedullary interstitial cell; type II, a mononuclear cell; and type III, a pericyte. The renomedullary (type I) cells are very prominent in the inner medulla, where they are arranged in rows between adjacent tubules and vessels resembling rungs on a ladder. These cells have numerous lipid inclusions or droplets, whose function is not known with certainty. The renomedullary cells are important sites of prostaglandin E_2 production.

H. Vasculature. The blood flow to the kidneys is large, amounting to approximately 1,200 ml/min (20–25% of cardiac output). The renal artery divides into anterior and posterior segmental branches at the hilus of the kidney (Fig. 1.1). From the segmental arteries, lobar arteries run toward the papillae, where they divide into interlobar arteries that ascend along the sides of the renal pyramids. At the corticomedullary junction, they continue into the arcuate arteries, which run parallel to the surface of the kidney. From the arcuate arteries, interlobular arteries ascend into the cortex, where they give off afferent arterioles to the glomeruli. Blood leaves the glomeruli through the efferent arterioles that form the peritubular capillary networks in the cortex. The efferent arterioles from juxtamedullary glomeruli descend into the outer medulla, where they form vascular bundles containing the vasa recta through which the outer and inner medullae are supplied. Blood from the capillaries drains into the interlobular, arcuate, and interlobar veins, which accompany arteries of the same name, and finally leaves the kidney through the renal vein. Networks of lymphatics are present in the renal cortex and the renal capsule, but lymphatics have not been described in the medulla. In the cortex, they follow the arteries and are embedded in the periarterial interstitial tissue.

I. Innervation. The kidneys are innervated mainly via the celiac plexus and the greater splanchnic nerves. Adrenergic nerve fibers follow the blood vessels throughout the cortex and outer stripe of the outer medulla. Nerve endings have also been described in contact with both proximal and distal tubules in the cortex and with various components of the juxtaglomerular apparatus.

III. Suggested Readings

Clapp WL, Abrahamson DL. Development and gross anatomy of the kidney. In: Tisher CC, Brenner BM, eds. *Renal pathology with clinical and functional correlations*, 2nd ed. Philadelphia: JB Lippincott, 1994:3–59.

Kriz W, Kaissling B. Structural organization of the mammalian kidney. In: Seldin DW, Giebisch G, eds. *The kidney: physiology and pathophysiology*, 3rd ed. Philadelphia: Lippincott Williams & Wilkins, 2000:587–654.

Madsen KM, Brenner BM. Structure and function of the renal tubule and interstitium. In: Tisher CC, Brenner BM, eds. *Renal pathology with clinical and functional correlations*, 2nd ed. Philadelphia: JB Lippincott, 1994:661–698.

Tisher CC, Brenner BM. Structure and function of the glomerulus. In: Tisher CC, Brenner BM, eds. *Renal pathology with clinical and functional correlations*, 2nd ed. Philadelphia: JB Lippincott, 1994:143–161.

Tisher CC, Madsen KM. Anatomy of the kidney. In: Brenner BM, ed. *The kidney*, 7th ed. Philadelphia: WB Saunders, 2004:3–72.

Evaluation of Kidney Structure: Radiology and Biopsy

C. Craig Tisher

The patient with kidney disease often presents with nonspecific signs and symptoms, including nausea, anorexia, lethargy, edema, dyspnea, and diminished urine output. Consequently, the physician must rely on laboratory studies to assist in the evaluation and diagnosis of kidney disease. This chapter reviews the use of radiologic procedures and the kidney biopsy to aid in the evaluation of the upper urinary tract.

I. **Radiologic Assessment**
   A. **Ultrasonography.** Ultrasound resolution is 1–2 cm. It is useful in the assessment of renal location, contour, and size. It can also be used to identify the cortex, medulla, renal pyramids, and a distended collecting system or ureter (Table 2.1). A kidney length of <9 cm or a size difference of >1.5 cm between the two kidneys is abnormal in an adult. *Simple cysts* are common and are uniformly benign. They contain no internal echoes, have a sharply defined smooth internal wall, and increase through transmission of posterior sound energy. Other hypoechoic renal mass lesions to consider include lymphoma, melanoma, infarct, hematoma, and xanthogranulomatous pyelonephritis. Complex cysts or solid lesions require further investigation with contrast computed tomography (CT), magnetic resonance imaging (MRI), or, possibly, angiography. Ultrasound has become the procedure of choice in the early diagnosis or screening of autosomal dominant polycystic kidney disease. *Hydronephrosis* appears as a multiloculated fluid collection within the renal sinus; however, ultrasound does not assess the functional importance of obstruction. An apparent obstruction can occur with anatomic variants such as an extrarenal pelvis, vesicoureteric reflux, and pregnancy. Hydronephrosis may persist after obstruction has been relieved. A furosemide renogram may document functional obstruction. Investigation of the renal vasculature is possible using color Doppler.
   B. **Intravenous Pyelography.** The intravenous pyelogram (IVP) provides an overview of the kidneys, ureters, and bladder. The nephrogram is formed by opacification of the renal parenchyma; its density depends on the glomerular filtration rate, rate of tubular fluid reabsorption, dose of radiographic contrast agent, and the rate of intravenous injection. The IVP can demonstrate gross differences in function between the kidneys from the nephrogram

TABLE 2.1. Indications for renal ultrasound

To quantify kidney size
To screen for hydronephrosis
To characterize kidney mass lesions
To evaluate perirenal space for abscess or hematoma
To screen for autosomal dominant polycystic kidney disease
To localize kidney for invasive procedures
To assess residual bladder volume in excess of 100 ml
To evaluate for renal vein thrombosis (Doppler)
To assess renal blood flow (Doppler)

phase. Renal insufficiency (serum creatinine >2–3 mg/dl) decreases the diagnostic value of the IVP and greatly increases the danger of causing acute renal failure. Normal renal size as measured by pyelography is approximately 11 cm, which exceeds that measured by ultrasound because of a magnification of approximately 10%. The left kidney is normally larger than the right. The IVP should be examined for renal size and position, calcifications, distorting intrinsic or extrinsic mass lesions, adequacy of parenchymal thickness, abnormalities of cortical contour or papillary appearance, dilation or blunting of calyces, abnormal position or course of the ureters, reflux, congenital variants, and completeness of bladder emptying (Table 2.2).

C. **Computed Tomography.** CT is useful for further investigation of abnormalities discovered on ultrasound or IVP. The CT is performed with contrast except when limited to demonstrating hemorrhage or calcification. The contrast media are filtered by the glomeruli and concentrated in the tubules, thus allowing parenchymal enhancement and visualization of neoplasms or cysts. The renal vessels and ureters can be identified. Spiral CT scan with intravenous radiocontrast injection, or *CT angiography*, is an emerging noninvasive procedure to evaluate renal vasculature, especially when renovascular hypertension is suspected. The CT is useful in the evaluation of mass lesions or fluid collections in the kidney or retroperitoneal space, particularly when ultrasound examination is hindered by intraabdominal gas or obesity (Table 2.3).

D. **Magnetic Resonance Imaging.** The loss of the corticomedullary demarcation in MRI is a nonspecific feature

TABLE 2.2. Indications for an intravenous pyelogram

To assess kidney size and contour
To investigate recurrent urinary tract infection
To detect and locate calculi
To evaluate suspected urinary tract obstruction
To evaluate cause of hematuria

TABLE 2.3.   Indications for computed tomography

To further evaluate a kidney mass
To display calcification patterns in a mass
To evaluate a nonfunctioning kidney
To delineate extent of kidney trauma
To guide percutaneous needle aspiration or biopsy
To diagnose adrenal causes for hypertension

of renal disease. Renal cysts are well visualized, but, unlike CT, MRI cannot accurately define foci of calcification. In the staging of solid renal lesions, MRI may be superior to CT because it can detect tumor thrombus in major vessels and can distinguish hilar collateral vessels from lymph nodes. However, some renal neoplasms appear homogeneous with surrounding normal renal parenchyma and therefore may be missed with noncontrast MRI. MRI can help in differentiating adrenal mass lesions because characteristic images may occur in pheochromocytoma; it is also useful to diagnose renal vein thrombosis (Table 2.4). MR angiography, especially when performed with intravenous contrast administration, is being used more commonly to evaluate renal arteries for the presence of stenosis. It is superior to digital subtraction angiography for the detection of renal artery stenosis and is less invasive than conventional angiography.

E. **Arteriography and Venography.** Contrast imaging of the arterial and venous vasculature is useful to assess renal artery stenosis, nephrosclerosis, renal vein thrombosis, renal infarction, or a renal mass. It is performed by percutaneous cannulation of femoral vessels and sometimes aided by digital subtraction techniques. *Arteriography* is useful in the evaluation of atherosclerotic or fibrodysplastic stenotic lesions of the renal arteries, aneurysms, arteriovenous fistulas, large vessel vasculitis, renal infarction, and renal mass lesions. It can be combined with selective renal vein renin sampling for evaluation of renovascular hypertension, percutaneous transluminal balloon angioplasty or stent placement, or renal ablation. *Venography* is performed to diagnose renal vein thrombosis.

TABLE 2.4.   Indications for magnetic resonance imaging

To serve as an adjunct to computed tomography in evaluating kidney masses
To serve as an alternative to computed tomography in patients who are intolerant of radiographic contrast agents
To evaluate suspected pheochromocytoma
To assess renal vein thrombosis

F. Summary. Radiologic tests can be very valuable diagnostic tools; however, they are expensive and carry a risk of adverse reactions. Proper patient selection and preparation can increase the value of the procedure and diminish toxicity. Although most contrast studies are now performed using low osmolar nonionic agents, they, too, can induce acute renal failure or vascular thrombosis. Prevention and management of radiocontrast-induced renal damage are discussed in Chapter 30. Consultation with the radiologist before selecting the test is often very helpful.

II. Renal Biopsy. Percutaneous needle biopsy of the kidney can be useful for establishing a diagnosis, assessing prognosis, monitoring disease progression, or selecting a rational therapy.

   A. Indications

      Acute Renal Failure

      When the underlying cause of acute renal failure is not evident initially, or recovery of renal function has not occurred after 3–4 weeks of supportive therapy, biopsy may be necessary to distinguish acute tubular necrosis from a host of other renal diseases that may require alternative management (see Chapter 30).

      Nephrotic Syndrome

      Renal biopsy is usually performed in the adult nephrotic patient without evidence of systemic disease to diagnose primary glomerular diseases. The most frequently encountered entities include membranous glomerulonephritis, focal segmental glomerulosclerosis, membranoproliferative glomerulonephritis, immunoglobulin A nephropathy, amyloidosis, and minimal change disease (see Chapters 6, 8, and 11).

      Proteinuria

      In the setting of persistent proteinuria of 2 g/24 hr/1.73 m^2 or more or when associated with an abnormal urine sediment or with documented functional deterioration, a renal biopsy may detect underlying kidney disease. Patients with orthostatic proteinuria do not require biopsy (see Chapter 6).

      Hematuria

      Renal biopsy may be helpful in patients with microscopic hematuria persisting longer than 6 months or in those with episodic gross hematuria or a family history of hematuria, particularly when there is an associated abnormal urine sediment or proteinuria. Secondary causes of hematuria must be excluded. Likely pathologic findings include benign essential hematuria, Alport's syndrome, thin basement membrane disease, and immunoglobulin A nephropathy. Usually, biopsy is not helpful in the clinical setting of isolated microscopic hematuria (see Chapter 5).

      Systemic Disease

      Various systemic disorders may have associated kidney involvement. These include diabetes mellitus, systemic lupus erythematosus, Schönlein-Henoch purpura, polyarteritis nodosa, Goodpasture's syndrome, Wegener's granulomatosis, and certain dysproteinemias. Biopsy is often performed to confirm the diagnosis, establish the extent of renal involvement, and guide management (see Chapters 9, 10, and 11).

Transplant Allograft

Biopsy of the allograft helps differentiate various forms of rejection from acute tubular necrosis, drug-induced tubulointerstitial nephritis or nephrotoxicity, hemorrhagic infarction, and de novo or recurrent glomerulonephritis (see Chapter 35).

B. Contraindications. Commonly accepted contraindications to percutaneous needle biopsy include a solitary or ectopic kidney (except transplant allografts), a horseshoe kidney, the presence of an uncorrected bleeding disorder, severe uncontrolled hypertension, small kidneys (usually indicative of chronic irreversible renal disease), renal infection, renal neoplasm, or an uncooperative patient.

C. Patient Preparation and Complications. Routine laboratory tests before biopsy should include a prothrombin time, partial thromboplastin time, complete blood count, platelet count, blood type, an antibody screen for possible crossmatching should the need for transfusion arise, and urinalysis to exclude a urinary tract infection. If coagulation parameters are abnormal, a bleeding time should be obtained. Patients should avoid ingestion of nonsteroidal antiinflammatory agents or aspirin in the week preceding biopsy. The percutaneous biopsy is usually performed with ultrasound or fluoroscopic guidance. After biopsy, the patient should remain on bed rest for up to 24 hours. Frequent vital signs are recorded to monitor evidence of hypovolemia as a result of hemorrhage. Hematocrits are obtained 4 hours after the biopsy and again the next morning. Aliquots of each voided urine are saved to observe for gross hematuria. Increasingly, percutaneous needle biopsy of the kidney is being performed in the outpatient setting in carefully selected patients.

The most frequent complication is bleeding, but that is usually self-limited. Significant bleeding requiring transfusion, percutaneous arterial embolization of a bleeding vessel, or nephrectomy is uncommon, with an occurrence rate of 2.1%. The mortality rate of 0.07% is comparable with that of percutaneous liver biopsy or coronary angiography. When percutaneous needle biopsy is technically not feasible and a histologic diagnosis is imperative, an open biopsy or a laparoscopic biopsy should be considered.

The tissue specimen should be submitted for light microscopy, immunofluorescence microscopy, and electron microscopy and evaluated by a pathologist experienced in interpretation of kidney biopsies.

III. Suggested Readings

Amis ED. Contemporary uroradiology. *Radiol Clin North Am* 1991;29:437–650.

Croker BP, Tisher CC. Indications for and interpretation of the renal biopsy: evaluation by light, electron and immunofluorescence microscopy. In: Schrier RW, ed. *Diseases of the kidney and urinary tract*, 7th ed. Philadelphia: Lippincott Williams & Wilkins, 2001:457–487.

Deininger HK, Beil D, Schmidt C, et al. Digital subtraction angiography and other noninvasive methods for evaluation of renal circulation and hypertension. *Uremia Invest* 1985;9:231–241.

Gimenez LF, Micali S, Chen RW, et al. Laparoscopic renal biopsy. *Kidney Int* 1998;54:525–529.

Haas M. A re-evaluation of routine electron microscopy in the examination of native renal biopsies. *J Am Soc Nephrol* 1997;8:70–76.

Olbricht CJ, Paul K, Prokop M, et al. Minimally invasive diagnosis of renal artery stenosis by spiral computed tomography angiography. *Kidney Int* 1995;48:1332–1337.

Parsons RB, Simpson WL Jr. Imaging. In: Johnson RJ, Feehally J, eds. *Comprehensive clinical nephrology*, 2nd ed. St. Louis: Mosby, 2003:47–62.

Tisher CC. Clinical indications for kidney biopsy. In: Tisher CC, Brenner BM, eds. *Renal pathology with clinical and functional correlations*, 2nd ed. Philadelphia: JB Lippincott, 1994:75–84.

Evaluation of Kidney Function: Biochemical and Nuclear Medicine Tests

Adam M. Pearlman and Joyce M. Gonin

This chapter reviews the basic biochemical studies and nuclear medicine tests used to assess renal function. See also Chapter 4.

I. Biochemical Tests

A. Assessment of Glomerular Filtration Rate. Estimating the glomerular filtration rate (GFR) is useful for measuring the overall functional capacity of the kidneys, as a predictor of time to the onset of end-stage renal disease, and for dosing medications appropriately.

B. Blood Urea Nitrogen. The normal blood urea nitrogen (BUN) range is 7–18 mg/dl or 2.5–6.4 mmol/L. Urea is freely filtered at the glomerulus but is up to 50% reabsorbed. The reabsorbed fraction is increased by volume depletion, which accounts for an elevated BUN level or creatinine ratio in this circumstance. Urea clearance is an imprecise estimate of GFR. Moreover, many conditions may affect BUN independent of the GFR:

- Increased BUN: High-protein diet or increased protein catabolism from gastrointestinal bleeding, corticosteroids, tissue trauma, burns, or tetracyclines
- Decreased BUN: Low-protein diet or decreased protein catabolism from liver disease or cachexia

C. Serum Creatinine. The upper limit of serum creatinine (S_{cr}) is 1.2–1.5 mg/dl or 106–133 μmol/L. Creatinine is freely filtered at the glomerulus, it is secreted at the proximal tubule, and some is reabsorbed. However, the S_{cr} normally provides a better estimate of the GFR than does the BUN because the degree of creatinine reabsorption and secretion is relatively small compared to the filtration. Thus, a rise in S_{cr} from 1.0–2.0 mg/dl normally indicates a decrease in GFR of approximately 50%. Several factors may affect S_{cr} independent of the GFR:

- Increased S_{cr}: Increased intake of creatine or creatinine from a recent meat meal or creatine supplements; decreased secretion because of competition from ketoacids, organic anions (in uremia), or drugs (e.g., cimetidine, trimethoprim, acetylsalicylic acid)
- Decreased S_{cr}: Decreased creatine intake or generation from diminished muscle mass associated with cachexia, aging, or a low-protein diet

- Variation in S_{cr}: Poor standardization between laboratories in calibration of S_{cr}

D. Creatinine Clearance. Creatinine clearance (C_{cr})can be directly measured from a timed urine collection (usually a 24-hour sample):

$$C_{cr} \text{ (ml/min)} = \text{urine creatinine (mg/dl)} \times \text{urine volume}$$
$$\text{(ml/24 hr)/ } S_{cr} \text{ (mg/dl)} \times 1{,}440 \text{ (min/24 hr)}$$

The normal ranges for adults aged 20–50 years are 97–137 ml/min/1.73 m^2 for men and 88–128 ml/min/1.73 m^2 for women. Values are often unreliable due to improper collection. Renal creatinine excretion should be 15–25 mg/kg/day in men and 12.5–20 mg/kg/day in women. These values decrease with advancing age and decreased muscle mass. Values outside the normal range should raise suspicion for an improper collection.

Tubular secretion of creatinine normally accounts for 10–40% of that excreted, but this percentage increases in those with chronic renal insufficiency disease. Thus, C_{cr} systematically overestimates the GFR, particularly in chronic renal insufficiency. Cimetidine blocks tubular secretion of creatinine. Therefore, loading with cimetidine before a 24-hour urine collection results in a more reliable estimate of the true GFR.

E. Cockcroft-Gault Formula and Modification of Diet in Renal Disease Abbreviated Equation. The Cockcroft-Gault (C-G) formula and Modification of Diet in Renal Disease (MDRD) formula are alternatives to a 24-hour urine collection to calculate the GFR. They are easier to obtain and give good accuracy.

The C-G formula is as follows:

$$GFR = [(140 - age) \times \text{lean body weight (kg)}]/(S_{cr} \times 72)$$
$$\times 0.85 \text{ in women}$$

F. The MDRD abbreviated equation is as follows:

$$GFR = 186 \times (S_{cr})^{-1.154} \times (age)^{-0.203} \times (0.742 \text{ if female})$$
$$\times (1.210 \text{ if African American})$$

G. Assessment of Tubular Function. A decline in GFR is normally matched by a proportionate decline in tubular function. This is apparent as a diminished ability to concentrate or dilute the urine or to conserve or eliminate acid, sodium, potassium, and other electrolytes. Therefore, patients with kidney disease are at special risk for developing disorders of water, electrolyte, or acid–base status.

Some patients have a more selective defect in tubular function, for example, a renal tubular acidosis. The specialized tests of urine concentration or dilution and of acid excretion are described in Chapters 15 and 17.

II. Nuclear Medicine Tests

A. Renogram. The renogram is used primarily to assess renal function although gamma camera pictures provide some information about renal size and shape. Several radionuclides are available: technetium-99m (Tc^{99m}) diethylenetriamine pentaacetic acid is freely filtered by the glomerulus and is not reabsorbed; it is used to estimate the GFR. Tc^{99m} dimercaptosuccinate is bound to the tubules and delineates the contours of functional renal tissue; it is used to assess cortical scarring from pyelonephritis or vesicoureteral reflux or to diagnose a renal infarct. Radioiodinated orthoiodohippurate (Hippuran) is secreted into the tubules; it is used to assess renal blood flow. Tc^{99m} mercapto-acetyl-triglycine combines the benefits of Tc^{99m} scanning with many of the characteristics of Hippuran. Currently, it is the agent of choice in most units.

A renogram is obtained by scanning over each kidney for 15–25 minutes after an intravenous (IV) injection of one of the above agents. The counts normally rise to a peak, reflecting filtration or secretion of the marker, and decline, reflecting elimination of the marker from the nephron. A delay in the time to peak and in elimination occurs in patients with renal parenchymal disease, renal artery stenosis, or outflow obstruction. In the latter case, IV furosemide, given halfway through the scan, fails to enhance elimination. This Lasix renogram is the most sensitive index of outflow obstruction. The delays in peak and decline in patients with renovascular hypertension are accentuated after blockade of angiotensin II generation with an angiotensin-converting enzyme inhibitor. This results from the withdrawal of angiotensin II–dependent tone in the efferent arterioles. The resultant sharp decrease in GFR reduces the rate of uptake and excretion of the marker. This angiotensin-converting enzyme inhibitor renogram is the most sensitive and specific test available to detect functionally important renovascular hypertension, as discussed in Chapter 22.

B. Nuclear Medicine Studies of Renal Function. The renal blood flow is quantified by Hippuran and the GFR

TABLE 3.1.   Indications for a renogram

Renogram type	Use
Furosemide renogram	Detects outflow obstruction
Angiotensin-converting enzyme inhibitor renogram	Detects renovascular hypertension
Technetium-99m dimercaptosuccinate scan	Detects cortical scarring or infarct
Hippuran or technetium-99m diethylenetriamine pentaacetic acid	Measures renal blood flow or glomerular filtration rate

by diethylenetriamine pentaacetic acid. Both agents are eliminated only by the kidneys. After IV injection, their plasma levels decline exponentially with a slope that is proportional to their clearances. The plasma disappearance method, combined with scanning over the kidneys, can be used to estimate the single-kidney GFR or renal blood flow. This is useful to predict the effects of a planned nephrectomy on overall kidney function. The indications for renography are summarized in Table 3.1.

III. Suggested Readings

Levey AS, Bosch JP, Lewis JB, et al. A more accurate method to estimate glomerular filtration rate from serum creatinine: a new prediction equation. *Ann Intern Med* 1999;130:461.

National Kidney Foundation. K/DOQI clinical practice guidelines for chronic kidney disease: evaluation, classification and stratification. *Am J Kidney Dis* 2002;39:S1.

Taylor A. Renovascular disease: functional testing: ACEI renography. *Semin Nephrol* 2000;20;437–444.

Wilcox CS. Use of angiotensin-converting-enzyme inhibitors for diagnosing renovascular hypertension. *Kidney Int* 1993;44:1379.

4

Clinical and Laboratory Evaluation of Renal Disease and Fluid Status

Wen-Ting Ouyang and Christopher S. Wilcox

I. **History and Physical Examination.** Kidney diseases may be part of a systemic, inherited, or drug-induced disease. Therefore, a comprehensive history including questions about over-the-counter medication and physical examination are essential. The physical examination is unreliable in complex intensive care unit situations where invasive procedures may be required to assess a patient's volume status. Whenever possible, an evaluation should include measures of blood pressure and heart rate while lying down and standing, funduscopic examination, and urinalysis.

A. **Clinical Assessment of Volume Status.** Orthopnea is a sensitive symptom of volume overload. Jugular venous distention is useful in assessing volume status and left ventricular failure. Distension of the internal or external jugular vein >3 cm above the sternal angle is an abnormal jugular venous distention. This is supported if there is abdominal-jugular reflux (hepatojugular reflux) or Kussmaul's sign. Jugular venous distention from congestive heart failure (CHF) must be differentiated from pure right-sided heart failure, which accompanies pulmonary hypertension from smoking or recurrent pulmonary emboli. These patients have an accentuated pulmonary second heart sound; an echocardiogram may be helpful for diagnosis. A third heart sound can be a normal finding in persons <45 years or may indicate CHF and fluid overload, idiopathic hypertrophic subaortic stenosis, or regurgitation of the mitral or tricuspid valves. A worsening of hypertension is a valuable clue to the presence of fluid overload in patients with chronic renal insufficiency or end-stage renal disease. The discovery of fine rales at the end of inspiration suggests pulmonary edema, fibrosis, or atelectasis. Peripheral edema implies renal fluid retention or fluid redistribution and suggests CHF, nephrotic syndrome, cirrhosis, cor pulmonale, malnutrition, or a complication of calcium channel blockade. Postural hypotension (fall in systolic blood pressure >10%) with reflex tachycardia indicates intravascular volume depletion. More severe dehydration reduces skin turgor and axillary sweating. Postural hypotension without an increase in heart rate indicates autonomic insufficiency, old age, or beta blocker therapy. Plasma levels of brain natriuretic peptide are helpful in assessing volume status but become unreliable in renal insufficiency, unless serial measurements can be obtained.

B. **Clinical Diagnosis of Uremia.** Initial symptoms of renal insufficiency are often nonspecific. Nocturia suggests a failure to concentrate the urine. Shortness of breath may indicate CHF, anemia, or metabolic acidosis. Anorexia, nausea, vomiting, diarrhea, and confusion in the presence of established renal insufficiency point to advanced uremia. Uremic encephalopathy alters mental status and may cause grand mal seizures. Uremic pericarditis causes a pericardial friction rub and may increase pericardial fluid accumulation that can be detected by an echocardiogram.

II. **Examination of the Urine.** A urine specimen obtained within the last 2 hours should first be tested with a dipstick. A 10-ml sample should be centrifuged at 3,000 revolutions/min for 3–5 minutes, and the sediment placed on a slide under a coverslip and examined under the microscope. It is often helpful to add one drop of methylene blue dye to the spun sediment.

A. **Color.** Urine is normally clear and yellow. A dark brown color suggests bilirubinuria. A red color suggests hemoglobinuria, myoglobinuria, porphyria, or drugs such as rifampin or phenazopyridine (Pyridium). A turbid white color suggests pyuria or crystalluria.

B. **Specific Gravity.** The normal range is 1.005–1.030. A specific gravity of 1.010 is isosthenuric and normally corresponds to a urine osmolality of approximately 300 mOsm/kg. Radiocontrast agents, protein, and glucose increase the specific gravity much more than osmolality because they are large, dense molecules. Otherwise, a high specific gravity suggests dehydration with a preserved concentrating function.

C. **pH.** The normal urine pH is 4.5–7.0. A persistent acidic pH is a normal finding. A persistent alkaline pH is found in vegetarians, in patients with classic distal renal tubular acidosis, in urinary tract infection with urease-producing proteus organisms, after administration of alkali or acetazolamide, in severe potassium depletion with excessive excretion of ammonia, in respiratory alkalosis, or during correction of metabolic alkalosis.

D. **Glucose.** A normal urine should contain no glucose. Urine glucose suggests either diabetes mellitus or decreased glucose reabsorption from the proximal tubule (renal glycosuria or proximal renal tubular acidosis). Pregnancy reduces the renal glucose threshold and can lead to glycosuria in otherwise normal women.

E. **Leukocyte Esterase and Nitrite.** A positive reaction for leukocyte esterase indicates pyuria. Nitrite suggests gram-negative bacteriuria. These tests lack sensitivity.

F. **Protein.** Normal urine contains no proteins. A positive test should be followed by a 24-hour urine collection for protein and microalbumin. Excretion of >150 mg/24 hr of protein (urine protein:creatinine ratio >150 mg/g) or >30 mg/24 hr of microalbumin (urine microalbu-

TABLE 4.1.   Urine casts

Type	Description and clinical relevance
Hyaline	Mucoprotein matrix without cellular elements; does not indicate renal disease
Red cell	Indicates glomerular bleeding
Leukocyte	Occurs in pyelonephritis, interstitial nephritis, and glomerulonephritis
Renal tubular epithelial	Occurs in acute tubular necrosis, glomerulonephritis, and tubulointerstitial disease
Granular, waxy	Represents degenerative cellular elements
Broad	Characteristic of chronic renal failure

min:creatinine ratio >30 mg/g) is abnormal. Pure tubular dysfunction should not result in proteinuria >1.5g/24 hr. Greater quantities of proteinuria indicate a glomerulopathy. Proteinuria >3.5 g/24 hr is termed *nephrotic range*. The dipstick test does not detect Bence Jones protein, which requires testing with sulfosalicylic acid and estimation by urine protein electrophoresis. A false-positive test for protein occurs with phenazopyridine, gross hematuria, or a very high pH.

    G. Examination of the Urinary Sediment. More than three red blood cells per high-power field is abnormal and should always be fully investigated to rule out glomerular, renal, or postrenal causes. Dysmorphic red blood cells indicate a glomerular source for bleeding. The presence of white blood cells suggests urinary tract infection or inflammation. Pyuria with a negative bacterial culture suggests prostatitis, chronic urethritis, renal tuberculosis, renal stone disease, or papillary necrosis. Wright's or Hansel's stain can identify eosinophils in the urine, which suggests drug-induced, allergic interstitial nephritis. Renal tubular epithelial cells are often seen in acute tubular necrosis, glomerulonephritis, or pyelonephritis. Table 4.1 details the types of casts.

III. Biochemical Analysis of Urine. See also Chapter 3.

    A. Urinary Sodium Concentration. A urinary sodium concentration (U_{Na}) <10 mEq/L in a patient with oliguric azotemia indicates a prerenal cause. A U_{Na} >40 mEq/L in an azotemic patient indicates acute tubular necrosis, diuretic use, or adrenal insufficiency (Table 4.2). Intermediate levels require the calculation of the fractional excretion of sodium (FE_{Na}):

$$FE_{Na} (\%) = (U_{Na}/S_{Na}) \times (S_{cr}/U_{cr}) \times 100$$

where S_{Na} indicates the serum sodium concentration, S_{cr} the serum creatinine concentration, and U_{cr} the urinary concentration.

TABLE 4.2. **Fractional excretion of sodium (FE_{Na}) in acute renal failure**

FE_{Na} <1%	FE_{Na} >1%
Prerenal azotemia	Diuretic use
Dehydration	Mineralocorticoid deficiency
Congestive heart failure	Chronic renal failure
Prior excessive diuresis	Acute tubular necrosis
Renal vasoconstriction	Acute interstitial nephritis
Ischemia	Severe ischemic nephropathy
Ischemic nephropathy	Nonreabsorbable solutes
Bilateral renal artery stenosis	Mannitol
Hepatorenal syndrome	Glucose
Sepsis	Radiocontrast agents
Early rhabdomyolysis	Anions such as HCO_3^-
Thrombotic thrombocytopenic purpura	Late obstructive uropathy
Contrast associated nephropathy	
Acute glomerulonephritis	
Nonoliguric acute tubular necrosis	
Early obstructive uropathy	

B. **Urinary Chloride Concentration.** This is valuable to diagnose the cause of metabolic alkalosis. A urinary chloride concentration (U_{Cl}) <15 mEq/L suggests chloride-responsive metabolic alkalosis. This is characteristic of extrarenal Cl^- loss, prior diuretic use, or severe volume depletion leading to contraction alkalosis. A U_{Cl}>15 mEq/L indicates chloride-resistant metabolic alkalosis. This is characteristic of Bartter's or Gitelman's syndrome, primary hyperaldosteronism, or current diuretic use (see Chapter 17).

C. **Urinary Anion Gap.**

$$UAG = (U_{Na} + U_K) - U_{Cl}$$

The urinary anion gap (UAG) represents unmeasured anions (mainly phosphate, sulfate, or bicarbonate) in excess of unmeasured cations (mainly NH_4^+). A normal gap is zero or negative. A positive number in an acidotic patient suggests a failure of NH_4^+ excretion because of renal tubular acidosis or administration of a carbonic anhydrase inhibitor. A strongly negative number suggests extrarenal losses of bicarbonate, which occurs in diarrhea or pancreatic drainage, and a preserved ability to generate and excrete NH_4^+.

D. **Assessing Glomerular Filtration Rate.** See Chapter 3.

IV. **Suggested Readings**

Corwin HL. Urinalysis. In: Schrier RW, Gottschalk CW, eds. *Disease of the kidney*, 6th ed. Boston: Little, Brown and Company, 1997:295–306.

Davidson AM, Grunfeld J-P. History and clinical examination of the patient with renal disease. In: Davidson AM, Camerson JS, Grunfeld J-P, et al., eds. *Oxford textbook of clinical nephrology*, 2nd ed. Oxford University Press, 1998:3–19.

Levey AS. Clinical evaluation of renal function. In: Greenberg A, Cheung A, Coffman T, et al., eds. *Primer on kidney disease*, 2nd ed. San Diego: Academic Press, 1998:20–26.

5

Hematuria

Kinjal R. Patel and Shakil Aslam

Hematuria can be classified by type (e.g., gross vs. microscopic) or cause (e.g., glomerular vs. nonglomerular). Gross hematuria is indicated by red, pink, or brown urine. Microscopic hematuria is two or more red blood cells (RBCs) per high-power field on the spun urine sediment. This is usually performed after an abnormal dipstick test that utilizes the reaction between orthotoluidine and hemoglobin or myoglobin.

I. **Evaluation.** Transient microscopic hematuria is relatively common. Up to 39% of adults between the ages of 18 and 33 may have microscopic hematuria at least once, and up to 16% on two or more occasions. Therefore, an extensive workup is not warranted except in high-risk patients, >50 years of age and those patients with other clinical or urinary abnormalities.

Figure. 5.1 summarizes a diagnostic approach to hematuria. A thorough history and physical examination should be performed initially. If gross hematuria is present, a urine specimen should be centrifuged. True hematuria is present if the color localizes to the sediment. It may be due to transient or persistent causes. If the supernatant remains discolored, the urine should be tested by dipstick. A positive result indicates hemoglobinuria or myoglobinuria, whereas a negative result suggests porphyria, use of the bladder analgesic phenazopyridine (Pyridium), or ingestion of beets.

If microscopic hematuria is detected, transient causes, such as vigorous exercise, sexual intercourse, menstrual contamination, infection, and instrumentation of the genitourinary tract, should be excluded by repeat dipstick when these circumstances no longer apply. If persistent, a glomerular etiology is suggested by dysmorphic RBCs and RBC casts on microscopy or proteinuria >500 mg/24 hrs. This should follow with a referral to a nephrologist and consideration of a renal biopsy.

An assessment of nonglomerular causes can include imaging by ultrasound, helical computed tomography, or intravenous pyelogram to detect strictures, cysts, neoplasms, or stones, whose presence should follow with a referral to a urologist. Urine cytology is a specific, but relatively insensitive, test for urothelial cancers.

II. **Differential Diagnosis**

A. **Glomerular Causes.** Primary glomerulopathies, such as immunoglobulin A nephropathy, commonly present with hematuria or RBC casts or both. The nephrotic syndrome with hematuria suggests focal and segmental glom-

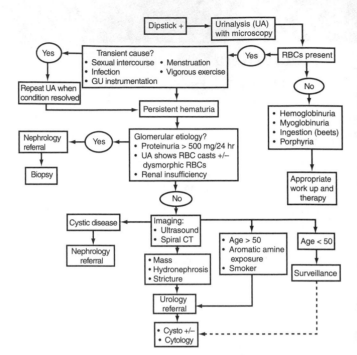

FIG. 5.1. Evaluation of hematuria. CT, computed tomography; GU, genitourinary; RBC, red blood cells.

erulosclerosis, membranoproliferative glomerulonephritis, membranous glomerulonephritis, or minimal change disease. Hematuria is associated with many systemic diseases that involve the kidney, such as systemic lupus erythematosus, cryoglobulinemia, or postinfectious glomerulonephritis. These patients usually have symptoms and signs of systemic illness—abnormal complement levels, abnormal hepatitis serology, or autoantibodies.

Rapidly progressive glomerulonephritis can progress to end-stage renal disease in weeks to months. It is classified into three types that are almost always accompanied by hematuria. Type I is antiglomerular basement membrane disease, with antiglomerular basement membrane disease antibodies in the serum or the kidney biopsy. Type II is associated with immune-complex diseases, including systemic lupus erythematosus, immunoglobulin A, and Henoch-Schönlein purpura, which can be diagnosed by history and a directed laboratory evaluation (see Chapter 7). Type III often is accompanied by a positive test for antineutrophil cytoplasmic antibodies; it is referred to as *pauci-immune* because of the relative lack of immune-complex deposition in the renal biopsy studied by immunofluorescence. Goodpasture's disease (type I) and Wegener's granulomatosis (type III) are often present with pulmonary involvement manifesting as hemoptysis or alveolar hemorrhage that can lead to pulmonary fibrosis.

Alport's syndrome and thin basement membrane disease frequently cause hematuria. Clinical clues of Alport's syndrome are a family history, ocular abnormalities, sensorineural hearing loss, and progressive renal insufficiency, especially in men. Thin basement membrane disease usually presents with isolated hematuria or loin pain hematuria syndrome and generally does not progress to renal insufficiency.

B. **Vascular Causes.** Renal vein thrombosis, which may complicate nephrotic syndrome, may present with hematuria. Renal venography, ultrasound with duplex Doppler velocimetry, or magnetic resonance venography, can secure the diagnosis.

Renal arterial embolism presents with flank pain and hematuria; it can complicate arrhythmias, recent myocardial ischemia, or aortic aneurysm. Renal angiography or magnetic resonance angiography is the tests of choice. Nonocclusive atheroemboli complicating trauma and cardiac or aortic catheterization can lead to hematuria that may be accompanied by renal insufficiency, livedo reticularis, digital gangrene of the lower limbs, proteinuria, eosinophilia, eosinophiluria, and complement consumption.

Malignant hypertension can cause hematuria or fibrinoid necrosis of capillaries resembling other forms of microvascular vasculitis (see Chapter 28).

C. **Cystic Disease.** Polycystic kidney disease can cause hematuria. The diagnosis is made by radiologic imaging of multiple cysts and large kidneys. A history of affected individuals in each generation may be evident in autosomal-dominant polycystic kidney disease, although the penetrance is variable (see Chapter 13).

D. **Tubulointerstitial Disease.** Hypersensitivity tubulointerstitial nephritis should be suspected in patients with rash, fever, eosinophilia, eosinophiluria, and pyuria who have had recent exposure to a drug known to cause this disease (see Chapter 12).

Papillary necrosis can complicate analgesic nephropathy, sickle cell crisis, or diabetes mellitus. It can cause gross hematuria, but microscopic hematuria is frequent.

E. **Infection.** Urinary tract infection is associated with transient hematuria that becomes persistent if complicated by pyelonephritis or abscess formation. Findings include dysuria, frequency and urgency of urination, pyuria, fever, and flank pain (see Chapter 20).

F. **Urologic Causes.** Renal cell carcinoma, transitional cell carcinoma, and other malignancies can present with hematuria. They should be investigated by ultrasound and computed tomography. Cytology is very specific but is not sufficiently sensitive for screening. Nephrolithiasis causes flank pain and hematuria. The stone can be identified by helical computed tomography or ultrasound. When the stone contains calcium, a plain abdominal film (see Chapter 19) can identify it.

G. Other Causes. Hematuria due to overanticoagulation is usually accompanied by abnormal bleeding from other sites. Therefore, isolated hematuria in such cases raises the possibility of an underlying disease that should be investigated. Severe hematuria may accompany cystitis, especially that caused by cyclophosphamide toxicity.

H. Treatment. Therapy should be targeted at the underlying disease. In severe cases, bladder catheterization with saline irrigation minimizes obstruction from blood clots.

III. Suggested Readings

Cohen RA, et al. Microscopic hematuria. *N Engl J Med* 2003; 348:2330–2338.

Grossfeld GD. Asymptomatic microscopic hematuria in adults: summary of the AUA best practice policy recommendations. *Am Fam Physician* 2001;63:1145–1154.

House AA. Nephrology: 2. Evaluation of asymptomatic hematuria and proteinuria in adult primary care. *CMAJ* 2002;166:348–353.

Van Savage JG, Fried FA. Anticoagulant associated hematuria: a prospective study. *J Urol* 1995;153:1594–1596.

6

Proteinuria and the Nephrotic Syndrome

Matthew Kapturczak and Anupam Agarwal

A healthy adult excretes <150 mg of protein per day in the urine. Excessive amounts of urine protein may denote the presence of a benign condition or represent evidence of a serious underlying disorder. If proteinuria is present, one must be careful not to label a patient with a serious disorder, because the prevalence of proteinuria on an initial screening urinalysis in healthy subjects can be as high as 25%, yet only a small percentage of these patients have underlying renal disease.

I. **Pathophysiology.** Each nephron has several grams of protein delivered to it each day, yet only a miniscule amount appears in the urine. The kidney processes approximately 150 L of filtrate containing 60–80 g/L of protein. This results in the excretion of about 1–2 L of urine per day, which contains <150 mg of protein. Two factors account for this: First, the glomerular filtration barrier, which comprises an endothelial layer, a basement membrane, and an epithelial cell layer, restricts the filtration of most proteins. Second, the proximal tubule reabsorbs and degrades much of the filtered protein.

   A. **Glomerular Proteinuria.** The glomerulus is a highly efficient filter that restricts the passage of molecules based on size and charge. Neutral dextrans with a radius <1.8 nm (18 Å) are freely filtered, whereas those that are ≥4.2 nm (42 Å) are excluded by the glomerular capillary wall. Molecules within these size limits have clearance rates that decrease progressively as their size increases. The glomerular capillary wall also carries a negative charge. This anionic state of the filtration barrier limits the filtration of molecules with a negative charge, whereas molecules carrying a more positive charge have a higher fractional excretion. This explains why albumin (5.5 nm or 55 Å), an anionic molecule, is not normally filtered across the glomerulus. In certain conditions, such as minimal change disease, the charge selective barrier is lost, resulting in a selective proteinuria that leads to the loss of albumin as the major filtered protein.

   B. **Tubular Proteinuria.** Many low-molecular-weight proteins that are filtered by the glomerulus are reabsorbed and degraded by the renal tubules, predominantly the proximal tubule. If the proximal tubule is damaged, as in tubulointerstitial disease, proteinuria can occur, but it is rarely >1,500 mg/24 hr unless accompanied by glomerular injury.

C. **Overflow Proteinuria.** Overflow proteinuria is usually seen in patients with no apparent renal disease but results from overproduction of immunoglobulin light chains and heavy chains or other small proteins. The overflow occurs because the amount of filtered protein exceeds the resorptive capacity of the tubules. This phenomenon can be observed in multiple myeloma.

II. **Interpretation of Proteinuria.** It is essential to determine the presence of albuminuria when protein is present. The presence of a positive dipstick suggests albuminuria and glomerular proteinuria. A negative dipstick in the presence of proteinuria suggests tubular or overflow proteinuria. Albuminuria can be further subdivided into several patterns.

A. **Intermittent Proteinuria.** Intermittent proteinuria may be a prelude to serious renal disease but is usually seen in patients with febrile illness, congestive heart failure, or stress or after heavy exercise. There is no long-term risk to developing renal insufficiency.

B. **Orthostatic Proteinuria.** Orthostatic proteinuria denotes the presence of proteinuria only in the erect position. Protein excretion rarely exceeds 1 g/24 hr, and it is a benign condition. There is no increased risk for developing renal insufficiency or hypertension.

C. **Persistent Proteinuria.** Persistent proteinuria is self-explanatory and denotes a sign of renal disease even with a normal glomerular filtration rate. The renal disease may be due to a primary glomerular disorder or to a renal process secondary to a systemic disease. Excretion of >3.5 g/1.73 m^2 of body surface area or 50 mg/kg of body weight denotes nephrotic-range proteinuria. On a random spot urine sample, a ratio of urine protein to urine creatinine (measured in mg) of >3.5 signifies nephrotic-range proteinuria. This determination is helpful in patients unable to collect a 24-hour urine sample.

III. **Nephrotic Syndrome.** The presence of nephrotic-range proteinuria with clinical and metabolic derangements denotes the nephrotic syndrome. Diagnostic features include proteinuria (>3.5 g/day/1.73 m^2 body surface area), hypoalbuminemia (<3.5 g/dl), edema, and hyperlipidemia. The common causes of nephrotic syndrome are listed in Table 6.1. Complications of nephrotic syndrome include increased risk of thrombosis, infections, severe edema, adverse effects of hyperlipidemia, hyponatremia, and acute renal failure. Thrombosis can occur in both the arterial and venous circulations with a predilection for renal veins. Disorders associated with higher risk for this complication include membranous nephropathy, lupus nephritis, and amyloidosis. A sudden increase in the degree of proteinuria, flank pain, or hematuria or worsening renal function in patients with nephrotic syndrome due to the above causes should raise a clinical suspicion of renal vein thrombosis.

IV. **Investigations.** The presence of proteinuria deserves a further workup, although the scope of investigations is

TABLE 6.1. Common causes of persistent proteinuria or nephrotic syndrome

Primary glomerular disorders
    Membranoproliferative glomerulonephritis
    Focal segmental glomerulosclerosis
    Immunoglobulin A nephropathy
    Minimal change disease
    Proliferative glomerulonephritis
    Fibrillary glomerulonephritis
Secondary disorders
    Hereditary–familial
        Diabetes mellitus
        Alport's syndrome
        Sickle cell disease
        Congenital nephrotic syndrome
    Autoimmune
        Systemic lupus erythematosus
        Goodpasture's syndrome
        Wegener's granulomatosis
        Polyarteritis nodosa
        Pauciimmune glomerulonephritis
    Infectious
        Postinfectious glomerulonephritis
        Endocarditis
        Hepatitis B and C
        Human immunodeficiency virus
    Drug-induced
        Nonsteroidal antiinflammatory agents
        Heroin
        Gold
        Mercury
        D-Penicillamine
        Captopril
    Neoplastic
        Hodgkin's disease
        Lymphoma
        Leukemia
        Multiple myeloma
    Miscellaneous
        Amyloidosis
        Preeclampsia–eclampsia
        Interstitial nephritis

determined by the clinical situation. A 24-hour urine collection should be obtained to quantify the protein excretion. To ensure an adequate urine collection, the creatinine excretion should also be measured. Men normally excrete 20–25 mg/kg of creatinine per day, and women excrete 14–22 mg/kg/day. The calculated and measured creatinine excretion should be compared to ensure a complete collection. The following formulas can be used to estimate creatinine excretion: (a) men: $(140 - \text{age in years}) \times (\text{weight in kg})/5,000$ and (b) women: $(140 - \text{age in years}) \times (\text{weight in kg})/5,000 \times 0.85$. Estimates of glomerular filtration rate can also be obtained using a web-based formula that uses the Modification of Diet in

Renal Disease glomerular filtration rate calculator available at http://www.kidney.org/professionals/kdoqi/gfrpage.cfm. A microscopic analysis of the urine sediment should be undertaken. The presence of hematuria and red cell casts suggests a glomerulonephritis. A renal ultrasound should be performed to assess the size of the kidneys, the degree of parenchymal echogenicity, and the presence of anatomical abnormalities. Renal vein Doppler studies should be performed if a renal vein thrombosis is suspected. Basic blood chemistries such as a creatinine, blood urea nitrogen, albumin, and cholesterol should be obtained. In selected patients, one may also obtain complement levels, antinuclear antibody pattern and titer, human immunodeficiency virus and hepatitis B and C serology, cryoglobulins, serum and urine electrophoresis, antineutrophil cytoplasmic antibodies, and antistreptolysin O and antihyaluronidase titers. In adults, a renal biopsy should be performed to confirm the diagnosis or assist in the management of the patient. A schematic approach to the clinical evaluation of proteinuria is depicted in Figure. 6.1.

V. **Management**

A. **Dietary Protein Restriction and Renin-Angiotensin System Inhibition.** Proteinuria is an independent risk factor for the progression of renal disease, and attempts to lower the level of proteinuria represent an important strategy in delaying the progression of underlying renal disease. The presence of proteinuria is also associated with a higher risk from cardiovascular mortality as reported in the Framingham study. Studies suggest that significant and prolonged proteinuria is associated with a proinflammatory state leading to the progression of renal disease. Therefore, reducing proteinuria is likely to improve patient outcomes. The management of a patient with proteinuria is twofold. If possible, one should treat both the underlying disease process and the complications of proteinuria. Treatment of the underlying disease depends on the type of renal lesion and may involve the use of corticosteroids, cytotoxic agents, or both. Although protein loss in the urine leads to hypoalbuminemia, it may also be compounded by an increased rate of renal albumin catabolism and an inappropriately low hepatic albumin synthesis rate. One way to reduce urinary protein loss is to affect renal hemodynamics by reducing intraglomerular pressure. This can be accomplished by decreasing the dietary protein intake, although this may sound counterproductive due to ongoing protein losses. However, high protein loads increase intraglomerular filtration pressure, which worsens proteinuria and promotes the progression of renal insufficiency.

In the presence of normal renal function, daily dietary protein intake should be approximately 0.8 g/kg body weight. With renal insufficiency, intake should be further reduced to 0.6–0.8 g of high-biologic-value protein/kg body weight per day. Allowance should be made for urinary losses, and this amount should be added to the daily

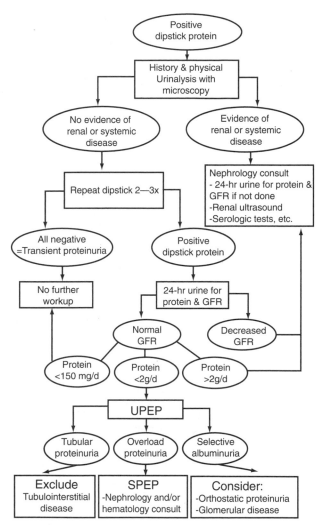

FIG. 6.1. Approach to the clinical evaluation of proteinuria. GFR, glomerular filtration rate; SPEP, serum protein electrophoresis; UPEP, urine protein electrophoresis. (Modified from Ibrahim H, Rosenberg M, Hostetter T. Proteinuria. In: Seldin D, Giebisch G, eds. *The kidney: physiology and pathophysiology*, 3rd ed. Philadelphia: Lippincott Williams & Wilkins, 2000:2269–2294.)

protein intake. Angiotensin-converting enzyme inhibitors also reduce intraglomerular pressure and can reduce proteinuria by up to 50%. These agents are now the drugs of choice for the treatment of both diabetic and nondiabetic renal disease–causing proteinuria. There is emerging evidence that angiotensin II receptor blockers may be equally effective in decreasing proteinuria. Moreover, the combination of angiotensin-converting enzyme inhibitors and angiotensin II receptor blockers has an additive effect on decreasing proteinuria. Drugs considered second-line agents include nondihydropyridine calcium channel blockers such as diltiazem.

B. Edema. Peripheral edema can be a medical as well as a cosmetic problem. Treatment consists of dietary salt and fluid restriction and the judicious use of diuretics. The complete and rapid correction of edema should be avoided because many patients with hypoalbuminemia and edema are intravascularly volume contracted. Diuretics in this setting may cause prerenal azotemia and worsen renal function. The use of diuretics is a delicate balance between providing patients with comfort, yet not worsening their renal function. The maintenance of trace to 1+ pitting edema of the ankles places the patient at less risk for intravascular volume depletion and its complications. The combination of a loop diuretic (e.g., furosemide) with a thiazide diuretic (e.g., metolazone) has additive effects and can be used in patients not responding to loop diuretics alone. Patients receiving these agents need to be monitored for hypokalemia. If this problem occurs, supplementation of potassium or the addition of potassium-sparing diuretics (amiloride or spironolactone) may be necessary.

C. Hyperlipidemia. Hyperlipidemia increases the risk for cardiovascular disease in the nephrotic patient. There is also evidence that hyperlipidemia may promote progressive renal injury, and, as a result, it is important to treat this condition. Initially, a diet low in saturated fat and cholesterol should be initiated; smoking should be discouraged and exercise should be encouraged. If the low-density-lipoprotein cholesterol continues to elevate despite dietary measures, the patient should begin therapy with a 3-hydroxy-3-methylglutaryl coenzyme A reductase inhibitor. A successful correction of hyperlipidemia helps preserve renal function and reduce proteinuria.

D. Hypercoagulability. The presence of thrombotic complications such as acute renal vein thrombosis in patients with nephrotic syndrome requires immediate hospitalization and heparin anticoagulation. Oral anticoagulation with warfarin should be continued for at least 6 months after initial heparin therapy. The treatment of other complications mentioned earlier can be found in the suggested readings list below.

VI. Suggested Readings

Bernard DB, Salant DJ. Clinical approach to the patient with proteinuria and the nephrotic syndrome. In: Jacobson HR, Striker GE, Klahr S, eds. *The principles and practice of nephrology*, 2nd ed. Philadelphia: Mosby, 1995:110–121.

Fogazzi GB. Urinalysis. In: Johnson RJ, Feehally J, eds. *Comprehensive clinical nephrology*, 2nd ed. St. Louis: Mosby, 2003:35–45.

Ibrahim H, Rosenberg M, Hostetter T. Proteinuria. In: Seldin D, Giebisch G, eds. *The kidney: physiology and pathophysiology*, 3rd ed. Philadelphia: Lippincott Williams & Wilkins, 2000:2269–2294.

II

Glomerular and Tubulointerstitial Diseases and Vasculitis

Diabetic Nephropathy

John R. Silkensen and Anupam Agarwal

Nephropathy is a serious complication of diabetes mellitus that often leads to end-stage renal failure or stage 5 chronic kidney disease and is a major cause of morbidity and mortality. In type I, or insulin-dependent diabetes mellitus (IDDM), 30–50% of the patients will develop nephropathy and renal failure, whereas in type II, or non–insulin-dependent diabetes mellitus (NIDDM), approximately 10–20% of patients will.

I. **Incidence.** Currently, approximately 6% of the U.S. population, or 18 million individuals, have diabetes mellitus. The yearly incidence of diabetes, which is the number of new cases diagnosed per year, is approximately 1.3 million in people over 20 years of age. In 2002, diabetes mellitus ranked fifth in causes of death by disease in the United States. At present, approximately 44% of all patients hospitalized for the treatment of end-stage renal failure have diabetes as the underlying cause. In fact, diabetes is the most common cause of end-stage renal disease in the United States. It is estimated that by the year 2006, diabetes will surpass all other causes contained in terms of incidence of chronic kidney disease. The prevalence of diabetic nephropathy increases with the duration of the disease. Poor glycemic control, hypertension, and genetic predisposition are all associated with a greater prevalence of renal disease.

II. **Clinical Presentation and Pathophysiology**

A. **Insulin-Dependent Diabetes Mellitus.** In 1984, Mogensen and Christensen described the progression of renal disease in IDDM and divided this evolution into five stages:

- Stage I: The hyperfiltration–hypertrophy stage is characterized by an increase in glomerular filtration rate (GFR) that is 20–50% above age-matched control subjects. Hypertrophy of the kidneys, visible on radiologic imaging, is also present. Functionally, glucosuria with polyuria and microalbuminuria (>20 but <200 µg/min) occur in this stage. With insulin treatment of several weeks' duration, the hyperfiltration and hypertrophy adjust in most patients, and the microalbuminuria falls below 20 µg/min.

- Stage II: This is a silent stage where the microalbuminuria is normal or near normal (<20 µg/min) and is usually seen from 1–5 years after diagnosis in 90–95% of patients with IDDM. The GFR is in the normal range in most patients. Features of early structural changes such as glomerular basement membrane thickening and mesangial expansion are evident in the kidney on histologic examination. Those patients destined to develop diabetic nephropathy often manifest a persistently elevated GFR (>150 ml/min), early hypertension, and poor metabolic control. Approximately 30–50% of diabetic patients will proceed into stage III and beyond and develop structural damage in the kidney.

- Stage III: This is also referred to as the *stage of incipient nephropathy* and occurs after 5–15 years of diabetes. There is further thickening of the glomerular basement membrane and mesangial expansion. The GFR starts to decrease in the later periods of this stage. Microalbuminuria (20–200 µg/min), which correlates with an excretion rate of 30–300 mg/24 hr if present, is a poor prognostic indicator. Hypertension develops early during this stage. This stage can last for several years. The level of protein excretion can be decreased, and the decline in GFR can be slowed with improved control of hyperglycemia and aggressive control of hypertension.

- Stage IV: This is the stage of overt nephropathy, or dipstick-positive proteinuria, and is characterized by fixed and reproducible proteinuria (>0.5 g/24 hr, detectable by dipstick). Hypertension is invariably present, and the GFR gradually declines. Histology reveals diffuse or nodular intercapillary glomerulosclerosis.

- Stage V: This is the stage of end-stage renal failure and on average occurs approximately 20 years from the time of diabetes onset in IDDM patients. In patients who progress to end-stage renal failure, the time required to develop overt diabetic nephropathy (stage IV) is highly variable but averages 15–17 years. However, subsequent progression to end stage (stage V) is relatively predictable and averages 5–7 years. The histology is characterized by glomerular sclerosis and obsolescence. Evidence of other complications of diabetes such as retinopathy, neuropathy, cardiac disease, and vascular disease is usually present at this stage.

B. Non–Insulin-Dependent Diabetes Mellitus. Far less is known regarding the development of diabetic nephropathy in NIDDM, or type II diabetes mellitus. At diagnosis, microalbuminuria is frequently present and often reversible with proper metabolic control. In contrast to insulin-dependent, or type I, disease, hyperfiltration is detected only rarely, and there is no evidence of glomerular hypertrophy. It is clear, however, that in comparison with an age-matched population, the presence of microalbuminuria in NIDDM carries a worse prognosis. Other risk factors for the development of nephropathy include hypertension, hyperglycemia, and cigarette smoking.

TABLE 7.1.   Features suggestive of nondiabetic renal disease in diabetic patients

Absence of diabetic retinopathy
Overt nephropathy with diabetes of less than 5 years' duration
Renal failure without significant proteinuria
Presence of red blood cell casts
Hypocomplementemia

Besides diabetic nephropathy, patients with diabetes mellitus are prone to an increased incidence of urinary tract infections (e.g., bacteriuria, cystitis, acute pyelonephritis), papillary necrosis, and neurogenic bladder with hydronephrosis. It is also important to consider other nondiabetic causes for renal disease in the diabetic patient, because many diabetics with renal disease are incorrectly labeled as having diabetic nephropathy. Table 7.1 summarizes features that, if present, may raise the suspicion of a nondiabetic cause for renal disease.

III. Pathology. The histopathologic alterations observed in diabetic nephropathy typically affect the glomeruli, vasculature, and tubulointerstitial compartment (Table 7.2). Nodular intercapillary glomerulosclerosis, although not pathognomonic of diabetic nephropathy, is the most characteristic of the renal lesions observed in this disease. However, a very similar lesion can be observed in light-chain deposition disease. Therefore, caution must be exercised when this lesion is found in patients with proteinuria in the absence of hyperglycemia or other signs and symptoms of diabetes mellitus.

IV. Pathogenesis. The pathogenesis of diabetic nephropathy is undoubtedly multifactorial and includes hemodynamic alterations, level of glycemic control, genetic predisposition, and race.

A. Hemodynamic Alterations. Both systemic and renal hemodynamics are critical determinants in the patho-

TABLE 7.2.   Histopathologic features of diabetic renal disease

Glomerular lesions
   Diffuse intercapillary glomerulosclerosis
   Nodular intercapillary glomerulosclerosis
   Capsular drop lesion
   Fibrin cap lesion
   Glomerular basement membrane thickening
Vascular lesions
   Subintimal hyalin arteriolosclerosis
   Benign arteriosclerosis
Tubular and interstitial lesions
   Hyalin droplets in proximal tubules
   Glycogen deposits (Armanni-Ebstein lesion)
   Tubular atrophy
   Interstitial fibrosis

genesis of diabetic nephropathy. Hypertension usually occurs before the onset of a decline in GFR and is associated with a higher incidence of developing nephropathy. Glomerular hyperfiltration occurs early in the disease and, if persistent, is more likely to be associated later with renal failure. Hyperglycemia is thought to be one of the mechanisms responsible for glomerular hyperfiltration.

B. Glycemic Control. An abnormal metabolic milieu must also be present for development of the characteristic renal lesions. The Diabetes Control and Complications Trial has clearly proven what many had long suspected—that glycemic control correlates with the appearance and progression of diabetic nephropathy. Improved control of hyperglycemia monitored by measurement of hemoglobin A_{1C} and reduction in intraglomerular and systemic hypertension can delay progression of the functional and histologic changes of diabetic nephropathy. Furthermore, normoglycemia after pancreas transplantation has been shown to reverse the lesions of diabetic nephropathy in native kidneys. The abnormal glycosylation of proteins that form the glomerular basement membrane and mesangial matrix, hyperperfusion of the glomerular capillaries with an associated increase in the transcapillary pressure gradient, and growth of the glomerular capillaries lead to progressive glomerulosclerosis.

C. Genetic Predisposition. Genetic susceptibility to diabetic nephropathy is supported by the association of a family history of hypertension and an increased incidence of nephropathy in siblings of affected individuals. Additionally, ongoing studies involving the renin–angiotensin system and its various components have provided further evidence for a genetic basis of diabetic nephropathy.

D. Race. Minority populations are more commonly affected with diabetic nephropathy. The incidence of diabetic nephropathy is two- to threefold higher in African Americans and six times higher in Native Americans and Hispanics compared to whites.

V. Evaluation. The presence of proteinuria, with or without hypertension and renal insufficiency, in a patient with diabetes mellitus of several years' duration indicates diabetic nephropathy until proven otherwise. The presence of diabetic retinopathy, which is observed in more than 90% of patients with diabetic nephropathy, strengthens the diagnosis. However, only one-fourth to one-third of those patients with diabetic retinopathy have clinically detectable renal disease. There are situations in which renal diseases other than diabetic nephropathy should be considered in the diabetic patient (Table 7.1). These include the absence of diabetic retinopathy, overt nephropathy with diabetes of less than 5 years' duration, renal failure without significant proteinuria, presence of an active urinary sediment, and low serum complements. In these situations, a percutaneous renal biopsy is often indicated to establish the diagnosis, determine the prognosis, and aid in management. A renal ultrasound should be obtained to exclude obstructive uropathy secondary to a neurogenic bladder.

VI. **Management.** Management of the renal disease associated with IDDM depends on the point in the disease at which the patient is encountered.

A. **Hypertension.** One of the most important factors in the management of diabetic renal disease is the control of hypertension. Lowering the blood pressure in the hypertensive diabetic patient can slow the rate of decline by 5–6 ml/min/yr. Intraglomerular hypertension is thought by many to cause progressive glomerular destruction. Although lowering systemic blood pressure can subsequently lower intraglomerular pressures, angiotensin-converting enzyme (ACE) inhibitors lower intraglomerular hypertension more predictably by reducing postglomerular vascular resistance. This accounts for some of the evidence showing a delay in progression of diabetic nephropathy in type I patients with diabetic nephropathy. The ACE inhibitors are considered drugs of choice on the basis of these findings. By extension, it is reasonable to assume that the newer angiotensin type I receptor blockers would be reasonable alternatives to the use of ACE inhibitors, especially when patients develop intolerable side effects from the latter agents. Recent clinical trials using combination therapy of ACE inhibitors with angiotensin receptor blockers have shown a synergistic effect with reduction in proteinuria and better blood pressure control compared to either agent used alone. Other useful agents to control hypertension include calcium channel blockers, α-receptor blockers, and cardioselective beta blockers.

B. **Hyperglycemia.** At the onset of diabetes mellitus, before insulin therapy is initiated (hyperfiltration–hypertrophy stage I), the GFR is elevated and the kidneys are enlarged. With insulin therapy and proper diet, both the GFR and the size of the kidneys usually decrease. Evidence suggests that failure to correct the elevated GFR increases the likelihood of the development of progressive renal disease later; thus, proper control of blood glucose levels early in the disease is important. Normalization of blood glucose levels will reduce microalbuminuria, especially in patients in the incipient nephropathy stage (stage III). Thus, proper control of blood glucose levels in any diabetic patient is an important treatment goal as demonstrated in the Diabetes Control and Complications Trial. With the development of progressive diabetic nephropathy and renal failure, close attention should be given to blood glucose levels because renal clearance of insulin is diminished and hypoglycemia is more common.

C. **Urinary Tract Infection.** In general, asymptomatic bacteriuria (>100,000 organisms/ml) should be treated in the diabetic patient. The development of acute pyelonephritis, especially if associated with obstruction, can result in papillary necrosis that can be life threatening.

D. **Renal Insufficiency.** Once it is established that renal insufficiency in a diabetic patient is secondary to the underlying disease and not to a superimposed or secondary problem that may be reversible, management is essentially the same as in any patient with renal insufficiency. Blood pressure control is essential, and ACE inhibitors have been established as the drugs of choice. Dietary protein restriction and a low-fat diet are important measures to slow progression of renal failure in diabetic nephropathy. Because of the high propensity for accelerated atherosclerosis in these patients, risk factors for coronary artery disease should be appropriately modified.

E. **Dialysis and Transplantation.** Hemodialysis and continuous ambulatory peritoneal dialysis offer a 3-year survival rate of approximately 50%. Patients should be educated to preserve one of their upper extremities for vascular access, which should be placed earlier in diabetic patients than in nondiabetic patients. In the younger diabetic patient, and especially in the absence of severe peripheral vascular disease, renal transplantation offers the best chance for survival. The 3-year patient survival with a living related donor allograft is close to 85%. The disease does recur in the transplanted kidney and can cause destruction of the graft in <5–10 years. The importance of glycemia control in transplant recipients is highlighted by clinical observations that patients with functioning islet transplants have significantly improved kidney survival. Unfortunately, the successful rehabilitation of the transplant patient often depends on the rate of progression of the disease in other organs.

VII. **Suggested Readings**

Caramori ML, Mauer M. Diabetes and nephropathy. *Current Opin Nephrol Hyperten* 2003;12:273–282.

Gaede P, Vedel P, Larsen N, et al. Multifactorial intervention and cardiovascular disease in patients with type 2 diabetes. *N Engl J Med* 2003;348:383–393.

Perkins BA, Ficociello LH, Silva KH, et al. Regression of microalbuminuria in type 1 diabetes. *N Engl J Med* 2003;348:2285–2293.

US Renal Data System. Excerpts from the USRDS 2003 Annual Data Report. *Am J Kidney Dis* 2003;42[Suppl 5]:S1–S230.

Wolf G, Ritz E. Diabetic nephropathy in type 2 diabetes prevention and patient management. *J Am Soc Nephrol* 2003;14:1396–1405.

Zandbergen AA, Baggen MG, Lamberts SW, Bootsma AH, et al. Effect of losartan on microalbuminuria in normotensive patients with type 2 diabetes mellitus. A randomized clinical trial. *Ann Intern Med* 2003;139:90–96.

8

Glomerular Diseases

Richard J. Johnson and C. Craig Tisher

Glomerular diseases may present clinically as acute glomerulonephritis (GN), nephrotic syndrome, or asymptomatic proteinuria or hematuria or both (Table 8.1). Some glomerular diseases appear limited to the kidney (primary glomerular diseases), whereas others may be part of a systemic process (secondary glomerular diseases). Diagnosis of the glomerular disease may be suggested by the type of clinical presentation, the presence or absence of systemic symptoms, and laboratory findings. A definitive diagnosis usually requires renal biopsy to define the disease based on its histologic pattern. However, it is becoming increasingly evident that a histologic pattern may have more than one etiology, and this may sometimes affect management. The basic clinical syndromes associated with the various glomerular diseases are shown in Table 8.1 and are discussed in detail below. Some of the common systemic causes of glomerular disease are discussed in Chapters 9, 10, and 11.

I. **Clinical Presentation and Laboratory Evaluation.** Patients with acute GN usually present with a "nephritic urinary sediment" characterized by hematuria, pyuria, red and white blood cells, granular casts, and varying degrees of proteinuria, often accompanied by hypertension, edema, and some degree of renal dysfunction. When the presentation is severe with acute renal failure, often with oliguria, then the clinical syndrome is called *rapidly progressive GN* (RPGN) and requires immediate treatment that usually includes hospitalization.

A second major presentation of glomerular disease is the nephrotic syndrome (see Chapter 6) in which patients manifest marked proteinuria (>3.5 g/day) with pitting edema, hypoalbuminemia, hyperlipidemia, and fatty casts in the urine. The most common cause is diabetic nephropathy, but there are also numerous diseases that appear to be specific to the kidney that can cause this syndrome. In contrast to the acute inflammatory or nephritic urinary sediment associated with acute GN, the sediment in subjects with nephrotic syndrome is characterized primarily by hyaline and granular casts and contains refractile fat bodies that show a characteristic "maltese cross" when examined under polarized light.

Finally, some subjects with glomerular disease may manifest asymptomatic micro- or macroscopic hematuria, especially those with immunoglobulin (Ig) A nephropathy or low-grade (<2 g/day) proteinuria. Patients with asymptomatic hematuria and an absence of other findings dictat-

TABLE 8.1. Definition and categorization
of glomerular diseases

Clinical syndrome	Manifestations	Major etiologies
GN	RBCs, RBC casts, proteinuria, hypertension, renal dysfunction	Acute poststreptococcal GN Other postinfectious GN (abscess, endocarditis) IgA nephropathy Lupus nephritis (WHO class III/IV)
Rapidly progressive GN	Presents as GN with acute renal failure (oliguria, rising serum creatinine)	Antiglomerular basement membrane nephritis (Goodpasture's) Vasculitis syndromes (Wegener's, microscopic polyangiitis, Henoch-Schönlein purpura, mixed cryoglobulinemia) Immune complex–associated (IgA, poststreptococcal GN)
Nephrotic syndrome	Proteinuria (>3.5 g/day), edema, high serum cholesterol, low serum albumin, urine lipids	Minimal change disease Focal segmental glomerulosclerosis MN MPGN Diabetic nephropathy Amyloid (myeloma, light-chain deposition disease) Fibrillary GN
Asymptomatic proteinuria	Urinary protein excretion <2 g/day	Low-grade glomerular disease (IgA nephropathy, MN, or MPGN) Hereditary glomerular disease (Alport's syndrome) Tubulointerstitial disease (see Chapter 6)
Asymptomatic hematuria	Urinary RBCs >2/high-power field (spun sediment)	Low-grade glomerular disease (IgA nephropathy, thin basement membrane disease) Other (see Chapter 5)

GN, glomerulonephritis; IgA, immunoglobulin A; MN, membranous neuropathy; MPGN, membranoproliferative glomerulonephritis; RBC, red blood cell; WHO, World Health Organization.

ing the presence of glomerular disease usually require a full workup to rule out other causes of bleeding in the urinary tract (see Chapter 5). Similarly, the spectrum of disease associated with low-grade proteinuria is wide and can include glomerular [e.g., membranous nephropathy (MN), Alport's syndrome], tubular (e.g., chronic tubulointerstitial disease), or other (e.g., myeloma) causes (see Chapter 6).

Table 8.2 presents recommendations for the initial workup of subjects presenting with either acute GN or nephrotic syndrome. The history and physical examination are critical because certain findings may suggest a particular diagnosis, such as the history of a streptococcal skin or throat infection (poststreptococcal GN), systemic symptoms such as alopecia, facial rash and arthritis (suggestive of lupus nephritis), or the triad of weakness, arthralgias, and palpable purpura [suggestive of vasculitis such as hepatitis C virus (HCV)–associated cryoglobulinemia]. Laboratory evaluation should include a careful examination of the urine sediment to determine the presence of glomerular disease. Marked proteinuria with hyaline casts and a sediment with minimal numbers of red cells and leukocytes should suggest nephrotic syndrome, whereas a sediment with red cells, white cells, and red and white cell casts ("full-house" sediment) suggests an acute GN such as that secondary to lupus nephritis or poststreptococcal GN. Red cells that are dysmorphic (showing irregular blebs) also suggest a glomerular cause of hematuria. Renal function is assessed by measurement of serum creatinine and a 24-hour creatinine clearance, but these tests are often unreliable in the setting of rapidly changing renal function. Specific serologic tests recommended in the evaluation of these subjects are shown in Table 8.2. In addition, a renal ultrasound examination should be ordered to assess renal size; large kidneys can be seen with diabetic nephropathy, amyloid, and human immunodeficiency virus nephropathy, whereas kidneys <9.5 cm in length suggest advanced or chronic disease and limit the possibility for biopsy due to the risk of bleeding and treatment because the disease is often too advanced at this stage.

Specific descriptions of the more common diseases presenting as acute GN or nephrotic syndrome are discussed below. Secondary causes of glomerular disease are discussed elsewhere, including systemic lupus erythematosus (Chapter 9), vasculitis (Chapter 10), and amyloid or plasma cell dyscrasias (Chapter 11).

II. Glomerulonephritis and Rapidly Progressive Glomerulonephritis

A. Acute Poststreptococcal and Other Postinfectious Glomerulonephritis.

Acute poststreptococcal GN is observed most commonly in children (ages 5–10 years), especially boys, after an untreated acute streptococcal infection. Individuals commonly present 2 weeks after a throat infection or 3 weeks after a skin infection with oliguria, weight gain, edema, and hypertension and are

TABLE 8.2.   General workup of patients suspected of having a glomerular disease

General recommendations

History: Family history of kidney disease and hearing loss (seen in hereditary Alport's syndrome); a history of medications associated with nephrotic syndrome (nonsteroidals, gold, penicillamine, captopril, mercury in skin-lightening creams); recent streptococcal (suggests poststreptococcal GN) or viral infections (seen with various GN, including Wegener's, anti-GBM, and immunoglobulin A nephropathy); history of cancer, such as solid tumors, Hodgkin's (minimal change), or non-Hodgkin's lymphoma (MPGN).

Physical examination: Look for features of nephrotic syndrome (pitting edema, xanthelasma); systemic features suggesting specific diagnoses, such as alopecia, arthritis, and facial rash (lupus); palpable purpura (suggests cryoglobulinemia, endocarditis-associated GN, or lupus); hepatomegaly and clubbing of the nails (HCV- or hepatitis B–associated nephropathy); livedo reticularis (vasculitis).

Laboratory examination: Routine electrolytes, glucose, liver function tests, albumin, cholesterol, 24-hr urine protein and creatinine clearance (may be inaccurate in subjects with RPGN), serum and urinary protein electrophoresis (in adults with >1 g/day proteinuria to rule out myeloma and plasma dyscrasias that can present with amyloid or light-chain deposition disease).

Radiologic studies: Renal ultrasound to assess kidney size (should be >10 cm to assure safe for biopsy).

Specific serologic tests

For nephrotic syndrome: Human immunodeficiency virus antibody (associated with focal segmental glomerulosclerosis), hepatitis B surface antigen (membranous), HCV antibody (membranous nephropathy, MPGN, and cryoglobulinemia), rheumatoid factor and serum cryoglobulins (both associated with cryoglobulinemia, usually secondary to HCV infection), antinuclear antibodies and anti-DNA antibody (lupus), serum protein electrophoresis (monoclonal band suggests myeloma or light-chain associated nephropathy), C3 and C4 (low levels suggest MPGN and/or cryoglobulinemia, or types III and IV lupus).

For acute GN or RPGN: Streptozyme or antistreptolysin-O titer (for poststreptococcal GN); blood cultures (for endocarditis and infection-associated GN), antinuclear antibodies, and anti-DNA antibody (lupus); anti-GBM antibody (Goodpasture's disease), antineutrophil cytoplasmic antibody (rule out Wegener's or idiopathic microscopic polyangiitis), C3 and C4 (low C3 suggests poststreptococcal or other postinfectious GN; low C3 and C4 suggests lupus, HCV-associated cryoglobulinemia, or MPGN type I).

anti-GBM, antiglomerular basement membrane; DNA, deoxyribonucleic acid; GN, glomerulonephritis; HCV, hepatitis C virus; MPGN, membranoproliferative glomerulonephritis; RPGN, rapidly progressive glomerulonephritis.

noted to have a nephritic urinary sediment. Subclinical cases are common, especially in household contacts of the index case. The pathogenesis appears to be due to an immune reaction to certain antigens, especially endostreptosin and pyrogenic exotoxin B, associated with specific serotypes (M-type 4, 12, and 49) of group A β-hemolytic streptococci. Throat cultures are usually negative when active GN is detected, but serologic tests including the streptozyme and the antistreptolysin O titer are positive in the majority of subjects, and low serum C3 levels characterize the disease.

Kidney biopsy should be reserved for patients with an atypical presentation or in whom the disease does not improve spontaneously over a 2- to 3-week period. The biopsy, if obtained, usually shows glomerular hypercellularity due to both an infiltration of leukocytes and proliferation of intrinsic glomerular endothelial and mesangial cells. Immune complexes are demonstrated in the capillary wall by immunofluorescence microscopy, and electron microscopy reveals irregular subepithelial deposits, or "humps," along the capillary loops.

Therapy is largely supportive with fluid and sodium restriction and administration of diuretics to control blood pressure and edema. Modest protein restriction may be useful in azotemic patients, and antihypertensive agents should be used to control blood pressure in those who do not respond to conservative measures. Immunosuppressive agents are not indicated in general, except possibly in patients with prolonged renal failure and a kidney biopsy with glomerular crescents (proliferation of extraglomerular cells within Bowman's space). In this situation, a trial of high-dose steroids may be considered.

Both the patient and family members should have throat cultures and those with streptococcal infection require antibiotic treatment. Children, even with severe disease, do well with supportive management; however, the presence of crescents on biopsy indicates a more guarded prognosis. Complete recovery is less certain in adults, particularly in those with a creatinine clearance of <40 ml/min/1.73 m^2, persistent proteinuria of >2 g/day, or increased age. Recurrence of acute poststreptococcal GN is rare.

Acute GN may also occur following, or concurrent with, other infections, especially in subjects with subacute or acute bacterial endocarditis, bacterial sepsis, visceral abscess, infected ventriculoatrial shunts, and osteomyelitis. Treatment aimed at eradicating the primary infection is usually associated with recovery of GN in these patients.

B. **Immunoglobulin A Nephropathy (Berger's Disease).** IgA nephropathy is the most common form of GN in Asia and in industrialized nations, comprising 15–40% of all biopsy-proven GN. In contrast, IgA nephropathy is distinctly uncommon in Africa and South America. Most cases occur in the second or third decade with a male predominance. The most common presentation is the discovery of microscopic hematuria and non–nephrotic-range proteinuria in an asymptomatic individual; however, the classic presentation observed 30–40% of the time is that of an episode of macroscopic hematuria that often occurs concurrently with an upper respiratory tract infection. Proteinuria is generally mild, but the nephrotic syndrome is occasionally present. Renal function is usually normal or only mildly depressed, but occasionally patients may present with RPGN or acute renal failure due to acute tubular necrosis resulting from gross hematuria. No serologic tests have been found to be consistently helpful, and a kidney biopsy is required for diagnosis.

Renal histology demonstrates a mild to moderate mesangial cell proliferation with extracellular matrix expansion. The diagnosis is confirmed by the demonstration of IgA deposits in the mesangium by immunofluorescence microscopy, often with coexistent IgG and C3 deposits. Electron microscopy usually demonstrates mesangial immune deposits.

IgA nephropathy is often slowly progressive, and by 20 years 50% of subjects either have developed end-stage renal disease or have substantial loss of renal function. An increased risk for progression is associated with proteinuria >1 g/day, an elevated serum creatinine at presentation, hypertension, or significant glomerular or interstitial fibrosis on biopsy. As with all types of GN, treatment should include aggressive blood pressure control and reduction of proteinuria with angiotensin-converting enzyme (ACE) inhibitors or angiotensin receptor blockers (ARBs). Some studies also suggest benefits from fish oil (omega fatty acids) and corticosteroids with or without azathioprine, especially in those with risk factors for progression, although such treatment is not currently universally accepted. However, subjects with IgA nephropathy who present with the syndrome of RPGN and are found to have crescentic nephritis on kidney biopsy should be treated aggressively with high-dose steroids with or without cyclophosphamide (see below).

C. **Rapidly Progressive Glomerulonephritis.** RPGN presents clinically as acute renal failure in the setting of a nephritic urinary sediment (e.g., red cell and white cell casts, microscopic hematuria). This is a medical emergency that requires immediate hospitalization and usually a kidney biopsy for specific diagnosis. Biopsy in these subjects reveals a crescentic GN in which there is proliferation of cells outside the glomerulus but within Bowman's space, often forming a crescent shape on histologic cross-section. Categorization is further defined by the immunofluorescence microscopic findings. The presence of IgG in a linear pattern along the glomerular basement membrane (GBM) defines Goodpasture's, or anti-GBM, disease. The presence of immunoglobulin and complement in a granular pattern on the capillary wall suggests an immune complex–associated disease such as lupus nephritis, IgA nephropathy, or acute poststreptococcal GN. The absence of immune deposits is observed with

TABLE 8.3.   Rapidly progressive glomerulonephritis: major categories

Immunofluorescence pattern of immunoglobulin G	Major etiologies	Serologic tests
Linear staining	Goodpasture's disease	Anti-GBM antibody positive
	Goodpasture's syndrome (with pulmonary hemorrhage)	
	Anti-GBM disease (restricted to the kidney)	
No staining	Vasculitis syndromes	
	Wegener's granulomatosis	C-ANCA positive
	Microscopic polyangiitis	P-ANCA positive
	Polyarteritis nodosa	ANCA negative
Granular staining	Immune complex diseases	
	Systemic lupus	Antinuclear antibody positive, low C3,C4
	Immunoglobulin A	Negative serologies
	Poststreptococcal glomerulonephritis	Streptozyme, low C3
	Membranoproliferative glomerulonephritis	Low C3, low C4

ANCA, antineutrophil cytoplasmic antibodies; anti-GBM, antiglomerular basement membrane.

the vasculitis syndromes, including Wegener's granulomatosis and microscopic polyangiitis, also known as *pauciimmune GN*. A description of each of the major categories of RPGN is shown in Table 8.3, and more details on lupus nephritis are provided in Chapter 9. Chapter 10 provides a description of the vasculitis syndromes.

A classic cause of RPGN is the autoimmune disease known as *Goodpasture's syndrome*. This disease typically presents in men in the second or third decade with a second peak in subjects older than 60 years of age. Some patients present with renal involvement only (e.g., anti-GBM or Goodpasture's disease), whereas others present with pulmonary hemorrhage and nephritis (e.g., Goodpasture's syndrome); rarely, subjects may present with only pulmonary involvement. Classically, patients manifest hemoptysis after an upper respiratory infection and have a nephritic urinary sediment. With pulmonary involvement, a history of smoking or hydrocarbon exposure is common.

The chest x-ray shows pulmonary hemorrhage, and laboratory tests usually demonstrate an iron deficiency anemia from blood loss and varying levels of renal dysfunction. Circulating anti-GBM antibodies are present, and the kidney biopsy reveals crescentic GN with linear staining of IgG and C3 along the GBM. The antibody has been shown to be directed against the α_3 chain of type IV collagen that is present in both the glomerular and alveolar basement membranes.

Treatment of Goodpasture's disease includes high-dose intravenous steroids [e.g., methylprednisolone sodium succinate (Solu-Medrol), 500 mg daily × 3 days] followed by a course of oral prednisone and cyclophosphamide. Plasma exchange is also conducted every other day until the anti-GBM antibody titer is no longer detectable. The prognosis is guarded, and patients presenting with oliguria, a serum creatinine >6.0 mg/dl, or severe scarring on the kidney biopsy frequently do not recover renal function. If kidney transplantation is necessary, the procedure should be delayed until anti-GBM antibody titers are low or undetectable to avoid rapid recurrence of the disease in the graft.

Treatment of other causes of RPGN such as immune complex– or vasculitis–associated disease also usually involves a short course of high-dose methylprednisolone (Solu-Medrol, 500 mg daily × 3 days) followed by oral steroids and cyclophosphamide (2–3 mg/kg/day for 3–9 months). Some authorities are now suggesting changing the cyclophosphamide to mycophenolate at 3 months to reduce the potential toxicity associated with long-term cyclophosphamide use that includes infertility, bladder cancer, and leukemia. Plasma exchange is reserved for severe cases in which dialysis is required.

III. **Nephrotic Syndrome.** The nephrotic syndrome may occur as a consequence of both systemic and renal-limited disease processes. In the Western world, the most common cause of the nephrotic syndrome is diabetic nephropathy (see Chapter 7). Another common cause, especially in the elderly, is amyloidosis, which often occurs secondary to multiple myeloma (see Chapter 11). Other plasma cell dyscrasias can result in the nephrotic syndrome, such as light-chain deposition disease (also discussed in Chapter 11). In the following sections, the other major diseases associated with the nephrotic syndrome are discussed.

   A. **Minimal Change Disease.** Minimal change disease (MCD), also called *nil disease* or *lipoid nephrosis*, is the most common cause of idiopathic nephrotic syndrome in children between the ages of 2 and 12 years but is also observed in 20% of adults with the nephrotic syndrome. The onset is often acute and may be precipitated by a viral infection, allergy, bee sting, or immunization. The nephrotic syndrome has been reported in adults with Hodgkin's lymphoma and other T-cell malignancies. A minimal change syndrome with interstitial nephritis and acute renal failure has also been reported as an idiosyncratic response to the use of nonsteroidal antiinflammatory drugs.

The primary clinical findings are dramatic weight gain and pitting edema, usually in the presence of a normal blood pressure. The urinary sediment classically shows proteinuria, hyaline casts, and oval fat bodies, and red cells are usually absent. The creatinine clearance is usually near normal; however, renal failure can be seen that may be due, at least in part, to volume contraction secondary to severe hypoalbuminemia, or *prerenal azotemia*. Children presenting with classic symptoms of MCD do not require biopsy and are treated empirically; however, the presence of hypertension or microscopic hematuria requires further evaluation.

The kidney biopsy shows normal-appearing glomeruli by light microscopy in the absence of immunoglobulin by immunofluorescence microscopy. Typically, the only abnormality noted by electron microscopy is fusion or effacement of the foot processes of the glomerular visceral epithelial cells.

Treatment consists of oral corticosteroids, typically prednisone, 2 mg/kg/day. More than 90% of children with MCD experience a complete remission within 4–8 weeks, but as many as 75% require repeated courses of therapy due to relapse. Patients who relapse three or more times within a year or who relapse before being tapered off steroids (steroid dependent) may require a 12-week course of oral cyclophosphamide therapy, or less commonly, chlorambucil. Children who do not respond to corticosteroids require a kidney biopsy to establish the diagnosis and possibly to be considered for another therapy. Prednisone is also effective in inducing remission in adults with MCD, albeit at a much lower success rate than in children. Treatment is frequently longer, and alternate-day administration of prednisone is often required. Treatment failures often respond to cyclophosphamide, but, again, the risk of using this agent in a benign disease must be considered carefully.

B. **Focal Segmental Glomerulosclerosis.** Focal segmental glomerulosclerosis (FSGS) is currently the most common cause of nephrotic syndrome in young adults, accounting for 20–30% of all cases in many series. Patients typically present with the classic features of nephrotic syndrome and small amounts of red cells in the urine; however, some patients have isolated proteinuria and, rarely, hematuria is more marked. There are several clinical settings in which FSGS can be observed. First, it may develop in a patient who is being treated repeatedly for MCD and becomes progressively resistant to corticosteroids. Second, it may occur as a consequence of heroin use (heroin nephropathy) or with human immunodeficiency virus infection. In these latter two conditions, there is a much higher frequency

(90%) in African Americans. Third, FSGS may be associated with a wide spectrum of other diseases, including morbid obesity, persistent reflux nephropathy, sickle cell disease, and cyanotic congenital heart disease.

Diagnosis is by kidney biopsy, which demonstrates a light microscopic pattern of segmental or total sclerosis of glomerular tufts, often with segmental increases in mesangial matrix and cellularity. Within any given tissue section, there are both normal-appearing and segmentally scarred glomeruli. There is a predisposition for involvement of juxtamedullary glomeruli. Often, both IgM and C3 deposits are present in the sclerotic segments of the glomeruli, where they are thought to be trapped passively rather than having a pathogenetic role in the disease.

Treatment consists of prednisone at an average dose of 1 mg/kg body weight per day. Prolonged treatment of 5–8 months is often required and, even then, partial (urinary protein excretion, <2 g/day) or complete remission is observed in only 50% of patients. Favorable prognostic indicators include absence of tubulointerstitial disease on kidney biopsy, a normal or only modestly elevated serum creatinine, and nonnephrotic proteinuria. Failure to observe a decrease in urine protein excretion after 12 weeks of prednisone therapy in adults or 8 weeks in children raises the likelihood of steroid resistance. As in all patients with the nephrotic syndrome, the use of ACE inhibitors or ARBs or both may help to reduce proteinuria and control hypertension.

C. **Membranous Nephropathy.** MN, or membranous GN, is the most common cause of nephrotic syndrome in the middle-aged adult (40–60 years of age). MN usually presents as frank nephrotic syndrome, often with low-grade microhematuria and relatively well-preserved renal function. However, some patients present with asymptomatic, low-grade or nephrotic-range proteinuria that is discovered on routine urinalysis. The peak age of incidence is 35–60 years, and men predominate by a ratio of 2:1. Patients can lose 10–20 g of protein per day and experience severe disability. Although most cases are idiopathic, MN can be associated with certain medications (especially penicillamine, gold, and, rarely, captopril or nonsteroidal agents), certain viral infections (especially chronic hepatitis B virus and HCV), and malignancies (classically solid tumors of lung, breast, and gastrointestinal origin). Occasionally, patients with systemic lupus erythematosus may develop MN (class V lupus glomerular disease, see Chapter 9). Rarely, MN may accompany other autoimmune diseases, particularly diabetes mellitus and autoimmune thyroiditis. In most cases of idiopathic MN, no serologic or clinical features are pathognomonic, and serum complement levels are normal.

Diagnosis is made by kidney biopsy. By light microscopy, the glomeruli typically appear normocellular with thickening of the GBM. Use of silver methenamine, which stains GBM, often reveals additional "spike-like" protrusions on the epithelial side of the GBM, which represents extensions of basement membrane–like material. Immunofluorescence microscopy demonstrates IgG and C3 along the capillary wall in a granular pattern, and electron microscopy reveals that the immune deposits are located on the outer side of the GBM under the epithelial foot processes (subepithelial region).

Management first involves ruling out secondary causes of MN. Supportive therapy includes controlling the manifestations of the nephrotic syndrome by reducing proteinuria with ACE inhibitors or ARBs or both, treating hypercholesterolemia with statins, and reducing blood pressure. In patients with markedly low serum albumin levels (<2.0 g/dl), there is a markedly increased risk for venous thromboses, especially of the renal vein, and some clinicians recommend prophylactic warfarin (Coumadin) therapy. More specific disease management is recommended for patients with MN who have features predictive of progression, including an elevated serum creatinine at presentation, urinary protein excretion >6.0 g/day, or presence of hypertension. In these patients, a regimen of prednisone (2 mg/kg/day for 1 month followed by slow taper over 6 months) with cyclophosphamide (2 mg/kg/day for 6 months) should be considered. Some recommend use of the Ponticelli regimen, consisting of prednisone and chlorambucil. For patients with none of these features, and particularly for women and children who have a better prognosis, only supportive therapy is recommended.

Frequently, patients with mild disease will not progress or may even spontaneously remit over a 5- to 10-year period. In contrast, subjects with marked proteinuria and an elevated serum creatinine frequently progress, and as many as 40% will eventually require dialysis in the absence of therapy.

D. **Membranoproliferative Glomerulonephritis.** Membranoproliferative GN (MPGN) is often associated with the nephrotic syndrome. When it presents between the ages of 10 and 30 years, it is usually idiopathic, but, between the ages of 35 and 60, it usually is associated with HCV infection. In both situations, the presentation is usually characterized by prominent hypertension, mild nephrotic syndrome, and microhematuria, with relatively preserved renal function. Patients with HCV infection may also manifest features of a systemic illness associated with circulating cryoglobulins, which includes the triad of weakness, arthralgias, and palpable purpura. Occasionally, there are symptoms suggestive of vasculitis that include livedo reticularis, leg ulcers, and pulmonary or cardiac involvement.

In children, two major forms are recognized: type I MPGN, which is thought to be mediated by circulating immune complexes that are passively trapped in glomeruli, and type II MPGN, in which the disease is associated with a circulating IgG, or the *nephritic factor* that activates complement via the alternative pathway. Type II MPGN is also termed *dense deposit disease*. Clinically, these diseases may appear identical, but in some patients with type II MPGN, there also is partial lipodystrophy of the face and upper body due to loss of adipocytes, and drusen bodies are rarely seen in the retina.

Diagnosis is facilitated by measuring serum complement levels and hepatitis serologies. Type I MPGN, both idiopathic and HCV associated, is usually associated with depression of both serum C3 and C4 documenting activation of the classic pathway, whereas type II MPGN is associated with the circulating nephritic factor and depression of serum C3 with normal C4 levels that is consistent with activation of the alternative pathway (Table 8.3). Depressed serum complement levels are observed in other glomerular diseases, including postinfectious GN, cryoglobulinemia, and systemic lupus erythematosus. Hence, diagnosis ultimately rests on performing a kidney biopsy. By light microscopy, glomeruli are hypercellular and often lobular in appearance due to increased extracellular matrix in the mesangium. Immunofluorescence microscopy demonstrates IgG and complement (C3 and C4), often lightly decorating the GBM in type I MPGN; in type II MPGN, only C3 is present. Finally, by electron microscopy, the presence of deposits between the endothelial cells and the GBM can be demonstrated in type I MPGN, whereas, in type II MPGN, areas of the GBM appear to be replaced by a homogeneous dense deposit of unknown etiology. A type III MPGN has also been described that is similar to type I MPGN, except the deposits are in both the subendothelial and subepithelial spaces, thereby having some features of an MN.

Treatment of MPGN consists of managing the hypertension and the nephrotic syndrome with ACE inhibitors, a low-salt diet, and diuretics. For children with MPGN, a trial of alternate-day prednisone is often recommended. In adults, treatment remains unclear, although there is some evidence that antiplatelet agents may provide some benefit. Patients with HCV-associated MPGN are usually treated with antiviral therapy consisting of interferon-α or pegylated interferon; in subjects with normal renal function, ribavirin is often added. However, ribavirin may cause significant hemolysis, particularly in the presence of renal insufficiency.

The natural history of MPGN is complex; some patients have chronic, smoldering disease, whereas others manifest a progressive course. As many as 50% may develop renal insufficiency after 15–20 years, and recurrence after transplantation is common.

E. **Fibrillary Glomerulonephritis.** Fibrillary GN is a recently recognized cause of the nephrotic syndrome that is observed primarily in adults between 40 and 60 years of age. It usually presents with nephrotic syndrome with or without microhematuria and a mild to moderately elevated serum creatinine. The clinical presentation is often similar to MPGN, and by biopsy the glomeruli may appear mildly hypercellular and contain IgG and C3 deposits. However, serum complement levels are normal, and electron microscopy reveals a characteristic finding of fibrillar deposits in the mesangium and subendothelial areas of the GBM. Immunofluorescence microscopy reveals immunoglobulins and C3 in the mesangium and capillary walls in a granular pattern. Amyloid is also characterized by fibrillary deposits, but, in fibrillary GN, the Congo red stain is negative and the fibrillar deposits are larger in diameter (12–22 nm) and randomly organized. No effective therapy has yet been described for fibrillary GN. The prognosis of fibrillary GN is guarded, and, in one small series, 50% progressed to end-stage renal disease. Another rare type of GN, so-called immunotactoid GN, is also similar to fibrillary GN in that it is negative for Congo red stain, but, in this disease, the fibrils are even larger (>30 nm), cylindric, and in parallel arrays; this latter disease may be associated with plasma cell dyscrasias and is particularly observed with chronic lymphocytic leukemia or non-Hodgkin's lymphoma.

IV. Suggested Readings

Cattran DC. Idiopathic membranous glomerulonephritis. *Kidney Int* 2001;59:1983–1994.

Choi MJK, Eustace JA, Gimenez LF, et al. Mycophenolate mofetil treatment for primary glomerular diseases. *Kidney Int* 2002;61:1098–1114.

Durkan AM, Hodson EM, Wiollis NS, et al. Immunosuppressive agents in childhood nephrotic syndrome: a meta-analysis of randomized controlled trials. *Kidney Int* 2001;59:1919–1927.

Imperiale TF, Goldfarb S, Berns JS. Are cytotoxic agents beneficial in idiopathic membranous nephropathy? A meta-analysis of the controlled trials. *J Am Soc Nephrol* 1995;5:1553–1558.

Johnson RJ, Rennke H, Feehally J. Introduction to glomerular disease: clinical presentations. In: Johnson RJ, Feehally J, eds. *Comprehensive clinical nephrology*, 2nd ed. St. Louis: Mosby, 2003:255–269.

Levin A. Management of membranoproliferative glomerulonephritis: evidence-based recommendations. *Kidney Int* 1999;55:S41–S46.

Madore F, Lazarus JM, Brady HR. Therapeutic plasma exchange in renal diseases. *J Am Soc Nephrol* 1996;7:367–386.

Nakao N, Yoshimura A, Morita H, et al. Combination treatment of angiotensin II receptor blocker and angiotensin converting enzyme inhibitor in nondiabetic renal disease: a randomized, controlled clinical trial. *Lancet* 2003;361:117–134.

Orth SR, Ritz E. The nephrotic syndrome. *N Engl J Med* 1998;338:1201–1212.

Ponticelli C, Altieri P, Scolani F, et al. A randomized study comparing methylprednisolone plus chlorambucil versus methylprednisolone plus cyclophosphamide in idiopathic membranous nephropathy. *J Am Soc Nephrol* 1998;9:444–450.

9

Renal Involvement in Systemic Lupus Erythematosus

Richard J. Johnson and C. Craig Tisher

Systemic lupus erythematosus (SLE) is an autoimmune disease chiefly affecting the skin, kidneys, joints, serous membranes, and blood vessels. It is seen primarily in young women (age 18–40 years), especially African Americans, but can occur at any age. It is particularly common in the southeastern United States. Diagnosis of SLE is made by confirming the presence of four or more criteria as established by the American College of Rheumatology (Table 9.1); this establishes the diagnosis with 96% sensitivity and specificity.

The hallmark of the disease is the presence of antinuclear antibodies (ANA) in the serum. However, this finding can be deceiving, as low titers (<1:40) are common in the normal population, particularly in older patients, and a positive ANA may also be observed in other collagen vascular diseases. In this regard, both the specific antigen and the pattern of staining (ANA are often detected by immunofluorescence microscopy using human cells as substrate) may be helpful in distinguishing the various collagen vascular diseases. SLE is frequently associated with a diffuse (homogeneous) or speckled pattern of staining, whereas scleroderma is associated with nucleolar staining, and the CREST syndrome (*c*alcinosis, *R*aynaud's phenomenon, *e*sophageal dysmotility, *s*clerodactyly, and *t*elangiectasia) is associated with a centromere pattern. Similarly, anti–double stranded DNA and anti-Smith antibodies are highly specific for SLE, whereas anti-Scl70 suggests scleroderma, and anti-Ro and anti-La antibodies suggest Sjögren's syndrome. Other antibodies often correlate with specific organ involvement, such as the presence of antiribosomal P antibodies (lupus cerebritis) and anti-Jo-1 antibodies (lung involvement). Antihistone antibodies suggest the presence of drug-induced lupus. Finally, antiphospholipid antibodies suggest potential thrombotic complications (see below).

Renal involvement is common in SLE and may occur in 30–50% of patients during the early course of their disease and in the majority (60–80%) if followed long term. There is a wide variety of clinical presentations (see below).

I. **Clinical Presentation of Lupus Nephritis.** Patients presenting with lupus nephritis often also have extrarenal manifestations. The most common extrarenal manifestations include low-grade fever, the classic malar or "butterfly" rash, Raynaud's phenomenon, hair loss, and arthralgias. Pleuritis, or pericarditis, or both, may be observed in up to 40% of patients. Other common findings include oral and skin ulcers, hepatosplenomegaly, normochromic anemia, mild leucope-

TABLE 9.1.   American College of Rheumatology criteria for diagnosis of systemic lupus erythematosus

Malar rash
Discoid rash
Photosensitivity
Oral ulcers
Nonerosive arthritis
Pleuropericarditis
Renal disease (proteinuria and/or granular casts)
Neurologic disorder (epilepsy, psychosis)
Hematologic disorder (hemolytic anemia, leucopenia or lymphope-
  nia, thrombocytopenia)
Positive LE preparation, raised anti-DNA antibody, anti-Smith present,
  false-positive venereal disease research laboratory (test)
Positive fluorescent antinuclear antibody

Note: Four criteria are required.

nia, and thrombocytopenia. While most cases are idiopathic, some cases of lupus are associated with certain drugs, including hydralazine, sulfonamides, procainamide, carbamazepine, and isoniazid. Renal involvement is rare in drug-associated lupus.

The renal manifestations of lupus are varied. Some patients have no evidence of renal involvement (class I lupus); in these patients, renal biopsy typically shows normal morphology, although some immune deposits may be present (Table 9.2). In contrast, others have minimal evidence of renal involvement, such as the presence of microscopic hematuria, low-grade (<2 g/day) proteinuria, and normal renal function. These patients typically have moderately elevated ANA titers and normal serum complement levels. Renal biopsy in these patients typically shows a mesangial pattern of disease (class II lupus nephritis) with immunoglobulin (Ig) G and C3 deposition in a mesangial pattern, and with mesangial hypercellularity with or without expansion of mesangial matrix. Both class I and class II variants of the disease are associated with a good renal prognosis, although, over the course of the illness, the renal disease could progress to a higher class with a worse prognosis.

The most serious presentation of lupus nephritis observed in 40% of patients includes severe hypertension, proteinuria (often, but not invariably, in the nephrotic range), deteriorating renal function, and an active or "full-house" sediment (red cells, white cells, and red and white cell casts). Some of these individuals are oliguric with acute (daily) increasing serum creatinine, thus manifesting as an acute renal failure. Extrarenal complications are also common, including cerebritis, pleuritis/carditis, and rash. In these patients, the ANA titer is often very elevated, and serum C3 and C4 levels are usually depressed. Antiphospholipid antibodies may be present and, if positive, can be associated with coexistent thromboses. Renal biopsy shows either class III or class IV

TABLE 9.2. Lupus nephritis according to World Health Organization classification

	Normal class I	Mesangial class II	Focal segmental proliferative class III	Diffuse proliferative class IV	Membranous class V
Overall incidence (%)	0–4	10–20	10–20	40–50	10–20
Light microscopy	Normal	Normal or diffuse mesangial proliferation	Focal (class III) or diffuse (class IV) mesangial and endothelial proliferation ± segmental necrosis ± hyaline thrombi		Diffuse thickening of the GBM and mild mesangial expansion
Immunofluorescence microscopy	Negative or positive IgG and C3 in mesangium	Granular deposits of IgG and C3 in mesangial areas	Diffuse deposits of IgG, C3, and C4 in mesangial and subendothelial areas of the GBM		Diffuse granular deposits of IgG and C3
Immune deposits by electron microscopy	Negative	Mesangial	Subendothelial, mesangial		Subepithelial, rare mesangial
Notes	Rarely seen; complete absence of any structural abnormality	May have no detectable clinical abnormality or mild abnormality on urinalysis only; excellent prognosis	Hematuria or proteinuria on urinalysis; rarely nephrotic; hypertension, renal insufficiency (usually indicates class IV); often high-titer antinuclear antibodies, low serum C3 and C4		Nephrotic syndrome; slowly progresses to renal failure

GBM, glomerular basement membrane; IgG, immunoglobulin G.

lupus nephritis (Table 9.2). Class III is characterized by focal proliferative changes, whereas class IV manifests diffuse proliferative changes that involve both a proliferation of endogenous glomerular cells as well as an infiltration of leukocytes. Focal necrosis, crescents, or both may be present in severe cases. Immunofluorescence microscopy usually shows diffuse granular deposits of IgG and C3, often with IgA, IgM, and C4. Electron microscopy reveals subendothelial and mesangial immune deposits. Although class III and class IV lupus nephritis were regarded as separate entities in the past, it is evident that class III is most likely a milder form of class IV disease, and, hence, treatment for both classes is the same.

A milder form of lupus nephritis presenting as nephrotic syndrome, often with only mildly reduced renal function, may also occur. These patients may not completely fulfill the criteria for SLE and often have only low-titer ANA antibodies and normal serum complements. The renal biopsy in these patients shows a pattern consistent with membranous nephropathy (see Chapter 8) with thickening of the basement membrane, the presence of IgG and C3 in a granular pattern on the capillary wall, and subepithelial immune deposits noted by electron microscopy (class V lupus; Table 9.2). Unlike idiopathic membranous nephropathy, there may also be some evidence of mesangial immune deposits.

In addition to the classic presentations of lupus nephritis (Table 9.2), some patients may manifest only tubulointerstitial involvement with low-grade proteinuria and microhematuria. Finally, some patients carry antiphospholipid or anticardiolipin antibodies; some of these patients may also manifest a lupus anticoagulant, as evidenced by a prolonged activated partial thromboplastin time. These patients may have a worse renal lesion with superimposed glomerular and peritubular capillary thromboses, and they are also at risk for large vessel thromboembolism.

II. **Management and Prognosis.** Patients presenting with mild lupus nephritis (class I and class II) are managed conservatively, usually limiting corticosteroids to the minimal dose that controls the extrarenal manifestations of their disease.

Patients presenting with acute lupus nephritis suggestive of class III or class IV disease are managed aggressively. If there is evidence of acute changes in renal function, the patient is hospitalized. Blood pressure is managed with sodium restriction, vasodilators, diuretics, and beta blockers. Angiotensin-converting enzyme inhibitors and angiotensin receptor blockers are avoided in the setting of acutely changing renal function because these agents may occasionally cause a temporary decrease in renal function. Managing electrolytes, especially hyperkalemia and hyponatremia, is often required (see Chapters 15 and 16), and, occasionally, acute dialysis is indicated. After diagnostic renal biopsy, disease-specific treatment is initiated. This usually consists of high-dose (or pulse) methylprednisolone sodium succinate (Solu-Medrol, 500 mg intravenously daily × 3 days) followed by oral prednisone (2 mg/kg/day that is gradually reduced beginning at 30 days). The National Institutes of Health protocol includes the use of pulse cyclophosphamide (0.5–1.0 g/m^2) monthly for 6 months, then every 3 months for a total of 2 years. However, due to the cumulative toxicity of cyclophosphamide, many authorities now recommend a shorter course of cyclophosphamide (3 months), followed by switching to a less toxic oral immunosuppressive agent such as mycophenolate mofetil or azathioprine.

Class V lupus nephritis, or membranous nephropathy, is usually managed in a manner similar to idiopathic membranous nephropathy, using a combination of corticosteroids and cytotoxic agents for patients with high-risk factors for progression (urinary protein excretion >6 g/day, hypertension, or reduced renal function).

Patients with antiphospholipid antibodies are also administered anticoagulants (warfarin), with the goal of maintaining the prothrombin time three times the international normalized ratio.

The overall prognosis of lupus varies, and 8–15% of patients develop end-stage renal disease. Interestingly, the clinical manifestations of lupus often are suppressed once the patient becomes uremic, and recurrence of lupus nephritis in the renal transplant is also rare.

III.   Suggested Readings

Balow JE, Boumpas DT, Austin HA III. New prospects for treatment of lupus nephritis. *Semin Nephrol* 2000;20:32–39.

Bono L, Cameron JS, Hicks JA. The very long term prognosis and complications of lupus nephritis and its treatment. *QJM* 1999;92:211–218.

Chan TMS, Li FK, Tang CSO, et al., for the Hong Kong-Guangzhou nephrology study group. Efficacy of mycophenolate mofetil in patients with diffuse proliferative lupus nephritis. *N Engl J Med* 2000;343:1156–1162.

Illei GG, Austin HA, Crane M, et al. Combination therapy with pulse cyclophosphamide plus pulse methylprednisolone improves long term outcome without added toxicity in patients with lupus nephritis. *Ann Intern Med* 2001;135:248–257.

Renal Vasculitis

Geraldine Shaw Bichier

Vasculitis is characterized by inflammation and necrosis of blood vessels, with subsequent tissue ischemia. Virtually any size or type of blood vessel, in any organ, can be affected. It may be primary or secondary. There is considerable overlap within the spectrum of the vasculitides, but certain patterns can be recognized. Although circulating immune complexes are implicated in the pathogenesis, they are rarely found in biopsy material, and this has lead to the term *pauciimmune*.

I. **Wegener's Granulomatosis.** Wegener's granulomatosis is an uncommon, primary systemic vasculitis predominantly affecting small and medium-sized arteries of the respiratory tract and kidneys.

A. **Clinical Picture.** Wegener's granulomatosis affects mostly middle-aged white people. The classic triad is of necrotizing granulomata of the upper and lower respiratory tract and necrotizing glomerulonephritis. Patients commonly present with epistaxis, hemoptysis, or painful sinusitis, and demonstrate pulmonary nodules on x-ray that may change or cavitate. Fever, rashes, arthritis, serositis, and neuritis occur with Wegener's granulomatosis. Antineutrophil cytoplasmic antibodies that react with proteinase 3 are highly specific in the right clinical setting and may be useful in monitoring disease activity for some patients.

B. **Renal Involvement.** Clinical renal disease is usually preceded by extrarenal manifestations, although there is evidence for renal involvement in approximately 85% of patients at presentation. Urinalysis reveals hematuria, red cell casts, and proteinuria. Renal function may be impaired in only a small proportion of patients initially but characteristically deteriorates in most. Biopsy usually shows focal segmental or diffuse necrotizing glomerulonephritis. Fulminant renal failure [rapidly progressive glomerulonephritis (RPGN)] can occur and is associated with crescents ("crescentic" glomerulonephritis). The pathognomonic granulomas as seen in the respiratory tract are typically absent. Immunofluorescence microscopy is usually negative, although immunoglobulin (Ig) G, IgM, and C3 may be seen along glomerular capillary walls.

C. **Management and Prognosis.** Early, aggressive treatment is indicated if there is evidence of major organ disease and should not be delayed until biopsy results are available. The need for dialysis does not preclude the use of aggressive therapy, as significant renal recovery can occur. The mainstay of therapy is methylprednisolone, 7 mg/kg/day intravenously, on 3 successive days followed by oral prednisone, 1 mg/kg/day. Steroids are tapered and discontinued after 6–12 months. Cyclophosphamide is given concurrently, either intravenously (0.5–1.0 g/m² in monthly pulses) or orally (starting at 2 mg/kg/day). Some form of immunosuppressive therapy is generally used for 6–12 months after remission. Adjunctive or alternative therapies include plasma infusion or plasmapheresis (particularly in patients with pulmonary hemorrhage or RPGN), trimethoprim-sulfamethoxazole, azathioprine, methotrexate, antilymphocyte globulin, and mycophenolate mofetil. Remission can be achieved in more than 90% of patients, although almost one-half relapse at some time. Treatment-related toxicity is a significant problem. Recurrence after transplantation is well documented.

II. **Polyarteritis Nodosa.** Polyarteritis nodosa (PAN) is a primary vasculitis of small and medium-sized arteries that involves many organs, notably the kidneys, nervous system, and heart. Aneurysms ("nodosa") form subsequent to healing and fibrosis.

    A. Clinical Picture. PAN is most common in men aged 35–50 years, often presenting as fever, weight loss, and visceral or joint pain. Renin-dependent hypertension due to glomerular ischemia is very common. Approximately 70% of patients develop cardiac disease, including ischemia and pericarditis; heart failure is a common cause of death. Lesions in one or more of the abdominal viscera, including the liver, mononeuritis multiplex, and polyneuropathy, occur frequently. Central nervous system involvement tends to occur late and may cause seizures and stroke. PAN is associated with hepatitis B antigenemia, intravenous drug abuse, and hairy cell leukemia. Biopsy of a clinically affected organ or celiac or renal arteriography may be used in diagnosis; arteriography shows characteristic aneurysms and irregular constrictions. Antibodies against myeloperoxidase are frequently detected but are not specific for PAN.

    B. Renal Involvement. Nearly all patients have some evidence of renal disease, ranging from minimal findings on urinalysis to gross hematuria and renal failure. The arcuate and interlobular arteries are primarily affected. Glomerular ischemia leads to fibrinoid necrosis, sclerosis, and patchy cortical infarction but little cell proliferation. The fall in the glomerular filtration rate generally results from reduced glomerular perfusion, although up to one-third of patients may also have glomerulonephritis. Necrotizing and crescentic glomerulonephritis are rare in PAN. Healing of the vessel wall leaves changes similar to hypertensive nephrosclerosis, but in PAN the elastic lamina is destroyed rather than reduplicated. Renal disease is the major cause of death.

C. **Management and Prognosis.** Early treatment is essential for renal disease. Treatment consists of cyclophosphamide and corticosteroids, and can succeed in increasing the survival rate to 80%. Plasmapheresis and a combination of lamivudine or interferon-α2b may be effective in hepatitis B–associated PAN.

III. **Microscopic Polyarteritis.** Microscopic polyarteritis may be considered a variant of PAN but tends to involve smaller arteries.

A. **Clinical Picture and Renal Involvement.** Microscopic polyarteritis may demonstrate multisystem involvement similar to PAN. However, hypertension is unusual and glomerulonephritis is very common. Inflammation of glomerular capillaries, interlobular arteries, and afferent arterioles is seen in combination with this disease. Glomerular capillaries manifest areas of fibrinoid necrosis and collapse, and there is basement membrane thickening and cellular proliferation of mesangial and endothelial cells. Crescents and RPGN may occur. The typical picture is of focal segmental glomerulonephritis with no immune deposits. Urinalysis shows protein, cells, and casts. Antimyeloperoxidase antineutrophil cytoplasmic antibodies are suggestive but not diagnostic.

B. **Management and Prognosis.** Microscopic polyarteritis is treated similarly to PAN and tends to have a better prognosis.

IV. **Henoch-Schönlein Purpura.** Henoch-Schönlein purpura is a vasculitis that involves small vessels (e.g., arterioles, venules). Immune complexes containing IgA are deposited in the skin and kidneys. Some believe that IgA nephropathy may be a renal-limited form of the disease.

A. **Clinical Picture.** Henoch-Schönlein purpura is relatively common and most often seen in young children. Its incidence increases in winter and spring, suggesting an infectious etiology in some patients. Skin involvement, seen in all patients, ranges from urticaria to palpable purpura. This classic "vasculitic rash" is usually seen over the buttocks and dependent extensor surfaces of the limbs. Skin biopsy reveals leukocytoclastic vasculitis with IgA deposits in new lesions. Abdominal pain, arthralgia, and edema are common.

B. **Renal Involvement.** Evidence of renal involvement is not universal, but ranges from microscopic or gross hematuria to acute nephritis with renal failure and hypertension. Proteinuria, sometimes in the nephrotic range, is common. Histologically, changes identical to IgA nephropathy are seen. There are IgA deposits in the glomerular mesangium and, usually, a mild focal segmental glomerulonephritis. Necrosis and crescents may be seen in severe cases. IgG and C3 deposition may also be detected, but serum complement is usually normal. The severity of glomerulonephritis does not correlate with the extent of extrarenal disease.

C. Management and Prognosis. Henoch-Schönlein purpura is usually self-limiting over weeks to months, although relapses that are milder than the initial episode occur. Supportive therapy, with fluid and sodium restriction and appropriate treatment of hypertension, is usually sufficient. Short courses of oral prednisone are often given to those with debilitating symptoms, although its efficacy is unproven. Plasmapheresis and prednisone combined with cyclophosphamide are recommended for crescentic nephritis. Risk factors for progressive renal disease include nephrotic syndrome, acute renal failure, and crescents on biopsy. The extent of renal disease generally determines the long-term prognosis. Usually, glomerulonephritis resolves, albeit with residual hematuria that does not necessarily have implications for future renal function. Recurrence after transplantation occurs, notably in living related donor allografts.

V. Suggested Readings

De-Groot K, Adu D, Savage C. The value of pulse cyclophosphamide in ANCA-associated vasculitis: meta-analysis and critical review. *Nephrol Dial Transplant* 2001;16:2018–2027.

Feehally J. IgA nephropathy and Henoch-Schönlein nephritis. In: Johnson RJ, Feehally J, eds. *Comprehensive clinical nephrology*, 2nd ed. Philadelphia: Mosby, 2003:319–330.

Jennette JC, Falk RJ. Renal and systemic vasculitis. In: Johnson RJ, Feehally J, eds. *Comprehensive clinical nephrology*, 2nd ed. St. Louis: Mosby, 2003:341–355.

Nachman PH, Falk RJ. Treatment of ANCA-associated small-vessel vasculitis. In: Brady HR, Wilcox CS, eds. *Therapy in nephrology and hypertension*. Philadelphia: WB Saunders, 2003:197–205.

Nachman PH, Jeanette JC, Falk JF. Vasculitic diseases of the kidney. In: Schrier RW, ed. *Diseases of the kidney and urinary tract*, 7th ed. Boston: Little, Brown and Company, 2001:1911–1938.

Renal Involvement in Thrombotic Microangiopathy, Scleroderma, Multiple Myeloma, and Amyloidosis

Geraldine Shaw Bichier

I. **Thrombotic Microangiopathy.** Thrombotic microangiopathy encompasses hemolytic uremic syndrome (HUS), thrombotic thrombocytopenic purpura (TTP), and the antiphospholipid syndrome. It is associated with preeclampsia, oral contraceptive use, and chemotherapeutic agents. The most common initial event is endothelial injury, resulting in platelet microthrombi, platelet consumption, hemolytic anemia, and variable renal and neurologic manifestations.

  A. **Clinical Picture.** The presentation of HUS and TTP correlates with the different distribution of the microangiopathic lesions. Typical HUS predominantly affects the kidneys of young children after an acute diarrheal illness. It is frequently associated with Shiga toxin–producing bacteria, usually *Escherichia coli* O157:H7, which can be identified on a stool culture. Atypical forms may be familial or associated with a variety of microbial agents. TTP, where microthrombi are mostly deposited in the brain, peaks in the third to fourth decade and is more common in women. It is associated with *ADAMTS13* deficiency. Neurologic symptoms that wax and wane include confusion, seizures, and paresis. However, both renal and neurologic manifestations can occur in either disease, and there is significant overlap between adult TTP and HUS.

  More than 90% of patients with TTP and HUS have purpura at presentation. Epistaxis, hematuria, gastrointestinal hemorrhage due to thrombocytopenia, and a Coombs'-negative hemolytic anemia are common. The peripheral blood smear shows schistocytes, burr, and helmet cells. Other complaints include fever, myalgia, and arthralgia.

  B. **Renal Involvement.** Approximately 90% of all patients have proteinuria, usually <2 g per day, and microscopic or gross hematuria. More than one-half will have renal failure of varying severity at some time, but renal involvement tends to be more common and more severe in HUS. Prolonged anuria, the need for early dialysis, and proteinuria that persists after recovery are risk factors for developing chronic renal failure.

  Histologically, there is endothelial cell hypertrophy and widening of the subendothelial space. Platelet and fibrin thrombi deposition are seen, occluding the glomerular capillaries and afferent arterioles and causing ischemia and necrosis. Immunofluorescence microscopy is usually negative.

C. **Management and Prognosis.** The typical Shiga toxin–associated form of HUS is usually self-limiting. Supportive therapy, including dialysis and bowel rest, is vital, but no specific therapy has been shown to affect the disease course. Antibiotics increase the risk of HUS if given for *E. coli* O157:H7.

Untreated TTP is almost invariably fatal within 3 months. Plasma therapy (either plasmapheresis or plasma infusion) is the only proven effective treatment and has improved the survival rate to 90%. Plasma therapy is also used for adult and atypical childhood HUS, although the latter is often refractory. Improvement in the platelet count and serum lactic acid dehydrogenase correlates with treatment response. Antiplatelet agents and corticosteroids have not been shown to be beneficial. Splenectomy and nephrectomy have occasionally been used in refractory or recurrent disease. Platelet infusions are given for life-threatening hemorrhages.

Overall, renal and neurologic sequelae are more likely in atypical and adult forms of HUS and in TTP. Relapses occur but are less common and milder in typical HUS. Recurrence after transplantation is more common in atypical HUS.

II. **Progressive Systemic Sclerosis (Scleroderma).** Progressive systemic sclerosis (scleroderma) is a systemic disease of collagen associated with obliterative vascular lesions. It mainly affects the skin, lungs, gastrointestinal tract, and kidneys.

A. **Clinical Picture.** Progressive systemic sclerosis is a relatively rare disease that is most common in middle-aged women. Arterial walls become inflamed, thus narrowing and eventually obliterating the lumen. Skin involvement is seen in 90% of patients: Ischemic ulcers, subcutaneous calcinosis, Raynaud's phenomenon, telangiectasia, and sclerodactyly may occur. Extradermatologic manifestations, which may predominate in some patients who experience an acute diffuse onset, include esophageal dysmotility, pulmonary interstitial fibrosis, cardiomyopathy, polymyositis, and arthralgia. Most patients demonstrate positive antinuclear antibodies. Anticentromere and anti-topoisomerase antibodies are highly specific for progressive systemic sclerosis. They are found in approximately 30% of patients and correlate with the CREST (calcinosis, *R*aynaud's phenomenon, *e*sophageal dysmotility, *s*clerodactyly, and *t*elangiectasia) syndrome or limited skin involvement and severe, diffuse disease, respectively.

B. **Renal Involvement.** Approximately one-half of all patients with progressive systemic sclerosis have some form of renal involvement, and renal failure accounts for more than one-third of deaths. Obliterative arterial lesions, mainly preglomerular, are seen on biopsy. There is concentric proliferation of smooth muscle cells in the media that migrate into the intima, producing an "onion skin" appearance. Basement membrane thickening and fibrinoid necrosis may be seen in the glomeruli and tubulointerstitium, along with immunoglobulin M and C3 deposition, tubular atrophy, and edema. Urinalysis is usually unremarkable, although ischemic glomerulosclerosis may cause hematuria.

An important complication is the scleroderma renal crisis, usually associated with hyperreninemic hypertension, which has an abrupt onset and the potential to progress to renal failure within weeks. It occurs in approximately 25% of patients and is more common in winter. Renal vasoconstriction, a consequence of cold-induced vasospasm, hypovolemia, or heart failure, is the postulated instigator.

C. **Management and Prognosis.** Prognosis and management are dependent on the pattern of organ involvement. Overall mortality from renal, cardiac, or respiratory failure approaches 65% 7 years after diagnosis, although the 1-year survival rate is now more than 75% with organ-specific treatment.

Immunosuppression does not change the course of the disease. Control of blood pressure is paramount: Scleroderma renal crisis was invariably fatal before the advent of angiotensin-converting enzyme inhibitors, but their use now controls hypertension in most patients. Early use of angiotensin-converting enzyme inhibitors can stabilize and improve renal function, and this improvement is often associated with extrarenal remission. Other therapy includes calcium channel blockers for Raynaud's phenomenon, proton pump inhibitors for esophageal reflux, and iloprost and endothelin receptor antagonists for pulmonary hypertension. Cold avoidance, good nutrition and skin care are also important. Poor vascular access may cause problems in hemodialysis. Continuous ambulatory peritoneal dialysis is often more successful, although compromised peritoneal vasculature may reduce efficiency.

III. **Multiple Myeloma.** Myeloma is a plasma cell tumor in the bone marrow that produces excessive immunoglobulin (M protein). The light chains of this immunoglobulin are detected in the urine as Bence Jones protein.

A. **Clinical Picture.** Multiple myeloma usually affects adults older than 50 years. The excess M protein causes erythrocyte sedimentation rate elevation, hyperviscosity, and renal failure. Bone pain, fractures, and hypercalcemia are common. Marrow infiltration causes anemia, thrombocytopenia, and immunoparesis.

B. **Renal Involvement.** More than one-half of all patients with myeloma have renal disease, and many of these develop progressive renal failure. Nephrotic-range proteinuria is common. The main pathology occurs in the tubules, where filtered proteins such as albumin, fibrin, and Tamm-Horsfall mucoprotein obstruct the lumen and form large eosinophilic casts. This "cast nephropathy" is accompanied by inflammation, interstitial fibrosis, and tubular atrophy. Nephrotoxic light chains spill into the urinary space and cause tubular dysfunction. Amyloid deposition complicates the picture. Renal failure may be precipitated by hypercalcemia and dehydration, chemotherapy, hyperuricemia, and nephrotoxins such as nonsteroidal antiinflammatory drugs.

C. **Management.** Renal involvement does not necessarily affect outcome and should not be a major obstacle to active treatment. Furthermore, renal impairment is often reversible with attention to hydration and other factors. Plasmapheresis, sometimes instituted for the hyperviscosity syndrome, may have a place in preventing or treating renal disease. Dialysis is used when indicated. Prednisone and melphalan have not improved the median survival beyond 3 years but are still used for patients older than 70 years. Vincristine, doxorubicin, and dexamethasone used in combination are effective at reducing tumor load in younger patients. High-dose melphalan with autologous hematopoietic stem-cell transplantation has greatly improved rates of remission and survival. Some centers reduce the melphalan dose in the face of renal failure.

IV. **Amyloid.** Amyloid is a fibrous protein that, when stained with Congo red, produces a bright green birefringence under polarized light. It is seen in two basic patterns: primary and secondary. Its deposition gradually destroys normal tissue.

A. **Clinical Picture.** Primary amyloid affects adults older than 40 years, two-thirds of whom are men. Cardiac failure and arrhythmias, peripheral neuropathy, fatigue, and orthostatic hypotension are common. Other features include hepatosplenomegaly and macroglossia. An M protein is found on serum protein electrophoresis in most patients: Transformation to myeloma may occur. Secondary amyloid is associated with chronic inflammatory disease, and deposits are principally seen in the kidneys, spleen, and liver.

B. **Renal Involvement.** The kidneys are involved in more than 90% of patients with primary and secondary amyloid. Nephrotic syndrome due to glomerular amyloid deposition is common. If tubular amyloid deposition is marked, nephrogenic diabetes insipidus, renal tubular acidosis, or hyperkalemia may predominate. Renal disease may be the only clinical manifestation of secondary amyloid (usually proteinuria), and progression tends to be slower than in primary renal amyloid. Amyloid should be considered in any patient with renal impairment or nephrotic syndrome who has an associated chronic inflammatory or multisystem disease.

C. **Management and Prognosis.** The course of renal amyloid may be reasonably stable for many years, but prognosis is poor once the nephrotic syndrome or azotemia appears. Amyloid should be confirmed by abdominal fat pad aspiration or biopsy of the kidney, tongue, or rectum. Treatment is problematic. Standard supportive therapy for nephrotic syndrome and renal failure is appropriate, although autonomic dysfunction or cardiac disease may compromise hemodialysis. Midodrine, an α-adrenergic agonist, may ameliorate orthostatic hypotension. Melphalan, prednisone, and other chemotherapeutic agents have been used with varying success in primary amyloid, although prognosis remains poor and measurable in months. Colchicine, which has demonstrated some benefit in secondary amyloid, may be tried. In secondary amyloid, treatment is directed at the underlying chronic disease, which also dictates the ultimate prognosis. Amyloid recurs in the transplanted allograft, but the decline in renal function is usually less severe than in native kidneys.

V. Suggested Readings

Goldschmidt H, Lannert H, Bommer J, et al. Multiple myeloma and renal failure. *Nephrol Dial Transplant* 2000;15:301–304.

Janson RW, Arend WP. Renal disorders associated with systemic sclerosis, rheumatoid arthritis, Sjögren's syndrome and polymyositis-dermatomyositis. In: Schrier RW, ed. *Diseases of the kidney and urinary tract*, 7th ed. Boston: Little, Brown, and Company, 2001:1861–1882.

Ring GH, Lakkis FG, Badr KF. Microvascular diseases of the kidney. In: Brenner BM, ed. *Brenner and Rector's the kidney*, 6th ed. Philadelphia: WB Saunders, 2000:1597–1620.

Ruggenenti P, Noris M, Remuzzi G. Thrombotic microangiopathy, hemolytic uremic syndrome, and thrombotic thrombocytopenic purpura. *Kidney Int* 2001;60:831–846.

Schwimmer JA, Joseph RE, Appel GB. Amyloid, fibrillary and other glomerular deposition diseases. In: Brady HR, Wilcox CS, eds. *Therapy in nephrology and hypertension*, 2nd ed. Philadelphia: WB Saunders, 2003:253–260.

Tubulointerstitial Nephritis

Awad A. El-Magbri and Shakil Aslam

I. **Definition and Description.** *Tubulointerstitial nephritis* refers to a group of disorders characterized by inflammation, cellular infiltration, and fibrosis of the renal tubules and interstitium with relative sparing of the glomeruli until late in the disease course. Tubulointerstitial inflammation may also be a feature of some glomerular diseases, such as nonsteroidal antiinflammatory drug–induced minimal change disease and focal segmental glomerulosclerosis, but glomerular abnormalities are predominant features of these conditions. Tubulointerstitial nephritis is a nonspecific clinicopathologic syndrome resulting from many diverse etiologic agents. The clinical presentation ranges from acute interstitial nephritis (AIN), with a sudden onset of acute renal failure requiring renal replacement therapy, to chronic interstitial nephritis, with a smoldering course leading to end-stage renal disease. Table 12.1 shows the causes of acute and chronic tubulointerstitial nephritis.

II. **Pathogenesis.** In most cases, drug-induced AIN results from cell-mediated hypersensitivity reactions. Renal biopsy generally does not show any immune deposits, and interstitial infiltrates are rich in T cells. The resulting interstitial inflammation is associated with damage to tubular cells, which plays a key role in pathogenesis of acute renal failure associated with AIN. Generally, this inflammation is reversible once the offending agent is withdrawn, but prolonged exposure may lead to irreversible and progressive renal insufficiency.

The lesions of tubulointerstitial nephritis result from direct interactions between inflammatory cells and tubular epithelial cells, causing release of soluble molecules or activation of the complement cascade or both. Tubular cells can also be activated to produce cell adhesion molecules, cytokines, and chemokines. Among these cytokines, transforming growth factor-β (TGF-β), endothelin-1, and platelet-derived growth factor-BB are potent fibrogens. TGF-β1 is probably the most important and best characterized. TGF-β1 is produced by many cells, including monocytes, macrophages, lymphocytes, fibroblasts, endothelial cells, and tubular cells. It acts as a chemoattractant for fibroblasts, induces proliferation of fibroblastic cells, and increases the transcription of genes encoding for proteins of the extracellular matrix. TGF-β1 also inhibits the production of metalloproteinases that degrade the matrix and increases the production of tissue inhibitors of metalloproteinases, which are their natural inhibitors. These reactions result in expansion of tissue matrix interstitial fibrosis, and tubular atrophy, leading to progressive renal insufficiency. Activation of

TABLE 12.1.   Causes of tubulointerstitial nephritis

Acute tubulointerstitial nephritis	Chronic tubulointerstitial nephritis
Hypersensitivity reactions (penicillin, sulfonamides, nonsteroidal antiinflammatory drugs)	Drugs (analgesics, lithium, cyclosporine, tacrolimus)
Immunologic disease (SLE, Goodpasture's syndrome)	Heavy metals (lead, cadmium, mercury)
Acute transplant rejection	Obstructive uropathy, nephrolithiasis, reflux disease
Infections	Immunologic diseases (SLE, Sjögren's syndrome, primary glomerulopathies, sarcoidosis)
Bacterial (associated with chronic obstruction or reflux)	Vasculitis (antineutrophil cytoplasmic antibody–associated, Wegener's granulomatosis)
Viral (BK polyoma virus, cytomegalovirus, hantavirus, human immunodeficiency virus, hepatitis B)	Chronic allograft nephropathy
Fungal (histoplasmosis)	Atherosclerotic kidney disease (ischemic nephropathy, cholesterol, microemboli)
Parasitic (leishmania, toxoplasmosis)	Metabolic diseases (hypercalcemia, cystitis, hyperoxaluria)
	Genetic diseases (Alport's syndrome, medullary cystic kidney)
	Miscellaneous (Balkan endemic nephropathy; Chinese herb, *Aristolochia* nephropathy)

SLE, systemic lupus erythematosus.

nuclear factor κB may cause transcription and release of proinflammatory cytokines in chronic tubulointerstitial nephritis associated with proteinuric kidney diseases. Activation of the renin–angiotensin system may also play an important role in maintaining this cycle of inflammation and fibrosis.

III. **Clinical Presentation and Diagnosis.** AIN accounts for 2–3% of all renal biopsies, and chronic interstitial nephritis accounts for 4.8% of end-stage renal disease cases in the United States. Drug therapy accounts for the majority of cases of AIN, although sarcoidosis, *Legionella*, leptospirosis, streptococcal, and viral infections may also be responsible. The major histologic changes are interstitial edema and a marked interstitial infiltrate consisting primarily of T lymphocytes and monocytes, but eosinophils, plasma cells, and neutrophils may also be found. Granuloma formation, a particular characteristic of renal disease in sarcoidosis, can occur in any form of AIN. Common clinical features are listed in Table 12.2. Fever, rash, eosinophilia, and eosinophiluria are typically absent in nonsteroidal antiinflammatory drug–associated AIN. Eosinophiluria (eosinophils >1% of urinary white cells by Hansel's stain) has a sensitivity and specificity of 67% and 83%, respectively, in AIN not caused

TABLE 12.2.   Clinical features of acute and chronic tubulointerstitial nephritis

Acute interstitial nephritis	Chronic interstitial nephritis
Begins abruptly with acute renal failure.	Insidious onset.
Occurs within days of exposure to offending drug or several months with NSAIDs.	Often diagnosed incidentally on routine screening or evaluation of hypertension.
Rash, fever, eosinophilia, eosinophiluria, and elevated immunoglobulin E.	Patients are usually asymptomatic.
	Hypertension is common.
Tubular function abnormalities ± Fanconi's syndrome.	Elevation in serum creatinine, tubular dysfunction (renal tubular acidosis), or Fanconi's syndrome.
Proteinuria is usually absent or mild ± microscopic hematuria ± sterile pyuria.	Proteinuria is usually mild (<1 g/day) and of low molecular weight.
Renal biopsy may be required to make a definitive diagnosis.	Renal biopsy shows: interstitial fibrosis, tubular atrophy, arteriolar sclerosis, and mononuclear cell infiltrate.
NSAID-induced tubulointerstitial nephritis may present with nephrotic range proteinuria from minimal change disease.	Papillary necrosis with analgesic nephropathy, causes gross hematuria, flank pain ± obstruction.

NSAID, nonsteroidal antiinflammatory drug.

by nonsteroidal antiinflammatory drugs. Eosinophiluria and hypocomplementemia are frequent findings in atheroembolic renal disease.

Chronic interstitial nephritis has an insidious onset and is commonly associated with evidence of tubular dysfunction such as Fanconi's syndrome, type IV renal tubular acidosis with hyperkalemia, and low-molecular-weight proteinuria. Analgesic nephropathy is 5–6 times more common in women. Atherosclerotic or ischemic kidney disease or both may occur in 5–22% of patients with advanced renal failure who are older than the age of 50. Metabolic disorders, such as cystinosis, oxalosis, and hypercalcemia, can occur in young individuals.

IV. Treatment of Acute Tubulointerstitial Nephritis. In most cases, cessation of the offending agent results in quick recovery and complete resolution of the renal disorder, although some patients progress to chronic renal insufficiency. If no sign of improvement is observed within a few days of discontinuation, renal biopsy or empiric therapy with steroids may be considered. Although controlled trials are lacking, many authors suggest using prednisone at 1 mg/kg for 2–6 weeks, with rapid tapering of the dose. This intervention may improve the outcome, speed renal recovery, and reduce the requirement for dialysis.

V. Treatment of Chronic Tubulointerstitial Disease.
Treatment depends on the etiology and generally consists of
supportive measures, such as adequate blood pressure control
and management of anemia. Treatment of lead nephropathy
by chelation therapy is of proven value and must be imple-
mented in lead poisoning. Chelation therapy with ethylenedi-
aminetetraacetic acid or succimer (Chemet) may slow down
the progression of chronic kidney disease, although its value
in reversing chronic renal insufficiency and hypertension is
questionable due to permanent scarring. The oral chelating
agent succimer has proved very successful in treating children; it has not been widely used in adults. Nevertheless, it
appears effective in reducing body lead stores. Because no
effective therapy reverses the long-term consequences of lead
poisoning, the best therapy is prevention and awareness of
potential environmental and occupational sources for lead
exposure. In patients with established lead nephropathy,
treatment consists of management of hypertension, gout, and
chronic renal insufficiency. Many patients with lead nephropathy progress to end-stage kidney failure and require dialysis.

VI. Suggested Readings

Haas M, Spargo BH, Wit EJ, Meehan SM. Etiologies and outcome of acute renal insufficiency in older adults: a renal
biopsy study of 259 cases. *Am J Kidney Dis* 2000;35:433.

Rossert J. Drug-induced acute interstitial nephritis. *Kidney Int*
2001;60:804.

Schwarz A, Krause PH, Kunzendorf U, et al. The outcome of
acute interstitial nephritis: risk factors for the transition
from acute to chronic interstitial nephritis. *Clin Nephrol*
2000;54:179.

Familial and Cystic Renal Diseases

Wen-Ting Ouyang and Christopher S. Wilcox

Renal cysts are fluid-filled cavities with epithelial linings. Simple renal cysts increase in frequency with age but are of little clinical importance. Ultrasound examination of simple renal cysts reveals a homogeneous pattern without internal echoes or calcium. Computed tomography scanning shows an attenuation value close to that of water, no enhancement with intravenous contrast, no thickening or irregularity of the cyst wall, and a smooth interface with the renal parenchyma. Cysts that lack these criteria are termed *complex* and require further evaluation.

Three adult cystic diseases cause significant complications: autosomal-dominant polycystic kidney disease (adult-type ADPKD), medullary sponge kidney, and medullary cystic disease (Table 13.1). Additionally, an autosomal-recessive polycystic kidney disease is encountered predominantly in children. It presents with abdominal mass, liver involvement that can include portal hypertension, and renal failure. Not all congenital disorders are inherited. Acquired cystic disease is encountered in patients who have received dialysis treatment for several years.

Renal cysts develop from tubules with which they may retain continuity. As the cysts accumulate glomerular filtrate, they enlarge and become isolated from the glomerulus. Thereafter, cyst expansion depends on transepithelial transport of solutes and fluid. The etiology of cyst formation may involve tubular obstruction that elevates intraluminal pressure, increased elasticity of the tubular basement membrane, proliferation of epithelial cells with production of excessive basement membrane, loss of polarity of the tubular cells, or cellular production of cytokines.

I. **Autosomal-Dominant Polycystic Kidney Disease**
   A. **Clinical Presentation and Diagnosis.** ADPKD is due to mutations in the polycystin gene that encodes a large protein expressed in the kidneys and blood vessels. ADPKD affects 1:400–1:1,000 Americans. It accounts for 8–10% of the cases of end-stage renal disease (ESRD). Approximately 85% of the cases are caused by a dominant gene located on the short arm of chromosome 16 (the ADPKD-1 gene). Approximately 5–10% of cases result from an abnormal gene located on the long arm of chromosome 4 (the ADPKD-2 gene), which causes a milder form of the disorder. ADPKD is associated with congenital hepatic fibrosis, hepatic cysts (in 50% of patients, and these increase with age), Caroli's disease, Budd-Chiari

TABLE 13.1.   Clinical features of major renal cystic disease

	Simple renal cysts	Autosomal-dominant polycystic kidney disease	Acquired cystic disease	Medullary sponge kidney	Medullary cystic kidney disease
Incidence	1:10	1:600	Common in dialysis patients	1:5,000	Rare
Typical age at presentation	Variable	20–40 yr	Variable	40–60 yr	Variable
Inheritance	None	Autosomal-dominant	None	None	Mainly autosomal-dominant
Cyst location	Variable	Proximal and distal tubules	Variable	Collecting duct	Corticomedullary
Flank pain or hematuria	Rare	Frequent	Rare	With stones or infection	None
Major complications	Rare	Hypertension UTIs Renal stones Aneurysm	Renal cell carcinoma	UTIs Renal stones	Salt wasting Polyuria
Renal failure	Absent	Inevitable over time	Associated with preexisting renal failure	Rare	Inevitable

UTIs, urinary tract infections.

syndrome, pancreatic cysts, and colonic diverticula. Cholangiocarcinoma and cysts in the gonads, epididymis, and central nervous system occur rarely. Cardiac valvular abnormalities are present in 25% of patients. Renal tubular dysfunctions manifest as impaired acidification and concentrating ability and diminished citrate excretion, predisposing to renal stones. Renal adenomas are present in 20% of patients but are rarely malignant. Cystic calcification is common. Proteinuria is usually mild (<1 g/day). Endothelial dysfunction of blood vessels contributes to hypertension, which is exacerbated by activation of the renin angiotensin and sympathetic nervous systems. Anemia is less common than anticipated from the degree of renal failure because of persistent erythropoietin production. A positive family history is present in only 60% of patients.

B. Screening. The test of choice for ADPKD is renal ultrasound. The diagnosis is effectively secured if more than three cysts are detected in an individual with a family history of ADPKD. The number of cysts also depends on age of screening. Fewer than 25% of ADPKD-1 gene carriers have detectable renal cysts before the age of 30 years. Gene linkage techniques can diagnose presymptomatic individuals if at least two affected and related persons are available for study. This test is useful for evaluating living related kidney donors among family members. DNA analysis with detection of mutants in the polycystin gene is available in specialized centers. Patients should be counseled before recommending presymptomatic diagnosis. The identification of a gene-carrier state does not predict the clinical course.

C. Complications and Management. Hypertension occurs early and is frequent. It usually responds to angiotensin-converting enzyme inhibitors or angiotensin receptor blockers, but an occasional patient develops acute renal failure. This may be because angiotensin II is required to maintain an adequate ultrafiltration pressure in glomeruli located downstream from a cyst causing vascular obstruction. Because diuretics may inhibit reabsorption of fluid from cysts, thereby leading to cyst expansion, they are best avoided when possible. Aggressive treatment of hypertension is warranted, especially because patients may have an undetected cerebral aneurysm, but this probably does little to delay the onset or progression of renal failure. Beta blockade is useful in patients with sympathetic overactivity.

Pain in the flank can indicate a cyst hemorrhage, which usually resolves with bed rest and analgesia. Cyst infection requires a careful choice of antibiotics. Drugs that penetrate into the cysts include trimethoprim-sulfamethoxazole or quinolones. Cyst infection should be differentiated from pyelonephritis, in which patients often have white blood cell casts on urinalysis. Some patients develop calcium oxalate or uric acid stones.

Patients with intractable pain from large cysts may require surgical decompression, percutaneous puncture and drainage, or laparoscopic unroofing.

Hematuria is usually self-limiting. Occasionally, it indicates malignant transformation. Nephrolithiasis should be excluded.

Renal insufficiency progresses to ESRD by age 60 in approximately one-half of patients. Women have a less aggressive course than men. ESRD develops earlier in blacks. Nephrolithiasis should be suspected in those with a rapid decline in renal function. Hemodialysis is often preferable to peritoneal dialysis because of the limited peritoneal space as a result of enlarged kidneys. Living related kidney donors must be screened carefully. Gene carriers may not show cysts even when they are 30 years old.

Headache of sudden onset in ADPKD suggests subarachnoid hemorrhage from rupture of an intracerebral aneurysm. The initial test is a noncontrast computed tomography scan of the head followed by a lumbar puncture if the computed tomography is negative and subarachnoid hemorrhage remains a possibility. Detection of cerebrospinal fluid xanthochromia indicates bleeding. Once the subarachnoid hemorrhage is diagnosed, conventional angiography is used to localize a bleeding intracerebral aneurysm. Early intervention by surgical clipping or coil embolization reduces recurrent bleeding.

Intracerebral aneurysm affects 5–10% of patients with ADPKD. Routine screening is not generally recommended, but opinions vary among centers. Screening with magnetic resonance imaging or angiography is reserved for patients with either a previous or family history of bleeding from a ruptured aneurysm or with uncontrolled hypertension. Aneurysms >5 mm require neurosurgical evaluation. Other causes of headache in these patients include ischemic or hemorrhagic stroke, hypertensive emergency, cervicocephalic artery dissection, and subdural hematoma.

D. **Counseling.** The patient's family members should be counseled after the diagnosis of ADPKD.

E. **Prognosis.** Once renal insufficiency is established, the creatinine clearance halves, on average, every 6 months. Not every carrier of an abnormal ADPKD gene progresses to ESRD.

II. **Acquired Cystic Disease.** Simple renal cysts are common and increase with age. Usually these are single, unilateral, and benign.

Acquired cystic disease in patients with ESRD can be benign, but malignant cysts occasionally develop. Ultrasound screening is recommended for patients on dialysis >7 years. Patients with tumors >2 cm should be referred for nephrectomy.

III. **Medullary Sponge Kidney.** Although medullary sponge kidney is a congenital anomaly, it does not usually present until age 40 to 60 years. There is marked enlargement of the medullary and inner papillary portions of the collecting ducts. Approximately one-fourth of patients have hemihypertrophy of the body.

Medullary sponge kidney is associated with recurrent hematuria and urinary tract infections, nephrolithiasis, polyuria from an inability to concentrate the urine, and distal renal tubular acidosis that may be completed by nephrolithiasis. Diagnosis is made by intravenous pyelography, which shows striations in the papillae or cystic collections of contrast medium in ectatic collecting ducts. Patients with renal tubular acidosis require treatment with alkali. Those with renal calculi should drink enough fluid to maintain at least 2 L of urine output per day. Those with hypercalciuria should receive a thiazide diuretic.

IV. **Medullary Cystic Disease.** Juvenile nephronophthisis is an autosomal-recessive defect in a gene on chromosome 2p.

Medullary cystic disease is an autosomal-dominant disease. *Renal–retinal dysplasia* refers to medullary cystic disease associated with retinal degeneration, familial retinitis pigmentosa, and pigmentary optic atrophy.

The kidneys have small, thin-walled cysts at the corticomedullary junction. The childhood form presents with polydipsia, polyuria, anemia, lethargy, and growth retardation. It usually progresses to ESRD before the age of 20. The adult form presents with salt-wasting nephropathy that may require large amounts of salt and fluid to combat orthostasis.

V. **von Hippel-Lindau Disease.** von Hippel-Lindau disease, an uncommon autosomal-dominant disorder, is associated with retinal angiomas, central nervous system hemangioblastomas, and pancreatic cysts. The development of renal cysts and bilateral or multicentric renal cell carcinomas mandates regular surveillance and early referral to surgery if detected. Pheochromocytomas occur in one-third of patients.

VI. **Tuberous Sclerosis.** Tuberous sclerosis is an uncommon autosomal-dominant disorder characterized by epilepsy, mental retardation, adenoma sebaceum, ash-leaf skin pigmentation, angiomyolipomas of the kidneys, renal cysts, and, occasionally, pheochromocytomas.

VII. **Sickle Cell Nephropathy.** Patients with sickle cell nephropathy can present with microscopic or gross hematuria from medullary congestion caused by sickling of erythrocytes at the low partial pressure of oxygen in the medulla; this can lead to papillary necrosis. Conservative treatment entails infusion of hypotonic fluid and diuretics. Patients may have tubular defects manifest as a concentrating defect, acidosis, hyperphosphatemia, hyperuricemia, or hyperkalemia. The development of focal segmental glomerulosclerosis with interstitial fibrosis is heralded by proteinuria and progresses to renal failure. Hypertension is infrequent in patients without nephropathy. Renal transplant can be successful, but nephropathy can reoccur.

VIII. Alport's Syndrome. Alport's syndrome is usually an X-linked disorder presenting with microscopic hematuria. ESRD can occur early. Men are more severely affected. Some families have high-frequency hearing loss. Anterior lenticonus, posterior polymorphous corneal dystrophy, and retinal flecks are rare diagnostic features. Kidney biopsy shows a thick glomerular basement membrane containing granules of varying density and sizes when the basement membrane is split. There is tubule dropout and interstitial fibrosis. Leiomyomatosis of the female genitalia or esophagus occurs in some families. Antiglomerular basement membrane disease occurs in 3% of transplant recipients.

 IX. Familial Thin Membrane Disease. Familial thin membrane disease, a benign condition, presents with hematuria. The thickness of the glomerular basement membrane is reduced by 75%. Renal failure does not occur. Renal biopsy is diagnostic.

  X. Nail-Patella Syndrome. Nail-patella syndrome is an autosomal-dominant condition with variable penetrance. Some children have nephritic syndrome and nail dysplasias.

 XI. Suggested Readings

Bogdanove N, Markoff A, Horst J. Autosomal-dominant polycystic kidney disease-clinical and genetic aspects. *Kidney Blood Press Res* 2002;25:265–283.

Chapman A. Renal cystic disorder. In: Brady HR, Wilcox CS, eds. *Therapy in nephrology and hypertension*. Philadelphia: WB Saunders, 2003:499–502.

Chesney RW. Noncystic hereditary diseases of the kidney. In: Brady HR, Wilcox CS, eds. *Therapy in nephrology and hypertension*. Philadelphia: WB Saunders, 2003:503–512.

Hudson BG, Tryggvason K, Sundaramoorthy M, et al. Alport's syndrome, Goodpasture's syndrome and type IV collage. *N Engl J Med* 2003;248:2543–2556.

Pirson Y, Chauveau D, Torres V. Management of cerebral aneurysms in autosomal-dominant polycystic kidney disease. *J Am Soc Nephrol* 2002;13:269–276.

HIV Infection and Kidney Disease

Richard J. Johnson and C. Craig Tisher

Patients infected with the human immunodeficiency virus (HIV) may develop numerous renal complications. The most important presentations are (a) the acute renal failure syndromes, (b) HIV nephropathy and other glomerular diseases, and (c) end-stage renal disease. These three entities are discussed below.

In addition, fluid and electrolyte abnormalities are common. In particular, hyponatremia is frequently observed and, in most cases, is due to volume depletion with water retention from the appropriate stimulation of antidiuretic hormone. Patients with HIV may also be at risk for developing the syndrome of inappropriate secretion of antidiuretic hormone in association with infection or drug use. Some patients manifest hyponatremia (often with hyperkalemia) as an indication of adrenal insufficiency secondary to HIV. Disorders of potassium, calcium, and magnesium may also be seen. Management of these disorders associated with HIV is discussed in Chapters 15–18.

I. **Acute Renal Failure in the HIV-Infected Patient.** Acute renal failure is a frequent complication in patients with HIV infection, especially those with the clinical picture of acquired immune deficiency syndrome (AIDS). Diagnosis is essentially the same as in any patient who manifests a rising level of blood urea nitrogen or serum creatinine (see Chapter 30). Ruling out prerenal causes is critical, because many patients with AIDS may develop volume depletion secondary to diarrhea and poor oral intake. The usual renal causes of acute renal failure, such as sepsis and the use of radiocontrast agents, are also common. Postrenal causes may also occur, secondary to obstruction from stones or tumors or autonomic dysfunction of the bladder.

There are also specific etiologies of acute renal failure that one should consider in the HIV-infected patient. A major category relates to nephrotoxicity of various antibiotics commonly used in HIV-infected patients, including the use of aminoglycosides, amphotericin B, foscarnet, and pentamidine. Acyclovir and valacyclovir, when used at high doses, and particularly in patients with preexisting renal insufficiency, may result in high urinary concentrations, leading to crystal formation and acute tubular obstruction (appearing as needle-like crystals on urinary sediment examination). Recently, certain protease inhibitors, notably indinavir and ritonavir, have been found to cause acute nephrotoxicity by forming intratubular crystals, leading to microscopic and occasionally gross hematuria and renal failure. The use of high-dose sulfadiazines to treat toxoplasmosis may be associated with crystalluria (appearing as "haystacks") in acute renal failure. Acute interstitial nephritis may also develop secondary to the use of rifampin, foscarnet, or the sulfa class of antibiotics.

In addition to drug toxicities, HIV can be associated with an acute thrombotic microangiopathy similar to thrombotic thrombocytopenic purpura or hemolytic uremic syndrome. Finally, HIV may be associated with a variety of glomerular diseases, some of which may present with a relatively acute deterioration in renal function (see below).

There is little doubt that acute renal failure contributes to mortality and morbidity in HIV-infected patients, although sepsis remains the leading cause of death. If these patients are hemodynamically stable, hemodialysis can be beneficial, and the decision to treat should be made using the same clinical criteria as in non–HIV-infected patients.

II. **Glomerular Diseases Associated with HIV Infection.**
HIV nephropathy refers to a specific form of glomerular disease that occurs in HIV-infected patients. The disease usually presents in patients with AIDS who have a CD4 cell count $<200 \times 10^3$ cells/ml, but it may occur at any stage, including the acute presentation of HIV infection. There is a disproportionate percentage (90%) of patients who are African American. Patients typically present with the acute nephrotic syndrome, often with massive (>6 g/day) proteinuria. Hypertension is rare, and edema may not be present, likely due to the frequent volume depletion associated with diarrhea and poor oral intake. The urinary sediment often shows granular casts and, occasionally, microscopic hematuria. Renal function is initially normal, but a rapid decline over months is common. Renal ultrasound often shows normal or enlarged kidneys.

Diagnosis is made by renal biopsy. By light microscopy, focal segmental glomerulosclerosis (FSGS) is present. Additional features suggest HIV nephropathy when compared to idiopathic FSGS. These include shrinkage of the glomeruli within Bowman's space (termed *glomerular collapse*), microcystic changes of the tubules, and tubuloreticular inclusions in the glomerular and peritubular capillary endothelial cells. The histologic lesion shows similarities to two other types of FSGS, namely, heroin nephropathy and collapsing FSGS, but, in these other entities, the subjects are HIV-negative.

Other glomerular disorders have also been reported in HIV-infected patients. These include membranoproliferative glomerulonephritis, membranous nephropathy, and immunoglobulin A nephropathy; some of these may be due to concurrent infection with hepatitis C virus (especially the membranoproliferative glomerulonephritis cases) or with hepatitis B virus (membranous nephropathy cases). These entities are also observed more commonly in white patients with HIV infection.

III. Management and Prognosis. The original prognosis for HIV nephropathy was dismal, with most patients reaching end-stage renal disease within 6 months. The prognosis has been improved by the advent of highly active antiretroviral therapy. Numerous case reports have found that proteinuria may improve and glomerular filtration rate may stabilize with highly active antiretroviral therapy. In addition, the judicious use of angiotensin-converting enzyme inhibitors or angiotensin receptor blockers, or both, will also slow the progression of the disease.

In the early days of HIV nephropathy, hemodialysis provided little long-term survival, as most patients died from the infectious complications of their HIV infection. However, with the use of highly active antiretroviral therapy, many HIV-infected patients do well on hemodialysis. Some universities are also performing kidney transplantation in selected HIV-infected patients who have maintained normal levels of CD4 cells. Although short-term survival has been reported to be acceptable in these small-scale studies, long-term studies are routinely necessary before transplantation is offered to these patients.

IV. Dialysis Procedures in HIV-Infected Patients. Because of the potentially lethal nature of HIV infection, there has been great concern among health care workers regarding the establishment of necessary and proper precautions for dialysis of patients who are known to be HIV positive. At present, the Centers for Disease Control and Prevention recommends that the universal precautions currently used in dialysis units to prevent hepatitis B transmission are adequate to prevent transmission of HIV. These include blood precautions, restriction of nondisposable supplies to a single patient, unless the items are sterilized between uses, and cleaning and disinfection of dialysis machines and surrounding surfaces. It has also been suggested that, to minimize blood spray from a dislodged needle, a transparent plastic bag should be placed over the patient's arm during dialysis.

In patients being treated for end-stage renal failure with peritoneal dialysis, it is recommended that bleach be added to each bag of dialysate effluent before disposal.

Protection of the staff is critical. Even though the current experience with HIV-infected patients suggests that the risk of infection to medical workers exposed to AIDS is extremely low, the lethal nature of the disease dictates extreme caution. Therefore, the policies developed by San Francisco General Hospital (refer to Humphreys and Schönfeld in Suggested Readings) for their personnel remain quite appropriate (Table 14.1).

Some controversy exists regarding the value of routine screening for HIV antibodies in patients with end-stage renal failure, especially for those not in the high-risk categories. Results of voluntary testing for HIV seropositivity in chronic hemodialysis patients who live in metropolitan areas reveal that, in high-risk patients, the prevalence of seropositivity is

TABLE 14.1. Precautions when caring for HIV-infected patients

Dispose of needles and syringes in puncture-resistant containers without breaking or recapping the needle.

Dispose of needles immediately after use; do not throw needles into regular trash; home dialysis patients should be provided with containers that are brought to the hospital for disposal with other contaminated waste.

Wear gloves for contact with blood or bodily substances.

Wear gloves to cover cuts, abrasions, ulcers, rash, or skin infections on your hands while working.

Wash hands as soon as possible after contact with blood or bodily substances or after touching objects that have been in contact with blood or bodily substances.

Wear protective eyewear when performing procedures that may result in splashes to the face (e.g., operative procedures, venous catheter placement, dialyzer reuse, endoscopies).

Wear a mask when patient is coughing and diagnosis of tuberculosis has not been excluded or when performing a procedure that may result in splashes of blood or bodily fluids to the face and mucous membranes; wear a mask when specified for communicable diseases that require respiratory precautions.

Wear a gown in anticipation of spills of blood or bodily fluids onto your clothing or when in contact with wounds or infected sites.

Contact your supervisor when you have had a needle stick or other exposure.

---

high (30–40%), whereas, in patients without such risk factors (intravenous drug use, male homosexuality, Haitian background, blood transfusion), the risk is negligible. It is argued that the low transmission rate of HIV in dialysis units and the apparent success of current precautions to prevent transmission of viral infections render routine screening unnecessary. In many states, routine screening is not permitted without the consent of the patient. However, all prospective transplant donors should be tested (see above), and a positive test usually precludes transplantation.

V. **Suggested Readings**

Ahuja TS, Borucki M, Grady J. Highly active anti-retroviral therapy improves survival of HIV-infected hemodialysis patients. *Am J Kidney Dis* 2000;36:574–580.

D'Agati V, Appel GB. HIV infection and the kidney. *J Am Soc Nephrol* 1997;8:139–152.

Dellow E, Unwin R, Miller R, et al. Protease inhibitor therapy for HIV infection: the effect on HIV-associated nephrotic syndrome. *Nephrol Dial Transplant* 1999;14:744–747.

Humphreys MN, Schönfeld PY. AIDS and renal disease. *Kidney* 1987;20:7–12.

Ifudu O, Mayers JD, Matthew JJ, et al. Uremia therapy in patients with end-stage renal disease and human immunodeficiency virus: has the outcome changed in the 1990s? *Am J Kidney Dis* 1997;29:549–552.

Rao TK. Acute renal failure syndromes in human immunodeficiency virus infection. *Semin Nephrol* 1998;18:378–395.

Stock P, Roland M, Carlson L, et al. Solid organ transplantation in HIV-positive patients. *Transplant Proc* 1999;33:3646–3648.

Winston JA, Burns GC, Klotman PE. The human immunodeficiency virus (HIV) epidemic and HIV-associated nephropathy. *Semin Nephrol* 1998;18:373.

III

Disorders of Water, Electrolytes, and Acid–Base Regulation

15

Disorders of Water Balance

Janet M. Caruso and Charles S. Wingo

Under physiologic conditions the osmolality of all body fluids is tightly regulated and maintained within a narrow range (285–295 mOsm/kg H_2O) by alterations in water intake and excretion. Water homeostasis is dependent on access to water and an intact thirst mechanism, appropriate renal regulation of solutes and water, the magnitude of extrarenal solute and water losses, and intact antidiuretic hormone (ADH) biosynthesis, release, and response to changes in serum osmolality. Derangements of water balance are reflected as changes in serum osmolality (S_{osm}), which are largely reflected as changes in serum sodium concentration (S_{Na}).

I. **Normal Water Balance.** Total body water (TBW) constitutes 60% of lean body mass (LBM) in men and 50% in women. The TBW is distributed between the intracellular compartment (two-thirds) and the extracellular compartment (one-third). Three-fourths of the extracellular fluid volume is interstitial lymph fluid and one-fourth is intravascular. Osmotic equilibrium is maintained between the intracellular and extracellular compartments by fluid shifts across cell membranes that are freely permeable to water.

Potassium salts are the predominant intracellular osmoles, and sodium salts are the major extracellular osmoles. Because cell membranes are freely permeable to water, S_{osm} is the same as extracellular fluid osmolality and intracellular fluid osmolality. Because S_{Na} is usually a major constituent of extracellular fluid osmolality, it directly correlates with S_{osm}. Derangements in blood urea nitrogen (BUN) or glucose concentrations can also alter S_{osm} and are included in the formal calculation of S_{osm}:

$$S_{osm} \text{ (mOsm/kg } H_2O) = 2\, S_{Na} \text{ (mEq/L)} + [\text{glucose (mg/dl)}/18] + [\text{BUN (mg/dl)}/2.8]$$

This calculation should approximate to within 10 mOsm/kg H_2O of the measured S_{osm}. A greater disparity (an "osmolar gap") could result from an error of measurement, pseudohyponatremia, or the presence of another osmotically active solute such as mannitol or ethylene glycol. Ineffective osmoles such as urea and ethanol can alter S_{osm} but do not affect water distribution between the intracellular and extracellular compartments because they are membrane permeable. Effective osmoles such as sodium, mannitol, and glucose are distributed for the most part extracellularly and can cause fluid shifts across the cell membrane.

Relatively small changes in S_{osm} are sensed by the hypothalamus, which stimulates thirst and ADH secretion. Hypotension and hypovolemia (>10% reduction of circulating plasma volume) can also stimulate thirst and ADH secretion through nonosmotic mechanisms. Thirst is the principal defense against hyperosmolality, whereas renal water excretion is the ultimate defense against hypoosmolality. ADH binds to specific receptors in the collecting duct to effect an increase in water permeability that promotes net water reabsorption into the interstitium. Maximal ADH action reduces urine volume to 500 ml/day and increases urine osmolality (U_{osm}) from 800 to 1,400 mOsm/kg H_2O. Complete absence of ADH results in a large diuresis (15–20 L/day) with a U_{osm} of 40–80 mOsm/kg H_2O. Any factor that impairs ADH release, tubular responsiveness to ADH, or medullary hypertonicity also limits urinary concentrating ability.

S_{Na} is a measurement that reflects the balance of body sodium and water. Changes in total body sodium alter effective circulating volume, whereas changes in S_{Na} usually reflect changes in water balance. Therefore, S_{Na} does not necessarily correlate with either effective circulating volume or with renal sodium excretion.

II. **Abnormal Water Balance.** Hyponatremia (S_{Na} <135 mEq/L), the most frequent electrolyte abnormality in hospitalized patients (incidence of 1–2%), occurs when water intake exceeds water excretion. This can occur by excessive water intake (water intoxication) with normal renal function or by normal solute-free water intake with decreased renal diluting capacity. Appropriate excretion of a water load requires adequate glomerular filtration, normal function of the diluting segments that are inhibited by loop diuretics, and suppression of ADH.

Hypernatremia (S_{Na} >145 mEq/L) is less frequent than hyponatremia (<1% of hospitalized elderly patients) and implies a relative deficiency of TBW compared with total body sodium. In general, this results from excessive water loss or from excessive sodium retention such as administration of hypertonic NaCl or $NaHCO_3$. Normally, a small increase in S_{osm} stimulates ADH secretion and thereby increases renal water retention. Because hypertonicity also stimulates thirst, even patients who are ADH deficient [central diabetes insipidus (DI)] can maintain their S_{osm} if they can drink and have access to water.

III. **Hyponatremia.** Most patients with hyponatremia are asymptomatic. Symptoms generally occur when significant hyponatremia (S_{Na} <125 mEq/L) has evolved in <24 hours (acute hyponatremia). Nausea, vomiting, and headache are common symptoms, but the clinical course can rapidly deteriorate to seizures, coma, and respiratory arrest. Severe acute hyponatremia (S_{Na} <120 mEq/L, developing over <24 hours) has a mortality of up to 50%, predominantly from complications of cerebral edema.

A diagnostic decision tree is presented in Figure 15.1. Initial evaluation of hyponatremia includes measurement of

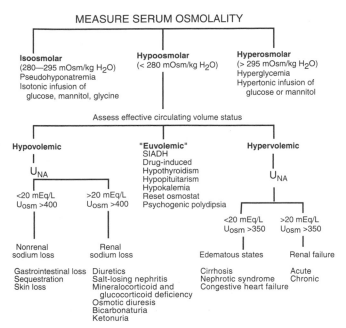

MEASURE SERUM OSMOLALITY

Isoosmolar
(280—295 mOsm/kg H$_2$O)
Pseudohyponatremia
Isotonic infusion of
glucose, mannitol, glycine

Hypoosmolar
(< 280 mOsm/kg H$_2$O)

Hyperosmolar
(> 295 mOsm/kg H$_2$O)
Hyperglycemia
Hypertonic infusion of
glucose or mannitol

Assess effective circulating volume status

Hypovolemic

U$_{NA}$

<20 mEq/L
U$_{osm}$ >400

>20 mEq/L
U$_{osm}$ >400

Nonrenal
sodium loss

Gastrointestinal loss
Sequestration
Skin loss

Renal
sodium loss

Diuretics
Salt-losing nephritis
Mineralocorticoid and
glucocorticoid deficiency
Osmotic diuresis
Bicarbonaturia
Ketonuria

"Euvolemic"
SIADH
Drug-induced
Hypothyroidism
Hypopituitarism
Hypokalemia
Reset osmostat
Psychogenic polydipsia

Hypervolemic

U$_{NA}$

<20 mEq/L
U$_{osm}$ >350

>20 mEq/L
U$_{osm}$ >350

Edematous states

Cirrhosis
Nephrotic syndrome
Congestive heart failure

Renal failure

Acute
Chronic

FIG. 15.1. Diagnostic algorithm for hyponatremia. SIADH, syndrome of inappropriate antidiuretic hormone secretion.

S$_{osm}$ and an assessment of the effective circulating volume (as an index of total body sodium). Accurate serial recordings of body weight and intake–output may be valuable. Signs of hypovolemia include poor skin turgor, dry mucous membranes, dry axillae, flat neck veins, tachycardia, and postural changes in vital signs (hypotension or relative tachycardia). Hemoconcentration (increased hematocrit and serum protein), an increased BUN to creatinine ratio, and urinary sodium concentration (U$_{Na}$) of <20 mEq/L are often seen. Hypervolemia is usually manifested by an elevated jugular venous pressure and peripheral or presacral edema. Hemodilution (decreased hematocrit and serum protein) and a decreased BUN to creatinine ratio are often observed, whereas the U$_{Na}$ is less helpful.

A. **Isoosmolar Hyponatremia.** Pseudohyponatremia (artifactual depression of the S$_{Na}$) can occur when the fraction of plasma that is water (normally 92–94%) is decreased by excessive amounts of lipids or proteins. This may occur with severe hyperlipidemias (usually triglyceridemia >1,500 mg/dl) or hyperproteinemias such as Waldenström's macroglobulinemia or multiple myeloma (serum protein >10 g/dl). In these instances, the measured S$_{osm}$ is normal, but the gap between measured and calculated S_{osm} is increased. Pseudohyponatremia must be distinguished from the true, potentially serious hyponatremia with normal S_{osm} that can occur with infusions of isosmotic, sodium-free solutions such as glycine in certain urologic procedures.

B. Hypoosmolar Hyponatremia. The initial assessment of hypoosmolar hyponatremia involves assessment of volume status.

Hypovolemia

Hypovolemic hyponatremia implies a total body sodium deficit in excess of water losses. The contracted effective circulating volume enhances isosmotic reabsorption of fluid in the proximal tubule and limits fluid delivery to the distal diluting segments. With significant hypovolemia, nonosmotic stimulation of thirst and ADH also occur.

Nonrenal sodium loss results from loss (vomiting, diarrhea) or sequestration (pancreatitis, peritonitis) of gastrointestinal fluids or from skin losses (burns).

Renal sodium loss results from a variety of mechanisms. Diuretic administration is most frequently seen in the elderly receiving thiazide diuretics, which can impair fluid delivery to the diluting segments (due to hypovolemia), inhibit NaCl reabsorption in the diluting segment, and potentiate ADH action and release. Salt-losing nephritis can occur in patients with chronic renal failure given a sodium-deficient diet or in patients with relatively preserved glomerular filtration rate but significant interstitial disease, such as polycystic kidney disease, medullary cystic disease, or chronic pyelonephritis. Mineralocorticoid and glucocorticoid deficiency result in a combination of volume depletion with enhanced proximal tubular reabsorption and nonosmotic stimulation of ADH. Osmotic diuresis, bicarbonaturia, and ketonuria result in excessive amounts of osmotically active solutes (glucose, bicarbonate, or ketones) in the urine, which cause excessive renal sodium and water excretion.

Euvolemia

Patients with euvolemia and hyponatremia generally have an increased TBW (by approximately 3–5 L) but normal total body sodium content and no edema. These disorders result primarily from nonphysiologic secretion, potentiation, or inappropriate action of ADH.

Syndrome of inappropriate ADH secretion is generally associated with malignancies (oat cell carcinoma of the lung, Hodgkin's and non-Hodgkin's lymphoma, thymoma, and other carcinomas), pulmonary disorders (tuberculosis, pneumonia, abscess, asthma, and acute respiratory failure), central nervous system disorders (tumors, head trauma, subarachnoid or subdural hemorrhage, meningitis, encephalitis, abscess, seizures, psychosis, and delirium tremens), and the postoperative period. Syndrome of inappropriate ADH secretion is a diagnosis of exclusion and requires that the patient has no causes for nonosmotic ADH release (hypovolemia, nausea) and no other cause of decreased diluting capacity (thyroid, renal, adrenal, cardiac, or liver disease). The urine is less than maximally dilute (>100 mOsm/kg H_2O) despite low serum osmolality, and U_{Na} is usually >20 mEq/L. Hypouricemia (<4 mg/dl) is a useful diagnostic clue. Because hyponatremia itself implies impaired urinary dilution, the diagnosis is confirmed by an elevated ADH level and does not require a formal urine dilution test.

Reset osmostat is most commonly seen in pregnant women and results from down-regulation of the central osmoreceptors. ADH release varies appropriately with changes in S_{osm}, but the S_{osm} threshold for ADH release is below normal. S_{Na}, although reduced, remains stable, because water excretion is normal.

Psychogenic polydipsia may be seen in psychotic patients who drink sufficient volumes of fluid to exceed their capacity to excrete solute-free water. In addition, these patients may have a subtle impairment in diluting capacity.

Drugs may potentiate ADH action (clofibrate, cyclophosphamide, nonsteroidal antiinflammatory agents, and ADH analogues), stimulate ADH release (vincristine, carbamazepine, narcotics, and barbiturates), or potentiate ADH action and stimulate its release (thiazide diuretics, chlorpropamide).

Hypervolemia

Patients with edema (congestive heart failure, nephrotic syndrome, and cirrhosis with ascites) can have an increased TBW that exceeds the increase in total body sodium. In these patients, a reduced effective circulating volume (from reduced cardiac output or peripheral arterial vasodilation) decreases filtrate delivery to the diluting segment and stimulates ADH release. In the absence of concomitant diuretic use, U_{Na} is usually <15 mEq/L, and U_{osm} is >350 mOsm/kg H_2O. In addition, acute or chronic renal failure can cause hyponatremia because renal diluting capacity is reduced.

C. **Hyperosmolar Hyponatremia.** Hypertonic infusions of glucose, mannitol, or glycine can cause shifts of intracellular fluid to the extracellular compartment with corresponding reduction in S_{Na}. In the case of hyperglycemia, for every 100 mg/dl glucose >100 mg/dl, S_{Na} will fall by approximately 1.6 mEq/L.

D. **Treatment.** Correction of hyponatremia in patients who are asymptomatic or who have only subtle neurologic dysfunction (and thus are likely to have chronic hyponatremia) should be gradual. Water restriction or the administration of a sodium chloride solution, if appropriate (described below), and frequent measurements of S_{Na} should be undertaken. Overzealous correction of S_{Na} in patients with chronic hyponatremia has been associated with the osmotic demyelination syndrome (central pontine myelinolysis), which can result in flaccid paralysis and death. Although the reasons are not clear, it appears that individual susceptibility to the osmotic demyelination syndrome may vary across patient populations. Specifically, malnourished individuals, particularly alcoholic patients, and premenopausal women appear to be at greater risk for residual neurologic injury. Caution should also be taken in treatment of the hypovolemic patient who is receiving isotonic saline, which restores normovolemia and causes loss of the hypovolemic stimulus to ADH release. In this setting, rapid correction of excess water can lead to overly rapid correction of hyponatremia. Suggested therapy for different clinical situations is described below.

Acute Symptomatic Hyponatremia

More rapid correction of hyponatremia is indicated if the risk of complications from cerebral edema outweighs the risk of aggressive treatment. The choice of 3% saline versus isotonic saline in the treatment of these patients remains controversial and should be guided by the severity of the clinical condition and the availability of intensive clinical monitoring. Symptoms attributable to acute severe hyponatremia may be subtle (lethargy, nausea, vomiting, agitation, hallucinations, weakness, headache) or severe (seizures, coma, Cheyne-Stokes respiration, pseudobulbar palsy). A well-designed treatment regimen may include

- Admission to an intensive care unit for monitoring of electrolytes, blood pressure, neurologic status, renal function, and frequent measurements of S_{Na} during its correction.
- A loop diuretic (such as furosemide, 1 mg/kg LBM) may be given to initiate and maintain a hypotonic salt and water diuresis.
- Hourly urinary sodium and potassium losses should be measured and replaced with isotonic saline or 3% NaCl (513 mEq sodium/L) and KCl until S_{Na} has increased by 10% or symptoms have stabilized. The rate of S_{Na} correction should not exceed 0.5 mEq/L/hr or 10 mEq/L/day.
- Thereafter, aim for slower correction of S_{Na} by water restriction. It is crucial to ensure that, during treatment of hyponatremia, the S_{Na} is raised gradually only to the normal range. The osmotic demyelination syndrome has been correlated both with too-rapid correction of the S_{Na} and with overcorrection.

Hypovolemic Hyponatremia

Initial therapy should include

- Discontinuation of diuretics
- Correction of nonrenal fluid losses
- Expansion of the effective circulating volume with 0.9% NaCl to replace one-third of the sodium deficit over 6 hours and the remainder over the next 24–48 hours, as dictated by the clinical condition.

A general estimate of the total body sodium deficit can be calculated as follows:

Sodium deficit (mEq) = $0.6 \times$ LBM (kg) $\times (140 - S_{Na})$

Euvolemic Hyponatremia

Euvolemic hyponatremia can usually be treated by water restriction to 1 L/day. The volume of excess water that must be excreted to normalize S_{Na} can be calculated as

Excess water (l) = current TBW – normal TBW

Current TBW (men) = $0.6 \times$ current LBM

Current TBW (women) = $0.5 \times$ current LBM

Normal TBW = current TBW $\times$ current S_{Na}/normal S_{Na}

A general estimate of LBM can be obtained after measurement of 24-hour urinary creatinine and can be calculated as

LBM (kg) = $7.138 + 0.02908 \times$ urine creatinine (mg)

When the cause of the syndrome of inappropriate ADH secretion is not reversible, medications may be used to create a state of drug-induced nephrogenic DI. These medications include demeclocycline, 600–1,200 mg/day, or lithium carbonate, 300 mg three times daily.

Hypervolemic Hyponatremia

Initial therapy should include salt and fluid restriction if the hyponatremia is caused by the primary disease. Therapy to improve the underlying disease should be undertaken (e.g., improve or optimize the cardiac output in patients with congestive heart failure). Vasopressin receptor antagonists may one day prove useful for the treatment of this type of patient.

IV. **Hypernatremia**
   A. **Clinical Presentation.** Signs and symptoms of hypernatremia include lethargy, restlessness, hyperreflexia, spasticity, and seizures, which may progress to coma and death. Patients with central or nephrogenic DI may have profound polyuria and polydipsia. Cerebral dehydration leads to capillary and venous congestion, cerebrovascular tears, venous sinus thrombosis, and subcortical subarachnoid hemorrhages. Mortality in infants and children is 43% in acute and 7–29% in chronic hypernatremia, whereas adults with acute hypernatremia have mortality rates as high as 60%.
   B. **Etiology and Treatment.** Hypernatremia can be classified according to the total body sodium content and the state of hydration.

Decreased Total Body Sodium

Loss of hypotonic body fluids results in effective circulating volume depletion and hypernatremia. The usual signs of hypovolemia are present: poor skin turgor, postural hypotension, tachycardia, dry mucous membranes, and flat neck veins. Extrarenal hypotonic fluid losses include dermal or gastrointestinal losses (vomiting, nasogastric suction, osmotic diarrhea). The renal response leads to a high U_{osm} (>800 mOsm/kg H_2O) and a low U_{Na} (<10 mEq/L). Hypotonic losses also occur from renal sources. Hypotonic polyuria can be produced by diuretics, osmotic diuresis (glucose, mannitol, or urea), or nonoliguric acute tubular necrosis. The urine may be either hypotonic or isotonic, and the U_{Na} is usually >20 mEq/L. More commonly, osmotic agents shift fluid to the extracellular compartment, resulting in hyponatremia.

Initial treatment includes isotonic NaCl until the effective circulating volume has been restored. Thereafter, hypotonic solutions (5% dextrose in water or 0.45% NaCl) can be used.

Normal Total Body Sodium

Losses of solute-free water can result in hypernatremia. Evidence of volume contraction is lacking unless the water losses are extreme. Extrarenal dermal and pulmonary losses of water can result in hypernatremia. In addition, water can be drawn from the extracellular compartment into damaged cells (rhabdomyolysis) with similar consequences. The U_{osm} is high, and U_{Na} reflects sodium intake. Renal water loss is more common and is usually related to partial or complete failure to synthesize or secrete ADH (central DI) or to a diminished or absent renal response to its action (nephrogenic DI). These disorders are characterized by an inability to concentrate the urine maximally, the result of both ADH deficiency (or resistance) and washout of the medullary osmotic gradient by chronic polyuria. Approximately one-half of the cases of central DI are idiopathic and are usually diagnosed in childhood. The remainder are caused by head trauma, hypoxic or ischemic encephalopathy, and central nervous system neoplasms. Patients with nephrogenic DI have impaired urinary concentrating ability despite maximal synthesis and release of ADH. Nephrogenic DI results from a failure of the countercurrent mechanism to generate a hypertonic medullary and papillary interstitium or a failure of ADH to increase the water permeability of the collecting duct. Nephrogenic DI may be congenital but more commonly is acquired. Chronic diseases of the renal medulla (medullary cystic disease, pyelonephritis), poor protein or salt intake, hypercalcemia, hypokalemia, various systemic diseases (amyloidosis, multiple myeloma), and numerous medications (demeclocycline, lithium, glyburide) have been implicated as causes of nephrogenic DI.

Central DI can be distinguished from nephrogenic DI by the fluid deprivation test (Table 15.1) followed by

TABLE 15.1.   Fluid deprivation test

During the test, urine output, weight, and vital signs must be strictly monitored to prevent severe volume contraction; weight loss should not exceed 3–5%.

Patients with mild polyuria (<6 L/day) should have fluids withheld the night preceding the test (e.g., 6 p.m.); patients with severe polyuria (>6 L/day) should be fluid deprived only during the day (e.g., 6 a.m.) to allow close observation. Time to achieve a maximal U_{osm} varies from 4–18 h.

S_{osm} should approach 295 mOsm/kg H_2O after fluid deprivation and before antidiuretic hormone administration.

U_{osm} is measured at baseline and every hour until two values vary by <30 mOsm/kg H_2O or 3–5% of body weight is lost.

Five units of subcutaneous aqueous vasopressin or 10 μg of intranasal deamino-8-D-arginine vasopressin are administered and, 1 hr later, a final U_{osm} is measured.

S_{osm}, serum osmolality; U_{osm}, urine osmolality.

exogenous ADH administration. Patients with severe central DI have baseline S_{osm} and S_{Na} that are high normal, and their urinary concentrating ability improves after ADH administration but not after water deprivation. In patients with severe nephrogenic DI, baseline S_{osm} is also increased, but they do not respond to either ADH treatment or water deprivation. A more direct approach to distinguish central DI is to measure plasma or urine ADH levels simultaneously with S_{osm} after either fluid restriction or hypertonic saline infusion. Patients with central DI have subnormal levels of ADH for the level of S_{osm}, whereas patients with nephrogenic DI exhibit normal or elevated values.

Treatment includes replacement of pure water loss with 5% dextrose in water. Free water deficit can be calculated as follows:

$$\text{Free water deficit (l)} = (0.6 \times \text{current LBM}) \times [(\text{measured } S_{Na} - \text{desired } S_{Na})/\text{desired } S_{Na}]$$

Usually the solute-free water deficit should be replaced over 48–72 hours with frequent monitoring of S_{Na} and S_{osm}. The S_{Na} should decrease by approximately 0.5 mEq/L/hr, with a goal to reduce S_{Na} by 10 mEq/L/day in patients with chronic hypernatremia or unknown duration of hypernatremia. Faster rates of correction can cause seizures.

The treatment of choice for central DI is intranasal deamino-8-D-arginine vasopressin, a synthetic analogue of ADH, 10–20 μg twice per day. Therapy for acquired nephrogenic DI should be directed toward the primary disorder. Thiazide diuretics and a low salt intake may decrease the polyuria.

Increased Total Body Sodium

Increased total body sodium is usually iatrogenic, resulting from administration of hypertonic sodium-containing solutions ($NaHCO_3$ given to patients with metabolic acidosis) or from inappropriate repletion of hypotonic insensible fluid losses with 0.9% saline in critically ill patients. Treatment includes discontinuation of hypertonic sodium-containing solutions and administration of diuretics to promote excretion of excess salt and water.

V. Suggested Readings

Adrogue HJ, Madias NE. Hypernatremia. *N Engl J Med* 2000; 342(20):1493–1499.

Adrogue HJ, Madias NE. Hyponatremia. *N Engl J Med* 2000; 342(21):1581–1589.

Berl T, Verbalis J. Pathophysiology of water metabolism. In: Brenner BM, ed. *Brenner & Rector's the kidney*, 7th ed. Philadelphia: WB Saunders, 2004:857–919.

Gross P, Reimann D, Henschkowski J, et al. Treatment of severe hyponatremia: conventional and novel aspects. *J Am Soc Nephrol* 2001;12:S10–S14.

Laureno R, Karp BI. Myelinolysis after correction of hyponatremia. *Ann Intern Med* 1997;126(1):57–62.

Moritz ML, Ayus JC. The pathophysiology and treatment of hyponatremic encephalopathy: an update. *Nephrol Dial Transplant* 2003;18:2486–2491.

Steele A, Gowrishankar M, Abrahamson S, et al. Postoperative hyponatremia despite near-isotonic saline infusion. *Ann Intern Med* 1997;126:20–25.

Potassium Disorders

Charles S. Wingo and Ronald M. Goldin

Disorders of serum potassium concentration (S_K) are common, silent, and potentially lethal. Hypokalemia (S_K <3.5 mEq/L) and hyperkalemia (S_K >5.0 mEq/L) may result from dietary or hormonal imbalance, pharmacologic effects, or abnormalities of renal or gastrointestinal function.

I. **Physiology.** Approximately 90% of the daily potassium intake of 50–150 mEq is excreted in the urine. However, up to 30% of daily potassium intake may be eliminated in the feces in the setting of reduced renal function. If diarrhea is present, enteric potassium losses can be substantial.

Because only 2% of total body potassium is in the extracellular fluid and 98% is intracellular, factors causing transcellular potassium shifts can lead to substantial changes in S_K. Potassium balance is closely regulated by several hormones, frequently via their effects on the ubiquitous Na^+/K^+-ATPase, as well as by the plasma potassium concentration itself.

Insulin promotes cellular potassium uptake by stimulating Na^+/K^+-ATPase, which has its greatest activity in skeletal muscle and liver. While basal insulin levels are key to potassium homeostasis, hyperkalemia appears to stimulate further insulin secretion, whereas hypokalemia inhibits its release.

Catecholamines have divergent effects on S_K, as α-agonists stimulate cellular potassium release and β_2-agonists promote cellular K^+ uptake. The effect of β_2 activity on plasma potassium levels also appears to be mediated by Na^+/K^+-ATPase.

Aldosterone is the major regulator of total body potassium through its effects on the renal collecting duct, colon, sweat glands, and muscles. Its release is exquisitely sensitive to changes in plasma potassium concentrations. Although aldosterone deficiency may lead to mild hyperkalemia, adrenal insufficiency more often causes hyponatremia; however, hyperkalemia may be more profound in the setting of renal dysfunction or restricted sodium intake.

Thyroid hormone is also known to stimulate Na^+/K^+-ATPase activity. No known feedback mechanism exists.

Dopamine has been shown to affect potassium via β-agonist–like activity, whereas the precise nature of the role of *parathyroid hormone* in potassium regulation has not yet been elucidated.

Metabolic acidosis promotes hyperkalemia, whereas alkalosis leads to hypokalemia. Alkali therapy has little effect on S_K in patients without endogenous renal function. This suggests that acid–base balance affects S_K primarily by altering renal potassium excretion. Specifically, exogenous mineral (but not organic) acid administration increases S_K largely by reducing renal potassium clearance, whereas exogenous alkali decreases S_K by increasing renal potassium excretion.

A. **Renal Regulation of Potassium.** The regulation of renal potassium excretion is primarily through active transport in the collecting duct. This segment has the capacity for active potassium secretion and absorption. Active potassium secretion occurs largely in the cortical collecting duct and its proximal extension, the initial collecting tubule. This secretory mechanism requires sodium absorption at the luminal membrane, which leads to basolateral sodium extrusion in exchange for potassium uptake by Na^+/K^+-ATPase. Potassium is secreted passively at the luminal membrane either via potassium channels or coupled to chloride. Potassium secretion may be stimulated by hyperkalemia, increased tubular flow, diminished luminal chloride concentration, and increased distal sodium delivery. Most diuretics (loop, thiazides, osmotic) enhance potassium secretion by increasing distal nephron luminal flow and sodium delivery.

Dietary potassium loading stimulates its secretion by the cortical collecting duct, and, when intake is reduced, the kidney is able to actively reabsorb potassium. This occurs primarily in the medullary collecting duct via a luminal H^+,K^+-ATPase.

II. **Hypokalemia**

A. **Evaluation.** Hypokalemia is a common electrolyte abnormality, occurring in up to 20% of hospitalized patients. Symptoms are uncommon (<50% of cases), typically are present at concentrations <2.5 mEq/L, and correlate with the rate of decline of S_K (Table 16.1). Hypokalemia can lead to hypertension due to the resultant sodium retention.

TABLE 16.1.   Clinical manifestations of hypokalemia

Cardiac
    Predisposition to digitalis glycoside toxicity
    Ventricular irritability
    Abnormal electrocardiogram (flattened T waves, U waves, ST segment depression)
    Coronary artery spasm
Neuromuscular
    Skeletal (weakness, cramps, tetany, paralysis, and rhabdomyolysis)
    Gastrointestinal (constipation, ileus)
    Encephalopathy
Renal
    Polyuria
    Increased ammoniagenesis
    Increased renal vascular resistance
Endocrine
    Carbohydrate intolerance
    Decreased plasma aldosterone concentration

TABLE 16.2. Differential diagnosis of hypokalemia

Artifactual (high white blood cell count)
Redistribution (cellular shift)
    β-Adrenergic agonists (epinephrine, terbutaline)
    Alkalosis
    Theophylline toxicity
    Refeeding (hyperalimentation)
    Insulin administration
    Periodic paralysis (familial, thyrotoxic)
    Barium poisoning
    Mineralocorticoid excess (both renal and extrarenal effects, see below)
Inadequate dietary intake
Gastrointestinal losses
    Diarrhea and chronic laxative abuse
    Ureterosigmoidostomy (urinary diversion)
    Villous adenoma
    Gastrointestinal fistulas
Renal losses
    Metabolic alkalosis (vomiting, nasogastric drainage)
    Diuretics
    Hypomagnesemia
    Antibiotics/antifungal/chemotherapeutic agents
        Penicillins (e.g., carbenicillin)
        Amphotericin B (renal tubular acidosis)
        Aminoglycosides
        Cisplatin
Glucocorticoids (increased cellular potassium loss and increased
    excretion)
Mineralocorticoid excess
    Adrenal adenoma or bilateral adrenal hyperplasia
    Glycyrrhizinic acid intoxication (licorice ingestion)
    Adrenal enzyme deficiency syndromes
Renal tubular acidosis (drug-induced, classic, distal, and proximal)
Acute renal failure syndromes (especially with recovery of renal
    function)
    Diuretic phase of acute tubular necrosis
    Postobstructive diuresis
    Interstitial nephritis
    Bartter's syndrome, Liddle's syndrome, Gitelman's syndrome
    Acute leukemia (lysozymuria)

    The evaluation should begin with a comprehensive history and physical examination and should particularly emphasize the drug history, volume status, and blood pressure. See Table 16.2 for a differential diagnosis.

    Figure 16.1 provides a diagnostic approach to hypokalemia, which should include analysis of serum and urine electrolytes. Initially, one must determine whether the hypokalemia is artifactual, due to redistribution, or represents evidence of true potassium depletion. Spuriously low values, or pseudohypokalemia, may be seen in conditions with markedly elevated white blood cell counts (>100,000–250,000) when the blood sample is stored for prolonged periods. This artifact can be avoided by separating the plasma from leukemic patients quickly after blood is col-

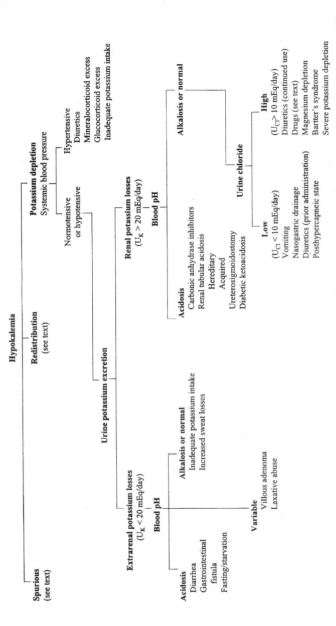

FIG. 16.1. Diagnostic approach in hypokalemic patients.

lected. Because more than 98% of total body potassium is located intracellularly, a small shift, or redistribution, of potassium can produce marked changes in its extracellular concentration. This may result from either drug or non-drug causes, some of which were discussed earlier.

True hypokalemia may be caused by either renal or extrarenal mechanisms. Renal conservation occurs during extrarenal potassium losses and is associated with urinary potassium excretion of <20 mEq over 24 hours. When potassium excretion equals or exceeds potassium intake during a period of hypokalemia, a renal component must exist.

Hypokalemia in the hypertensive patient can be caused by diuretics, potassium depletion, and primary mineralocorticoid excess (e.g., hyperaldosteronism). Cushing's syndrome is less frequently associated with hypokalemia. Thiazides and loop diuretics commonly cause hypokalemia, but rarely is it severe (S_K < 3.0 mEq/L) without other compounding factors such as increased sodium intake, reduced potassium intake, magnesium depletion, or hyperaldosteronism. Renin values may help distinguish hypertensive patients with diuretic-induced hypokalemia (elevated renin activity) from those with mineralocorticoid excess (suppressed renin activity).

B. Treatment. S_K is not an exact indicator of the total body potassium deficit, but, excluding transcellular shifts, the magnitude of hypokalemia generally correlates with the degree of potassium depletion. For a typical adult, S_K decreased by an average of 0.3 mmol/L for each 100 mmol of potassium depletion. S_K levels below 3.0 mEq/L reflect potassium deficits of >300 mEq, whereas S_K levels of <2.0 mEq/L may reflect deficits of >1,000 mEq. The following factors should be considered in the correction of hypokalemia.

- Acid–base status: Potassium chloride is generally the preferred means of replacement. Patients with hypokalemia often have coincidental metabolic alkalosis, and the use of chloride enables the maintenance of electroneutrality in the collecting tubule, avoiding a rise in H^+ secretion. In patients with hypokalemia and metabolic acidosis, potassium bicarbonate or potassium citrate may be used as alternate replacement therapies.
- Initial intravenous (IV) potassium replacement should be given in dextrose-free solutions, because the increase in serum insulin levels induced by dextrose may transiently lower serum potassium levels.
- Overzealous administration of potassium is the most common cause of hyperkalemia. This is especially evident in patients with either impaired renal function or long-standing potassium depletion, which has led to suppression of aldosterone release, causing altered extrarenal and renal potassium homeostasis.
- Coexisting hypomagnesemia can prevent correction of hypokalemia, because it is believed to lead to increased urinary potassium losses.

Potassium replacement may be administered either orally or intravenously. Oral replacement over several days is safe and rarely causes hyperkalemia in patients with normal renal function when given in doses up to 120 mEq/day. The wax-matrix KCl tablets are preferred because of the rare gastrointestinal ulcerations associated with sustained-release tablets. Over-the-counter salt substitutes contain 15–40 mEq/teaspoon of potassium chloride and are inexpensive and well tolerated.

IV replacement of potassium more often leads to hyperkalemia and should be reserved for those patients unable to take oral supplements, with electrocardiographic (ECG) changes, or in life-threatening situations (e.g., paralysis, digitalis intoxication with arrhythmias). Rates of up to 10 mEq/hr are safe without ECG monitoring. Doses up to 40 mEq/hr may be delivered via central venous catheter with ECG monitoring for S_K <2.5 mEq/L when associated with ECG changes or symptoms; however, these doses are rarely necessary. S_K should be checked at least every 4–6 hours during high-dose replacement.

Treatment of ongoing potassium depletion, as seen with diuretic therapy, may require 40–120 mEq/day. Combining a potassium-sparing diuretic with a loop or thiazide agent to limit potassium loss may be useful, but, in these cases, potassium supplementation should generally be held. However, with intractable chronic hypokalemia (as seen in Gitelman's or Bartter's syndrome), potassium-sparing diuretics may be used in conjunction with a high-potassium diet or oral supplements.

III. Hyperkalemia
A. Evaluation.
As with hypokalemia, the initial step in the evaluation of hyperkalemia is to determine whether the alteration in serum potassium is the result of a spurious value (pseudohyperkalemia), a redistribution between intracellular and extracellular compartments, or a true change in the total body potassium content. This requires a complete history, including diet, medications, and individual or family history of renal disease. Symptoms of hyperkalemia are uncommon but may include weakness and paresthesias. However, life-threatening hyperkalemia can be silent, so any of the classic ECG findings (Table 16.3) should be treated emergently, as progression to ventricular fibrillation may be rapid and unpredictable.

TABLE 16.3.   Electrocardiographic findings in hyperkalemia

Peaking or tenting of T waves
Flattening of P waves
Prolongation of PR interval
Widening of QRS complex (to sine wave)
Ventricular fibrillation, asystole, or both

TABLE 16.4. Causes of hyperkalemia

Spurious
    Hemolysis
    Thrombocytosis
    Leukocytosis
    Ischemic blood drawing
    Familial hyperkalemia
Redistribution
    Increased cellular release
        Exercise
        Tissue necrosis or trauma (rhabdomyolysis, hematoma)
        Hyperkalemic periodic paralysis, succinylcholine
        Hyperosmolality
    Decreased cellular potassium uptake
        Insulin deficiency (e.g., diabetic ketoacidosis)
        Aldosterone deficiency or blockade (spironolactone)
        β-Adrenergic blockers (e.g., propranolol)
        Digitalis poisoning
    Other
        Exogenous potassium administration
        Arginine and lysine administration
        Fluoride intoxication
        Acidosis
Decreased renal clearance
    Acute or chronic renal failure
    Hyperkalemic renal tubular acidosis
    Drug-induced hyperkalemia (see Table 16.5)
    Mineralocorticoid deficiency (acquired and hereditary forms)
    Hyperkalemic hypertensive syndromes (pseudohypoaldosteronism)

The most common cause of pseudohyperkalemia is hemolysis, which can be ruled out by obtaining a fresh blood sample in a heparinized tube through a large-bore needle while avoiding a prolonged tourniquet time. Pseudohyperkalemia can also occur due to potassium released during clotting, when either the platelet count is >1,000,000/mm^3 or the white blood cell count is >70,000/mm^3. This false elevation can be excluded by simultaneously measuring plasma and serum potassium concentrations, as the serum potassium concentration should not exceed that in the plasma by >0.3 mEq/L. If the clinical and initial laboratory findings suggest the need for urgent treatment, ECG confirmation of hyperkalemia may often be quicker than confirmation by measurement of plasma potassium. Rarely, pseudohyperkalemia may be caused by "leaky" erythrocytes of either acquired (infectious mononucleosis) or hereditary etiology.

In the absence of pseudohyperkalemia or potassium redistribution (Table 16.4), a S_K >5.0 mEq/L reflects reduced renal potassium clearance. Excessive potassium intake does not usually cause hyperkalemia in situations when renal potassium excretion is normal. Diminished renal potassium clearance may be due either to severely compromised renal function (glomerular filtration rate

TABLE 16.5.   Drug-induced hyperkalemia

Common
  Potassium-sparing diuretics (amiloride, triamterene)
  Nonsteroidal antiinflammatory drugs
  Cyclosporine and tacrolimus
  Heparin
  Angiotensin-converting enzyme inhibitors and angiotensin II receptor blockers
  Pentamidine
  Sulfamethoxazole-trimethoprim (high-dose)
Uncommon
  β-Adrenergic antagonists
  Succinylcholine
  Digitalis poisoning

<20 ml/min) or to impaired collecting duct function. In the latter case, either hyperaldosteronism or a decrease in distal sodium and water delivery is usually seen. Many medications (Table 16.5) may interfere with collecting duct potassium secretion via their effect on aldosterone synthesis (nonsteroidal antiinflammatory drugs, cyclosporine, heparin) or its action (spironolactone, amiloride, trimethoprim).

Hyperkalemic distal renal tubular acidosis (RTA) is believed to be due to a defect in sodium reabsorption in the collecting duct and is most often associated with obstructive uropathy or sickle cell disease. Type IV RTA develops due to aldosterone deficiency or resistance and results in diminished potassium secretion in the collecting duct. This disorder is found most commonly in patients with diabetic nephropathy or chronic interstitial nephritis, most of whom have modest renal failure. In those patients with type IV RTA who have true hyporeninemic hypoaldosteronism, plasma renin and aldosterone levels are decreased, whereas cortisol levels are normal. Mineralocorticoid replacement therapy should thus restore S_K to normal, but this may aggravate the fluid retention and hypertension that is present in most of these patients. Hyperkalemic RTA is therefore best managed with the combination of a loop diuretic, dietary potassium restriction, and alkali.

Patients with adrenal cortical insufficiency (Addison's disease) may develop mild degrees of hyperkalemia, but impairment of renal sodium conservation is usually the predominant clinical finding. Although these individuals typically exhibit hyperpigmentation, hypotension, hyponatremia, and acidosis, intrinsic renal parenchymal function is preserved. Hyperkalemia can, however, be severe during periods of volume depletion or during an Addisonian crisis. Treatment consists of saline and both glucocorticoid and mineralocorticoid replacement therapy.

Table 16.6 lists laboratory and diagnostic tests that are helpful in establishing the etiology of hyperkalemia.

TABLE 16.6. Laboratory and diagnostic tests to evaluate hyperkalemia

Urinalysis
Bladder catheterization
Renal ultrasound
Electrocardiogram
Urine and serum electrolytes
Serum creatinine and blood urea nitrogen
Arterial blood gases and pH
White blood cell count
Platelet count
Hematocrit (if low, may indicate chronic kidney disease)

The presence of "muddy-brown" casts in the urine sediment may suggest the diagnosis of acute tubular necrosis. Bladder catheterization (to eliminate bladder neck obstruction) and renal ultrasonography (to rule out hydronephrosis or small, end-stage kidneys) should also be considered.

B. **Treatment.** Hyperkalemia is life threatening because of its effects on cardiac conduction. Drug therapy for the acute treatment of hyperkalemia is listed in Table 16.7. Simultaneous use of several, or all, of these measures may be indicated if ECG abnormalities exist. With the exception of Na^+/K^+ exchange resins, none of the treatments removes potassium from the body, and they should be considered temporary measures. Severe hyperkalemia may require emergent dialysis.

IV calcium is the most rapid form of treatment for hyperkalemia, but its specific potassium-antagonizing effects on cardiac muscle last only 30–60 minutes. A second dose may be given if no resolution of ECG changes is seen in 5–10 minutes, but additional doses are generally less effective. Slow infusions should be given over

TABLE 16.7. Drug therapy for hyperkalemia

Drug	Dose	Onset of action (min)
Calcium gluconate or chloride	10–30 ml (10% solution) IV	1–3
Glucose/insulin	25–50 g glucose IV/5–10 U regular insulin (repeat every 30–60 min)	15–30
Albuterol	10 mg nebulized	30
$NaHCO_3$	50 mEq IV	See text
Sodium polystyrene sulfate (Kayexalate)	Oral, 30 g, or enema, 60 g	60–120

20–30 minutes in patients on digitalis to prevent myocardial digitalis toxicity. Intravenous calcium should not be given in $NaHCO_3$-containing solutions to prevent precipitation.

Insulin acts to enhance cellular potassium uptake and is the second most rapid method of treatment, with an onset of action of 15–30 minutes. Ten units of regular insulin given intravenously will reliably decrease the S_K and should be accompanied by 1 ampule of 50% dextrose in water to avoid hypoglycemia. Effects of insulin and glucose last 4–6 hours and may be repeated every hour as needed to reverse ECG changes. Alternatively, 25–50 units of regular insulin may be mixed with 1 L of 10% dextrose in water, and one-third may be infused over 20 minutes with the remainder infused as needed to maintain S_K.

β_2-Agonists also reduce S_K, although not as reliably as insulin. Nebulized albuterol, 10–20 mg (2–8 times the usual dose), has an onset of action in 30 minutes and can decrease the S_K by up to 1 mEq/L. The major limitation of β-agonist therapy is tachycardia.

The use of $NaHCO_3$ (1–2 ampules given intravenously) should be reserved for patients with frank acidosis, as its action depends on residual renal function. Blumberg et al. have shown that $NaHCO_3$, because of its hypertonicity, may precipitate volume overload and should therefore be used cautiously in chronic renal failure.

Definitive therapy of hyperkalemia requires potassium removal. This may be accomplished by loop or thiazide diuretics when renal function is adequate; otherwise, and in cases in which more rapid elimination is needed, sodium polystyrene sulfate (Kayexalate) may be used. This Na^+/K^+ exchange resin binds approximately 1 mEq potassium/gram resin when administered orally and approximately 0.5 mEq/g resin when used rectally. The full effect with either means of administration is observed in 2–4 hours. Clinical volume overload is rare despite the 2–3 mEq Na^+/g resin load. Sorbitol is often added orally to improve intestinal transit, but it should not be given rectally due to the risk of colonic perforation. Retention enemas using Kayexalate alone are the preferred method of rectal administration. Dosing may be repeated every 4–6 hours until S_K normalizes.

Hemodialysis is the most rapid and effective method of potassium removal and should be considered primarily when hyperkalemia is complicated by volume overload, acidosis, and renal failure. Potassium can be removed at a rate of 25–30 mEq/hr on hemodialysis, whereas peritoneal dialysis can remove just 10–15 mEq/hr. Rapid removal may be problematic in the setting of digitalis intoxication, as this can accentuate the effects of digitalis toxicity. The use of a dialysate bath without potassium should be avoided in most cases, because the rate of potassium removal is only marginally better than with 1 or 2 mEq/L K^+ baths, and a zero K^+ bath has a greater risk of provoking life-threatening hypokalemia.

Chronic hyperkalemia is rare unless renal function is impaired. In these cases, dietary potassium intake should be restricted to 40–60 mEq/day, and loop diuretics may be helpful. Oral $NaHCO_3$ can be used in an effort to maintain serum bicarbonate in the 22–24 mEq/L range. Kayexalate, 15–60 g/day, is also effective. Finally, and particularly in patients with hyperkalemic RTA, fludrocortisone acetate (Florinef) can be given in initial doses of 0.1–0.3 mg/day when patients have no evidence of hypertension or circulatory overload.

IV. Suggested Readings

Blumberg A, Weidmann P, Shaw S, et al. Effect of various therapeutic approaches on plasma potassium and major regulation factors in terminal renal failure. *Am J Med* 1988; 85:507–512.

Genarri FJ. Hypokalemia. *N Engl J Med* 1998;339:451–458.

Greenberg A. Hyperkalemia: treatment options. *Semin Nephrol* 1998;18:46–57.

Halperin M, Kamel K. Potassium. *Lancet* 1998;352:135–140.

Malnic G, Bailey MA, Giebisch G. Control of renal potassium excretion. In: Brenner BM, ed. *Brenner and Rector's the kidney*, 7th ed. Philadelphia: Saunders, 2004:453–495.

Weiner ID, Linas SL, Wingo CS. Disorders of potassium metabolism. In: Johnson RJ, Feehally J, eds. *Comprehensive clinical nephrology*, 2nd ed. St Louis: Mosby, 2003:109–121.

Acid–Base Disorders

I. David Weiner and Charles S. Wingo

Acidosis is the manifestation of a disease process that, if left unopposed, results in acidemia (blood pH <7.35). *Alkalosis* is the manifestation of a disease process that, if left unopposed, results in alkalemia (blood pH >7.45).

Acidosis can be subdivided into metabolic (a primary reduction in plasma bicarbonate concentration) and respiratory [a primary increase in the partial pressure of CO_2 (PCO_2)]. Likewise, alkalosis can be divided into metabolic (a primary increase in plasma bicarbonate concentration) and respiratory (a primary decrease in PCO_2). Simple acid–base disorders are caused by a *single* primary change in either PCO_2 or bicarbonate concentration. In most cases, simple acid–base disorders result in an abnormal blood pH. Certain terms that are frequently confused are defined below.

- pH: A measure of acidity, equal to $-\log[H^+]$.
- PCO_2: Partial pressure (mm Hg or Torr) of CO_2 in a solution; concentration of CO_2 in blood, $[CO_2]$ (in mmol/L), is equal to $PCO_2 \times 0.03$, which is approximately 1.2 mM for a PCO_2 of 40 mm Hg.
- Total CO_2: Moles of CO_2 that can be released from a solution by adding a strong acid; plasma bicarbonate concentration approximates plasma total CO_2.

The simple acid–base disorders are listed in Table 17.1 with the primary causes and compensatory changes.

I. Pathophysiology. Acid–base homeostasis is maintained within a narrow range through a series of reversible chemical buffers and physiologic pulmonary and renal compensations. Intracellular and extracellular buffers that counteract changes in pH include CO_2/bicarbonate, phosphate, proteins (particularly hemoglobin), and bone. Although all body buffers participate in acid–base regulation, it is convenient to think in terms of the bicarbonate buffer system, because all extracellular buffers are in equilibrium. This relationship may be expressed in terms of the Henderson-Hasselbalch equation as follows:

$$pH = 6.10 + \log \{[HCO_3^-]/(PCO_2 \times 0.03)\}$$

A normal blood pH is 7.40 ± 0.05 and is equivalent to an H^+ concentration of 40 ± 5 nM. Between pH 7.20 and 7.50, each 0.10 increase in pH is equivalent to a decrease in the hydrogen ion concentration of approximately 10 nM. Because the pH is the negative logarithm of $[H^+]$, a 0.3 decrease in pH is equal to a doubling of the H^+ concentration.

TABLE 17.1. Simple acid–base disturbances and predicted compensations

Disorder	Mechanism	Primary change	Compensatory change	Expected compensatory response[a]
Metabolic acidosis	Excessive acid production or retention, or excessive base loss	↓ $[HCO_3^-]$	↓ PCO_2	$PCO_2 = 1.5 \times [HCO_3^-] + 8\ (\pm 2)$ or $PCO_2 = $ last two digits of pH
Metabolic alkalosis	Excessive base intake or retention, or excessive acid loss	↑ $[HCO_3^-]$	↑ PCO_2	$PCO_2 = 0.9 \times [HCO_3^-] + 16\ (\pm 5)$ or $PCO_2 = $ last two digits of pH
Respiratory acidosis				
Acute	Decreased CO_2 elimination	↑ PCO_2	↑ $[HCO_3^-]$	$\Delta[HCO_3^-] = 0.1 \times \Delta PCO_2$
Chronic	Decreased CO_2 elimination	↑ PCO_2	↑ $[HCO_3^-]$	$\Delta[HCO_3^-] = 0.4 \times \Delta PCO_2$
Respiratory alkalosis				
Acute	Increased CO_2 elimination	↓ PCO_2	↓ $[HCO_3^-]$	$\Delta[HCO_3^-] = 0.2 \times \Delta PCO_2$
Chronic	Increased CO_2 elimination	↓ PCO_2	↓ $[HCO_3^-]$	$\Delta[HCO_3^-] = 0.5 \times \Delta PCO_2$

↑, increased; ↓, decreased.

[a]These equations can predict expected steady-state relations between a primary and a compensatory change. For example, a decrease in $[HCO_3^-]$ to 15 mEq/L (metabolic acidosis) produces a secondary change in PCO_2. With 95% confidence, PCO_2 will be $PCO_2 = 1.5 \times 15 + 8\ (\pm 2) = 30.5 \pm 2$ or 28.5–32.5 mm Hg. By coincidence, the last two pH digits approximate the predicted PCO_2.

Under normal conditions, the body produces both volatile and nonvolatile acids. The volatile acid produced is CO_2, which is produced by metabolism from the cellular metabolism of carbohydrates and lipids. CO_2 is excreted by the lungs in the normal process of respiration. The nonvolatile acids include all other acids produced by the body. These include phosphoric, sulfuric, and hydrochloric acid, which are produced by cellular metabolism of proteins and amino acids. The nonvolatile acids are buffered by the body's intracellular and extracellular buffers, resulting in decreases in the alkali component of these buffer systems. Under normal conditions, the kidney produces bicarbonate in the process of net acid excretion; the bicarbonate produced replenishes the buffer systems consumed in buffering nonvolatile acid production.

A. Compensation for Primary Acid–Base Disorders. Physiologic compensation for changes in systemic pH involves changes in alveolar ventilation (P_{CO_2}) or renal acid and alkali excretion, or both. Changes in pulmonary ventilation cause parallel changes in the rate of CO_2 excretion and thus alter systemic CO_2 levels. Respiratory compensation begins within seconds and is predominantly completed within minutes. The kidney reacts more slowly to changes in systemic pH to alter net acid excretion. Renal excretion of an alkali load may require 24–48 hours, whereas full renal adaptation to an acid load may require 5–7 days or more.

B. Approach to Acid–Base Disorders. Evaluating a patient with an acid–base disturbance requires consideration of both the clinical presentation and the laboratory data. A carefully taken history can simplify a complex set of blood gas and electrolyte data. The arterial blood gas (ABG) is the cornerstone of the diagnosis of most acid–base disturbances, but several caveats should be considered.

- Systemic pH, P_{CO_2}, bicarbonate, and electrolytes should be evaluated simultaneously. We emphasize that the ABG provides a calculated, not measured, HCO_3^- concentration. A measured HCO_3^- concentration is obtained from serum or plasma electrolyte measurements.
- The pH should be independently calculated from the P_{CO_2} measured in the ABGs and the bicarbonate measured in the serum electrolytes using the Henderson-Hasselbalch equation. If the calculated pH differs from the measured pH by more than 0.04 pH units, then a laboratory error should be considered and all measurements repeated before corrective therapy is begun.
- A blood gas value represents a specific point in time; identical values can be obtained for different acid–base disturbances moving in opposite directions.
- Nomograms may lead to the wrong diagnosis if the clinical presentation is ignored.
- Physiologic compensation for a primary acid–base disorder seldom normalizes systemic pH. Metabolic

acidosis represents a primary decrease in plasma bicarbonate concentration, which decreases blood pH.

II. **Metabolic Acidosis.** Metabolic acidosis occurs through one of four general mechanisms:

1. Net acid production or net acid intake increases, thereby exceeding renal net acid excretion (e.g., ketoacidosis or lactic acidosis).
2. Renal net acid excretion fails to match endogenous net acid production [e.g., renal tubular acidosis (RTA) or administration of carbonic anhydrase inhibitors].
3. Bicarbonate loss via the gastrointestinal tract (e.g., diarrhea, fistula).
4. Extracellular fluid being diluted by a non–bicarbonate-containing solution (e.g., rapid saline administration).

The *compensatory response* to metabolic acidosis is an increase in ventilation that returns pH toward normal. When fully compensated, the PCO_2 closely approximates the last two digits of the serum pH. If this is not the case, a mixed acid–base disturbance should be considered.

A. **Clinical Presentation.** Metabolic acidosis can present with rapidly developing symptoms, or it can be insidious in onset, avoiding detection for months or years before being recognized. Acute metabolic acidosis is typically associated with florid symptoms related to the underlying disease. For example, nausea, vomiting, and abdominal pain are frequent with diabetic ketoacidosis. Patients with ischemic lactic acidosis may have abdominal pain (mesenteric ischemia) or hypotension (tissue hypoperfusion), and the person with methanol or ethylene glycol poisoning may present with symptoms of alcohol abuse, nausea, and vomiting. In contrast, chronic metabolic acidosis is typically more insidious. Associated symptoms such as recurrent renal stones, hypoalbuminemia, hypokalemia, osteomalacia or osteoporosis, or failure to thrive in children are common findings that bring this condition to medical attention.

The normal compensation to metabolic acidosis is respiratory hyperventilation, leading to increased CO_2 excretion, a decrease in the PCO_2 and compensatory respiratory alkalosis. Respiratory compensation produces rapid, deep (Kussmaul) respirations. Severe acidosis can be associated with mildly decreased myocardial contractility, hypotension, pulmonary edema, and tissue hypoxia. The ABG reveals the reduced pH, plasma bicarbonate concentration, and reduced PCO_2.

The anion gap helps in determining the etiology of metabolic acidosis. It is calculated from the following formula:

$$\text{Anion gap} = [Na^+] - ([Cl^-] + [HCO_3^-])$$

A normal anion gap ranges between 8 and 16 mM, provided that plasma albumin and globulin concentrations

TABLE 17.2.   Differential diagnosis of elevated anion gap metabolic acidosis

Etiology	Clinical features	Laboratory features	Treatment
Diabetic ketoacidosis	Fruity breath	Increased glucose >300 mg/dl; serum or urine ketones	Intravenous insulin and saline
Uremia	Oliguria, uremic breath, pericarditis	Increased blood urea nitrogen and creatinine; low urine output	Consider dialysis
Salicylate intoxication	Tinnitus, hyperventilation	Positive urine ferric chloride test; increased serum salicylate	Diuresis and alkalinization of urine; hemodialysis
Starvation ketosis	None	Serum or urine ketones	Refeeding
Methanol	"Blind drunk"	Elevated osmolal gap	Ethanol infusion and dialysis
Alcohol ketoacidosis	Ethanol abuse, often with binge drinking	Increased alcohol level; serum lactate increased	Glucose and saline; phosphorus and potassium
Ethylene glycol	May have accompanying renal failure	Elevated osmolal gap; calcium oxalate crystals in urine	Consider ethanol infusion plus dialysis
Lactic acidosis	Shock, tissue hypoperfusion	Lactate level	Correct underlying cause

are normal. When the anion gap is elevated above the normal range, the condition is referred to as an *anion gap metabolic acidosis*. Table 17.2 provides the differential diagnosis of an elevated anion gap acidosis, key clinical features, supporting laboratory data, and a brief outline of treatment options. When the anion gap is normal, the condition is termed a *non–anion gap metabolic acidosis*. The most common causes of non–anion gap metabolic acidosis are gastrointestinal tract bicarbonate loss from diarrhea and RTA.

The primary therapy for these disorders is to treat the primary process. Alkali administration to correct the systemic pH should be undertaken only after the risks related to the acidosis are balanced against the risks of therapy.

In acute metabolic acidosis, there is limited to no benefit of alkali therapy for severe metabolic acidosis on either systemic hemodynamics or mortality. Furthermore, alkali therapy of acute metabolic acidosis is associated with a substantial cation load, typically Na^+, which can lead to volume overload, pulmonary edema, or hypernatremia. However, if intravascular volume depletion is present, then administration of fluids containing dextrose 5% in water solution plus three ampules (150 mEq) of $NaHCO_3^-$/L can both increase intravascular volume and contribute to correction of the metabolic acidosis.

Chronic metabolic acidosis, in contrast to acute metabolic acidosis, leads to a wide variety of well-characterized sequelae. A few examples include protein degradation, growth retardation, malnutrition, skeletal bone demineralization, and recurrent renal stone disease. In most cases of chronic metabolic acidosis, therapy can be administered with chronic, low doses of alkali (see following discussion) with little risk of volume overload or hypertension from the sodium load. Treating chronic metabolic acidosis with alkali, if the underlying condition cannot be treated, is generally beneficial.

If alkali therapy is initiated, then the dose should be estimated based on the period over which correction of the acidosis is desired. If rapid correction of acute metabolic acidosis is desired, then the base deficit should be calculated using the formula

$$\text{Base deficit (mEq } HCO_3^-) = 0.6 \times \text{lean body weight (kg)} \times (24 - [HCO_3^-])$$

In severe metabolic acidosis, with plasma bicarbonate concentrations <5 mEq/L, the correction factor of 0.6 increases to 1.0 or more. For acute settings, 25% of the base deficit should be administered over the first 8 hours, with an additional 25% administered over the subsequent 16 hours, for a total dose of 50% over the first 24 hours. The response to therapy should be reevaluated after 24 hours, and dose adjustments made appropriately.

For chronic metabolic alkalosis, a replacement dose of 1–2 mEq/kg administered orally in two or three divided doses per day is frequently effective. However, proximal RTA requires much larger doses [e.g., 10–25 mEq/kg/24 hr (see below)].

B. Non–Anion Gap Metabolic Acidosis. The primary causes of a non–anion gap metabolic acidosis are bicarbonate loss in gastrointestinal fluids, such as diarrhea, and RTA. In theory, the two can be easily differentiated from the history and physical examination. However, some patients with chronic diarrhea may be receiving medications or have underlying conditions associated with RTA. Also, the patient may not admit to the diarrhea. The latter case is sometimes true in young adults who are self-inducing diarrhea through cathartic administration to control body weight.

Differentiating between these two conditions can be assisted by measuring the urine pH and the urine anion gap (UAG). If the urine pH is >6 in the presence of a non–anion gap metabolic acidosis, then RTA can be diagnosed. If the urine pH is <6, then the UAG is helpful. This is measured using the following formula:

$$UAG = U_{Na} + U_K - U_{Cl}$$

where U_{Na}, U_K, and U_{Cl} are the urinary concentrations of sodium, potassium, and chloride, respectively. If the UAG is either positive or between 0 and –5 to –10, then the patient is likely to have RTA. If the UAG is less than –20, then the patient is likely to have gastrointestinal bicarbonate loss and not an RTA.

C. **Renal Tubular Acidosis.** RTA is caused by the kidney's inability to maintain a normal plasma bicarbonate concentration in the absence of exogenous acid or alkali loads. Other causes of normal anion gap acidosis are listed in Table 17.3. The metabolism of a typical Western diet results in approximately 0.8 mEq/kg/24 hr of acid formation, predominantly in the form of hydrochloric, sulfuric, and phosphoric acid. This acid load is buffered by endogenous buffer systems, resulting in minimal effect, over short periods, on systemic pH. However, the buffers consumed in this process must be replenished by the kidneys, or progressive metabolic acidosis develops. When this occurs, it is termed an *RTA*. The RTAs can be divided into three types.

Classic or distal (type I) RTA is accompanied by hypokalemia, and the metabolic acidosis may be severe, with an $[HCO_3^-]$ of 5–10 mEq/L. Nephrocalcinosis or recurrent kidney stones may be present. It is caused by defective collecting duct acidification, resulting in a persistently high urine pH, ≥ 6. This disorder can occur as either an autosomal-dominant or an autosomal-recessive inherited disease, or it can be acquired. Acquired forms

TABLE 17.3.   Differential diagnosis of normal anion gap metabolic acidosis

Gastrointestinal tract bicarbonate loss from diarrhea, pancreatic or biliary fistulas, or an immature ileostomy yields fluid losses with a higher bicarbonate concentration than that of serum and produces potassium depletion.

Ureterosigmoidostomy with urine retention in the colon causes chloride and water reabsorption with bicarbonate secretion.

Ingestion of chloride salts or chloride-containing anion-exchange resins (i.e., $CaCl_2$, $MgCl_2$, or cholestyramine) causes chloride to exchange for bicarbonate across the gastrointestinal tract.

Renal tubular acidosis may be associated with frank renal bicarbonate loss or failure to match net acid intake and production.

are frequently associated with autoimmune diseases (e.g., systemic lupus erythematosus, pernicious anemia, or Sjögren's syndrome), nephrocalcinosis (e.g., hyperparathyroidism), or toxins (e.g., amphotericin B, lithium, or toluene). The inherited forms are due to genetic abnormalities leading to either lack of production or nonfunctional proteins required for urine acidification, including proteins such as H^+–adenosine triphosphatase and Cl^-/HCO_3^- exchange. Patients often present with musculoskeletal weakness or with nephrolithiasis. Severe distal RTA can present as a medical emergency with hypokalemic paralysis, coma, or shock.

Some patients have an incomplete distal RTA. These patients are typically not frankly acidemic, are generally asymptomatic, except for possible renal stone disease, and usually are detected only by formally testing urine acidification. These patients fail to reduce urine pH below 5.5 after administration of an oral acid load with NH_4Cl. Small amounts (1–2 mEq/kg/24 hr) of oral alkali are usually sufficient to correct the acidosis and, given sufficient time, will increase serum bicarbonate to normal levels. Alkali therapy can improve the hypokalemia if K^+ is given as the associated cation. Sources of alkali include the following:

- Sodium bicarbonate (325 mg = 4 mEq alkali).
- Shohl's solution (Bicitra) (1 ml = 1 mEq alkali and 1 mEq sodium).
- Polycitra (1 ml = 2 mEq alkali, 1 mEq potassium, and 1 mEq sodium).
- Polycitra-K (1 ml = 2 mEq alkali and 2 mEq potassium).
- Other potassium citrate preparations include K-Lyte (25 mEq potassium and alkali), K-Lyte DS (50 mEq potassium and alkali), and Urocit-K (5 mEq potassium and alkali).

Proximal (type II) RTA is characterized by moderate degrees of non–anion gap metabolic acidosis and an acid urine pH in the presence of metabolic acidosis but bicarbonaturia in the presence of a normal systemic pH. Type II RTA is caused by a proximal tubular defect and can be observed with acetazolamide administration or with Fanconi's syndrome. In the latter case, glycosuria, phosphaturia, and aminoaciduria are present. Medullary cystic disease, multiple myeloma, nephrotic syndrome, and renal transplantation can also lead to proximal RTA.

Proximal RTA is the result of the proximal tubule being unable to reabsorb adequate amounts of filtered bicarbonate. This leads to increased bicarbonate delivery to the distal nephron, exceeding the distal nephron reabsorptive capacity and resulting in bicarbonaturia. Eventually, the ongoing bicarbonate loss depletes total body bicarbonate stores, leading to metabolic acidosis. As the plasma bicarbonate decreases, the filtered bicarbonate load ($[HCO_3^-]$ × glomerular filtration rate) decreases until it is within the reabsorptive capacity of the proximal tubule. This permits normal urine acidification by the distal nephron.

As a result, patients with proximal RTA typically exhibit mild to moderate acidosis, with a plasma bicarbonate concentration of 15–18 mEq/L. The urine pH is generally below 6 in the absence of alkali therapy and increases above 6 when alkali is administered.

Proximal RTA usually occurs in children and presents as failure to thrive, growth retardation, vomiting, volume depletion, and lethargy. X-rays may reveal features suggestive of rickets in children and osteopenia in adults. Serum potassium is low or normal.

The fractional excretion of bicarbonate (FE_{HCO_3}) can be used to distinguish between proximal and distal RTA. It is calculated as

$$FE_{HCO_3} = (U_{HCO_3}/P_{HCO_3})/(U_{Cr}/P_{Cr})$$

It is important to emphasize that FE_{HCO_3} can be interpreted only when the plasma bicarbonate is normal. Under these conditions, FE_{HCO_3} is <5% in distal RTA but >15% in proximal RTA.

Proximal RTA can be difficult to treat, requiring 10–25 mEq/kg/24 hr of oral alkali. Large doses of alkali are required, because increasing the plasma bicarbonate causes increased bicarbonaturia as a result of the proximal tubular defect. Increased distal delivery of bicarbonate promotes potassium secretion that can lead to severe hypokalemia. Thus, approximately 50% of the alkali therapy should be given as the potassium salt. Osteomalacia may require vitamin D and calcium supplements, whereas rickets can be corrected with vitamin D and 1.6 g/day of sodium phosphate.

Hyperkalemic (type IV) RTA is the most commonly encountered RTA. It is characterized by hyperkalemia and a mild, non–anion gap metabolic acidosis; urine pH is frequently <6, indicating a retained ability to acidify the urine. Although type IV RTA frequently coexists with chronic renal insufficiency and diabetes mellitus, the hyperkalemia and metabolic acidosis are out of proportion to the degree of renal insufficiency. Occasionally, this disorder occurs in the presence of normal renal function. In this case, a primary defect in aldosterone production or action is usually responsible for both the hyperkalemia and the acidosis.

Most cases of type IV RTA are related to impaired ammonium excretion that is the direct result of the hyperkalemia. The ammonium excretion defect leads to inadequate net acid excretion, resulting in RTA. In these cases, the ability to acidify the urine is normal.

The hyperkalemia reflects either impaired potassium secretion (primarily in the cortical collecting duct) or enhanced potassium reabsorption (primarily in the medullary collecting duct). Treating the hyperkalemia restores the normal ability to excrete ammonium and corrects the RTA and the metabolic acidosis.

Some cases of type IV RTA are secondary to impaired aldosterone production and respond well to mineralocorticoid replacement therapy [fludrocortisone acetate (Florinef), 0.1–0.2 mg/day]. These cases are characterized by impaired urine acidification, intravascular volume depletion, and hypotension.

However, hyperkalemic RTA typically coexists with renal insufficiency, hypertension, and extracellular fluid volume expansion, features that are not typically associated with mineralocorticoid deficiency. In this latter group, mineralocorticoid therapy usually fails to restore serum potassium or plasma bicarbonate to normal and may worsen the hypertension and NaCl retention. Hyperkalemic RTA is especially common in diabetic nephropathy, interstitial nephritis, and obstructive uropathy and after renal transplantation. Most patients with hyperkalemic RTA are best treated with a loop diuretic (e.g., furosemide, 20–80 mg by mouth, two to three times per day); generally, sodium bicarbonate (0.5–1.0 mEq/kg/ 24 hr) can be reserved for refractory cases.

III. **Respiratory Acidosis.** Respiratory acidosis represents a primary increase in PCO_2, which decreases systemic pH. The increased PCO_2 is generally caused by failure of CO_2 excretion that results from decreased alveolar ventilation. Abnormalities in CO_2 production are rare. Respiratory acidosis frequently occurs with diseases involving the central nervous system, lungs, and heart. Chronic obstructive pulmonary disease that results in loss of alveolar surface is the most common cause of respiratory acidosis. Sedatives and opiates that depress central nervous system centers of respiration are common iatrogenic causes of respiratory acidosis. Severe electrolyte abnormalities (hypokalemia or hypophosphatemia) that impair muscle function, impaired mechanical ventilation, and bronchopulmonary diseases are other common causes of respiratory acidosis (Table 17.4).

The retained CO_2 results in an increased carbonic acid concentration that is buffered, primarily, by intracellular buffers such as hemoglobin or phosphate, resulting in a small increase in plasma bicarbonate concentration. The kidneys compensate by increasing net acid excretion, which generates new bicarbonate that is returned to the blood. Enhanced urinary acidification also increases urinary chloride excretion, resulting in a decreased plasma chloride concentration. The renal response usually takes longer than 24 hours to develop fully.

Because the renal compensation to respiratory acidosis requires 1–3 days or more to become maximal, it is possible to differentiate between acute and chronic respiratory aci-

TABLE 17.4.   Causes of respiratory acidosis

Decreased alveolar ventilation and CO_2 removal
    Obstruction (e.g., bronchospasm, emphysema, or aspiration)
    Primary depression of respiratory center (e.g., drugs, trauma, neo-
        plasm, or infection)
    Mechanical or structural defect (e.g., pneumothorax, hemothorax, or
        adult respiratory distress syndrome)
    Mechanical or neuromuscular defect (e.g., primary muscular disease,
        neuromuscular diseases, drugs, botulism, or tetanus)
    Decreased stimulation of respiratory center (sleep apnea)
Decreased capillary exchange of CO_2
    Cardiac arrest
    Circulatory shock
    Severe pulmonary edema
    Massive pulmonary embolus

dosis. In acute respiratory acidosis, <24 hours in duration, the serum bicarbonate can be calculated using the formula

$$\Delta[HCO_3^-] = 0.1 \times \Delta P_{CO_2}$$

In contrast, in chronic respiratory acidosis, the serum bicarbonate can be calculated using the formula

$$\Delta[HCO_3^-] = 0.4 \times \Delta P_{CO_2}$$

Patients with respiratory acidosis may present with respiratory distress, dyspnea, or obtundation if the disease is acute in onset. They may complain of headaches or show signs of increased intracranial pressure caused by cerebral vasodilation produced by CO_2. The P_{CO_2} is increased, and the blood pH is decreased. In contrast, chronic respiratory acidosis typically produces few symptoms. The treatment for both acute and chronic respiratory acidosis is restoration of adequate ventilation.

IV. **Metabolic Alkalosis.** Metabolic alkalosis is due to a primary increase in plasma bicarbonate concentration, resulting in an increase in blood pH. This increase in plasma bicarbonate concentration can result from addition of bicarbonate or its precursors to the extracellular fluid or loss of fluid with a chloride to bicarbonate ratio greater than that of serum.

The kidney's ability to excrete an alkali load depends on several factors, including aldosterone and total body chloride stores. Hyperaldosteronism, whether primary or secondary, directly increases renal net acid excretion, thereby impairing the ability to excrete bicarbonate. When total body chloride stores are normal, the kidney is able to rapidly excrete bicarbonate, whereas when chloride depletion is present, the kidneys are unable to excrete bicarbonate.

Metabolic alkalosis is frequently related to loss of either chloride salts or acid. Certain diuretics and gastrointestinal diseases (e.g., vomiting or nasogastric suction) cause greater chloride than bicarbonate losses. This leads to extracellular fluid volume contraction and an increase in bicarbonate concentration. Alveolar hypoventilation leading to an increased P_{CO_2} is the compensatory respiratory response to this primary disturbance; however, this compensation is usually limited to a rise in P_{CO_2} to a maximum of approximately 55–60 mm Hg. P_{CO_2} at this level can lead to hypoxia, which stimulates ventilation and prevents further P_{CO_2} increases. Volume depletion, if present, increases renal bicarbonate retention by decreasing the glomerular filtration rate, thereby decreasing the filtered bicarbonate load. Volume depletion also reduces luminal chloride delivery to the collecting duct, thereby inhibiting bicarbonate excretion by the collecting duct. Hyperaldosteronism, whether primary or secondary, further contributes to metabolic alkalosis by stimulating renal bicarbonate generation. In this condition, the increase in plasma bicarbonate reflects the generation and retention of bicarbonate by the kidney as a consequence of increased net acid excretion.

A. **Clinical Presentation.** The clinical presentation of most common causes of metabolic alkalosis can be divided into those with and those without volume depletion. Metabolic alkalosis associated with volume depletion is invariably related to chloride depletion. Such individuals may exhibit orthostatic hypotension, tachycardia, azotemia, and other features of reduced effective circulating volume. Unless a renal mechanism is responsible for the volume and chloride depletion (e.g., diuretics), these patients exhibit intense chloride conservation, and the urinary chloride concentration is <10 mEq/L. Table 17.5 lists some common causes of chloride-responsive metabolic alkalosis.

In contrast, the most common cause of chloride-resistant metabolic alkalosis is excessive mineralocorticoid action. Blood pressure is usually increased, and volume depletion is not present. Urinary chloride excretion typically reflects intake and is usually >20 mEq/L.

Hypokalemia is a common feature of metabolic alkalosis unless frank renal insufficiency is present. The hypokalemia and decreased ionized calcium may contribute to muscle cramps, weakness, and hyperreflexia. Plasma bicarbonate concentration and pH are increased, and the compensatory alveolar hypoventilation increases P_{CO_2} but decreases O_2 partial pressure that can lead to signs of hypoxia. Severe alkalemia can lead to cardiac arrhythmias.

B. **Therapy.** Chloride-responsive metabolic alkalosis corrects with administration of chloride, usually provided as 0.9% NaCl (saline), but coexisting depletion of potassium, magnesium, and phosphate must also be sought and corrected if detected. Chloride-resistant alkalosis is usually caused by mineralocorticoid excess and coexisting hypokalemia. Both of these disorders must be corrected

TABLE 17.5. Causes of metabolic alkalosis

Chloride-responsive metabolic alkalosis: frequently observed with extra-
cellular fluid contraction (urine [Cl⁻] <10 mEq/L without diuretics)
  Vomiting/nasogastric suction
  Villous adenoma
  Diuretic therapy (urine [Cl⁻] <10 mEq/L)
  Posthypercapnia state
Chloride-resistant metabolic alkalosis: frequently observed with exces-
sive mineralocorticoid effect and hypokalemia (urine [Cl⁻] >20 mEq/L
and typically reflects intake)
  Primary hyperaldosteronism
    Bilateral adrenal hyperplasia
    Aldosterone-producing adenoma
  Secondary hyperaldosteronism
    Congestive heart failure
    Nephrotic syndrome
    Renal artery stenosis
  Other causes of excessive mineralocorticoid effect
    Glycyrrhizic acid (licorice)
    Cushing's syndrome or disease
    Congenital adrenocorticoid excess or ectopic adrenocorticotropic
      hormone
  Potassium depletion
  Bartter's syndrome
  Milk-alkali syndrome
  Acute alkali load

for acid–base balance to be restored. Spironolactone can be used to treat some causes of primary hyperaldosteronism; otherwise, the underlying causes of secondary hyperaldosteronism should be identified and treated. In particular, angiotensin-converting enzyme inhibitor administration to patients with congestive heart failure may be helpful.

V. **Respiratory Alkalosis.** Respiratory alkalosis results from a primary decrease in PCO_2 caused by alveolar hyperventilation. Pain, anxiety, hypoxia, severe anemia, progesterone and other drugs, endotoxin, and primary pulmonary disease can increase ventilation and lead to hypocapnia (Table 17.6). The initial response to alkalemia is buffering by intracellular protons. The renal compensation, which occurs over several days, is decreased net acid excretion, thereby decreasing plasma bicarbonate concentration and restoring pH toward normal. Patients often present with hyperventilation, perioral and extremity paresthesias, muscle cramps, hyperreflexia, seizures, or cardiac arrhythmias.

The ABG reveals a decreased PCO_2 and an increased pH. Plasma bicarbonate concentration is decreased, and the serum chloride concentration is usually increased. Some electrolyte changes of chronic respiratory alkalosis may mimic a non–anion gap acidosis. The only effective therapy is to eliminate the cause of the hyperventilation.

TABLE 17.6. Causes of respiratory alkalosis

Increased central nervous system drive for respiration
  Anxiety
  Central nervous system infection, infarction, trauma
  Drugs: salicylates, nicotine, aminophylline
  Fever, sepsis, especially gram-negative sepsis
  Pregnancy, progesterone
  Liver disease
Increased stimulation of chemoreceptors
  Anemia
  Carbon monoxide toxicity
  Pulmonary edema, pneumonia
  Pulmonary emboli
  Reduced inspired O_2 tension: high altitude
Increased mechanical ventilation
Iatrogenic

VI. Mixed Acid–Base Disorders. Patients may present with two or even three primary acid–base disorders. The first step in diagnosis is to define the primary disorder and the pulmonary or renal compensation (Table 17.1). Identification of the primary disturbance can be made from the pH. A pH <7.35 indicates a primary acidosis, whereas a pH >7.45 indicates a primary alkalosis. Overcompensation does not occur for primary acid–base disturbances.

A reduced plasma bicarbonate concentration indicates a metabolic acidosis or respiratory alkalosis. A bicarbonate concentration <15 mEq/L is typically a result of metabolic acidosis. A bicarbonate concentration >45 mEq/L occurs most commonly with metabolic alkalosis. Use of the formulas in Table 17.1 assumes adequate time for compensation.

The most common clinical settings for mixed acid–base disorders appear in Table 17.7. Severe acidemia can result from combined metabolic and respiratory acidosis. Even though the P_{CO_2} and bicarbonate concentration may be only moderately abnormal, the resulting acidemia is quite severe because of the lack of compensatory processes.

A mixed *metabolic acidosis* and *metabolic alkalosis* can be difficult to diagnose, because both disorders affect the plasma bicarbonate concentration. The pH and bicarbonate concentration can be increased, decreased, or normal. An elevated anion gap with an increased or normal bicarbonate concentration is the key to recognizing this diagnosis, as an elevated anion gap almost always indicates the presence of an anion gap metabolic acidosis. Many causes of metabolic acidosis are accompanied by vomiting, so this mixed disorder is not uncommon.

A *combined metabolic alkalosis* and *respiratory acidosis* is characterized by an increased bicarbonate concentration and increased P_{CO_2}. Based on the formulas in Table 17.1, the elevation in bicarbonate concentration is greater than predicted for compensation caused by respiratory acidosis.

TABLE 17.7. Common causes of mixed acid–base disorders

Disorder	Example	Clinical features
Metabolic acidosis/ respiratory acidosis	Cardiopulmonary arrest, severe pulmonary edema	Lactic acidosis with decreased ventilation.
Metabolic acidosis/ respiratory alkalosis	Salicylate intoxication	Elevated anion gap acidosis and central respiratory stimulation.
	Sepsis, severe liver disease	Lactic acidosis with respiratory stimulation.
Metabolic acidosis/ metabolic alkalosis	Renal failure with vomiting; alcoholic or diabetic ketoacidosis with vomiting; critically ill patients on gastric suction	Sepsis, renal failure, or diabetic ketoacidosis accompanied by gastric suction.
Metabolic alkalosis/respiratory acidosis	Chronic obstructive pulmonary disease with vomiting; adult respiratory distress syndrome with gastric suction	Often caused by theophylline toxicity; found in patients with cor pulmonale; can be exacerbated with chloride depletion from low NaCl intake.
Metabolic alkalosis/respiratory alkalosis	Inappropriate mechanical ventilation with gastric suction	Frequently seen in intensive care units.
	Pregnancy with vomiting	Pregnancy normally induces a chronic respiratory alkalosis.

Severe alkalemia can result from a *combined metabolic* and *respiratory alkalosis*. A mixed disorder is present if a respiratory alkalosis is not accompanied by the appropriate decrease in bicarbonate concentration or if metabolic alkalosis is not accompanied by the appropriate increase in PCO_2. This combination occurs frequently in critically ill patients because of excessive mechanical ventilation and diuretic use.

Finally, a triple acid–base disturbance can exist. This is *combined metabolic acidosis* and *metabolic alkalosis* accompanied by either respiratory acidosis or respiratory alkalosis. It frequently occurs in an alcoholic or diabetic patient with vomiting (metabolic alkalosis), lactic or ketoacidosis (metabolic acidosis), and a respiratory alkalosis caused by sepsis or liver disease. As with mixed metabolic acidosis and metabolic alkalosis, this diagnosis should be considered whenever an elevated anion gap is present and the serum bicarbonate is either normal or elevated. Alternatively, knowledge of previous laboratory values showing a chronic metabolic alkalosis, frequently as compensation for chronic respiratory acidosis, that is now apparently normalized should raise the consideration of a triple acid–base disorder.

VII. Suggested Readings

Adrogué HJ, Madias NE. Respiratory acidosis, respiratory alkalosis, and mixed disorders. In: Johnson RJ, Feehally J, eds. *Comprehensive clinical nephrology*, 2nd ed. St. Louis: Mosby, 2003:167–182.

Borthwick KJ, FE Karet. Inherited disorders of the H^+-ATPase. *Curr Opin Nephrol Hypertens* 2002;11:563–568.

Gauthier PM, Szerlip HM. Metabolic acidosis in the intensive care unit. *Crit Care Clin* 2002;18:289–308.

Kraut JA, Madias NE. Approach to patients with acid-base disorders. *Respir Care* 2001;46:392–403.

Lemann J Jr, Bushinsky DA, Hamm LL. Bone buffering of acid and base in humans. *Am J Physiol Renal Physiol* 2003; 285:F811–F832.

Calcium, Phosphorus, and Magnesium Disorders

Connie C. Mere and Francisco Llach

I. Disorders of Calcium Homeostasis

A. Regulation of Serum Calcium. There is approximately 1,000 g of calcium (Ca^{2+}) in the body, of which 99% is in the skeleton, where approximately 1% is freely exchangeable and serves as a buffer or storehouse of Ca. There are three definable fractions of Ca in serum calcium (S_{Ca}): ionized Ca^{2+} (approximately 50%), protein-bound Ca^{2+} (approximately 40%), and Ca^{2+} that is complexed, mostly to citrate and phosphate ions (approximately 10%). Approximately 90% of the protein-bound Ca^{2+} is bound to albumin. The ionized Ca^{2+} is maintained rigidly by the combined effects of parathyroid hormone (PTH) and 1,25 dihydroxyvitamin D [$1,25(OH)_2D$] (Fig. 18.1).

The Ca^{2+}-sensing receptor on the parathyroid chief cell is exquisitely sensitive to ionized S_{Ca}. Hypocalcemia stimulates PTH secretion, which increases renal distal tubular Ca^{2+} reabsorption and osteoclastic bone resorption. PTH also increases renal $1,25(OH)_2D$ synthesis, which, in turn, increases intestinal Ca^{2+} absorption (Fig. 18.2). These actions restore S_{Ca}. The action of PTH on distal tubular Ca^{2+} reabsorption provides the major acute regulation of S_{Ca}, whereas the action of $1,25(OH)_2D$ on intestinal calcium absorption requires 24–48 hours to become fully operative and provides the major chronic regulation (Fig. 18.1).

Hypercalcemia suppresses PTH secretion and thereby decreases osteoclastic bone resorption, renal tubular Ca^{2+} reabsorption, $1,25(OH)_2D$ synthesis, and intestinal Ca^{2+} absorption.

B. Vitamin D Metabolism. Vitamin D is a secosteroid that is converted by sunlight in the skin from 7-dehydrocholesterol (provitamin D_3) to previtamin D_3, which is rapidly transformed into vitamin D_3. Vitamin D_3 must undergo two successive hydroxylations to become biologically active (Fig. 18.2). The renal production of $1,25(OH)_2D$ is tightly linked to S_{Ca} through actions of PTH and phosphorus (Fig. 18.1). $1,25(OH)_2D$ maintains S_{Ca} by increasing intestinal Ca^{2+} absorption and recruiting bone stem cells as osteoclasts, which, in turn, mobilize bone Ca^{2+} into the circulation.

C. Factors Affecting Calcium Concentration or Measurement. [Ca^{2+}] in mg/dl (mg%) can be converted to molar units by dividing by four. The normal value of S_{Ca} is 8.5–10.5 mg/dl, and that of ionized S_{Ca} is

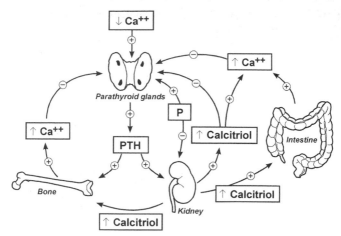

FIG. 18.1. Parathyroid hormone (PTH) feedback loop.

1.17–1.33 mmol/L. Each g/dl of albumin binds 0.8 mg/dl of Ca^{2+}. Thus, the total S_{Ca} can be corrected by adding 0.8 mg/dl for every 1 g/dl fall in albumin below 4 g/dl. Alkalosis enhances Ca^{2+} binding to albumin. A 0.1 pH unit reduces ionized S_{Ca} by 0.12 mmol/L.

D. Hypercalcemia. Hypercalcemia is diagnosed with S_{Ca} >10.5 mg/dl or ionized Ca^{2+} >1.33 mmol/L (Table 18.1).

Etiology and Differential Diagnosis of Hypercalcemia

- *Primary hyperparathyroidism* due to adenoma (85%), hyperplasia (15%), or parathyroid malignancy (1%). All are accompanied by elevated PTH.
- *Malignancy* due to (a) osteoclastic activating factor seen in multiple myeloma; (b) PTH-related peptide production by solid tumors, such as squamous cell carcinomas and carcinomas of the kidney, ovary, or bladder; or (c) ectopic vitamin D production by some hematopoietic tumors, such as B-cell lymphomas.

| Vitamin D$_3$ | Liver → | 25-Hydroxyvitamin D$_3$ | Kidney → | 1,25-Dihydroxyvitamin D$_3$ |
| (Cholecalciferol) | | | | (Calcitriol) |

FIG. 18.2. Biosynthesis of vitamin D.

TABLE 18.1.   Presentation of hypercalcemia

Grade of hypercalcemia	Serum calcium (mg/dl)	Symptoms
Mild	10.5–13.0	Asymptomatic, nausea/vomiting, constipation, polyuria, polydipsia, dehydration
Moderate	13–15	Bone pain, pseudogout, nephrolithiasis, acute renal failure, peptic ulceration, depression, psychosis, reduced cardiac conduction, arrhythmias
Severe	>15	Coma, cardiac arrest
Other	—	Weakness, hypertension, confusion, metastatic calcification, enhanced digitalis toxicity

- *Granulomatous conditions*, including sarcoidosis and mycobacterial infections that stimulate vitamin D (calcitriol) generation by activated macrophages.
- *Thyroid disease* that increases bone turnover by elevated triiodothyronine in thyrotoxicosis or by reduced renal Ca^{2+} excretion in hypothyroidism.
- *Vitamin D intoxication* during therapy for end-stage renal disease or osteoporosis.
- *Immobilization* with high bone turnovers, in Paget's disease, malignancy, adolescence, or a combination of these.
- *End-stage renal disease* with vitamin intoxication, secondary hyperparathyroidism, or aluminum toxicity.
- *After renal transplantation* in patients with preexisting parathyroid hyperplasia.
- *Milk-alkali syndrome* from ingestion of milk, Ca^{2+} (>5g/day), and alkali (e.g., antacids).
- *Rhabdomyolytic acute renal failure* that leads to Ca^{2+} and total body phosphorus (P) deposition in soft tissues that can be mobilized during the oliguric phase.
- *Lithium*, which alters the set point for Ca^{2+} inhibition of PTH secretion.
- *Familial hypercalcemic hypocalciuria*, an autosomal-dominant activating mutation of the Ca^{2+}-sensing receptor, causing mild hypercalcemia, hypophosphatemia, and reduced renal Ca^{2+} excretion. PTH is normal.

Evaluation of Hypercalcemia

Figure 18.3 summarizes the workup of hypercalcemia. Hypercalcemia associated with hyperparathyroidism is chronic and asymptomatic, whereas that associated with malignancy is acute and symptomatic (Fig. 18.3).

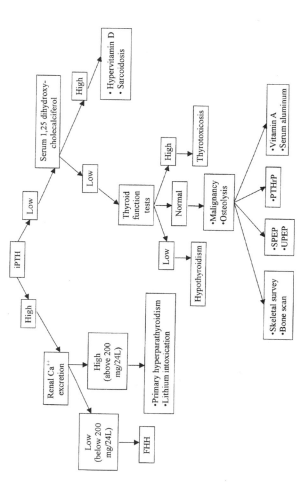

FIG. 18.3. Evaluation of hypercalcemia. FHH, familial hypercalcemic hypocalciuria; iPTH, intact parathyroid hormone; PTHrp, parathyroid hormone–related peptide; SPEP, serum protein electrophoresis; UPEP, urine plasma electrophoresis.

Treatment of Hypercalcemia

Asymptomatic hypercalcemia usually requires only evaluation, whereas symptomatic hypercalcemia (S_{Ca}, >13 mg/dl or $Ca^{2+} \times P$ product, >80 mg/dl) requires treatment. Most present with volume depletion and require vigorous replacement with NaCl and water followed by a diuresis that enhances Ca^{2+} excretion. A loop diuretic enhances Ca^{2+} loss but may exacerbate volume contraction and thus paradoxically enhance tubular Ca^{2+} reabsorption. Patients with adequate renal function who have been fully volume replaced benefit from a loop diuretic and large volumes of saline (e.g., normal saline at 100–200 cc/hr with furosemide, 20 mg). Saline diuresis usually reduces the S_{Ca} by 2–3 mg/dl within 24 hours.

If the S_{Ca} remains elevated, treatment with hypocalcemic agents or dialysis is required. Etidronate, pamidronate, and clodronate are diphosphonates that inhibit osteoclasts. Pamidronate can be given intravenously as a single infusion of 30–90 mg over 2–24 hours. Pamidronate is excreted intact primarily via the kidney and should be avoided in patients with severe renal impairment. A low dose (30 mg) in a large volume of infusion (>500 ml) given over 24 hours with monitoring of renal function should be used for those with less severe renal impairment. Bisphosphonates are useful in patients with hypercalcemia of malignancy, who usually respond within 7 days. The effect lasts 2–4 weeks. Side effects include fever and leukopenia. Plicamycin (Mithramycin) reduces osteoclast activity but is not recommended because of toxicity. Calcitonin (4–8 IU/kg intramuscularly or subcutaneously every 6–8 hours) can lower S_{Ca} by 1–3 mg/dl in hours, but tachyphylaxis develops within days. Side effects include flushing, nausea, and allergic reactions. Glucocorticosteroids reduce S_{Ca} in those with vitamin D intoxication or granulomatous diseases. The usual daily dose is 200–300 mg intravenously of hydrocortisone for 3–5 days.

Dialysis is reserved for those who are refractory to other measures or have renal insufficiency. Peritoneal dialysis or hemodialysis with a low or zero Ca^{2+} dialysate lowers S_{Ca} rapidly. These causes of renal failure in hypercalcemia are shown in Table 18.2.

TABLE 18.2.   Causes of renal failure in the setting of hypercalcemia

Vasoconstriction
Dehydration
Acute interstitial nephritis
Intratubular obstruction
Chronic interstitial nephritis
Renal calculi

TABLE 18.3. Presentation of hypocalcemia

Acute: paresthesias, tetany, seizures, hypotension, prolonged QT, atrioventricular block, ventricular fibrillation
Chronic: depression, dementia, dry and coarse skin, brittle nails, eczema, candidiasis, cataracts
Other features: asymptomatic, laryngospasm, muscle spasm
Chvostek's sign: facial twitch during tapping on the facial nerve; present in 25% of healthy patients
Trousseau's sign: carpal spasm 3 min after inflation of blood pressure cuff above systolic pressure

E. **Hypocalcemia.** Hypocalcemia is an S_{Ca} <8.5 mg/dl when corrected for serum albumin or an ionized S_{Ca} <1.17 mmol/L. The presentation and findings are shown in Table 18.3 and in Figure 18.4.

- *Hypoparathyroidism* may be idiopathic or from thyroid, parathyroid, or neck surgery.
- *Hypomagnesemia*: A low serum magnesium (Mg) concentration (S_{Mg}) inhibits PTH secretion and causes skeletal resistance to PTH. The hypocalcemia is refractory to treatment with calcium, vitamin D, and PTH and always requires Mg replacement.
- *Vitamin D deficiency* occurs in (a) sunlight deprivation; (b) malabsorption (gastric surgery, intestinal resection, celiac disease, steatorrhea); (c) liver disease (impaired 25-hydroxylation, reduced synthesis of vitamin D–binding protein); (d) nephrotic syndrome (urinary losses of vitamin D and vitamin D–binding protein); and (e) chronic renal insufficiency (impaired production of 1,25 dihydroxycholecalciferol, hyperphosphatemia, chronic metabolic acidosis).
- *Respiratory alkalosis* increases binding of Ca^{2+} to albumin and decreases ionized Ca^{2+}.
- *Acute pancreatitis* causes precipitation of calcium salts in the pancreas.
- *Enhanced bone turnover*, or hungry bone syndrome, can occur after surgical treatment of hyperparathyroidism or during rapid new bone formation.
- *Miscellaneous*: in critically ill patients with sepsis, in those with tumor lysis syndrome or rhabdomyolysis, and from albumin infusion and the use of foscarnet.

Evaluation of Hypocalcemia
The following are useful clues to the cause of hypocalcemia:

- *Normal S_{Ca} but low ionized Ca^{2+}*: hyperventilation/respiratory alkalosis
- *Low S_{Mg}*: hypomagnesemia
- *Low serum phosphorus*: vitamin D deficiency, poor intake, malabsorption, liver disease
- *High serum phosphorus*: rhabdomyolysis, tumor lysis, renal failure

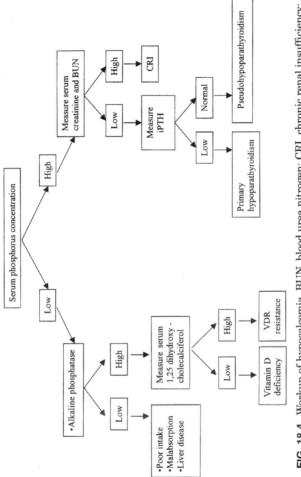

FIG. 18.4. Workup of hypocalcemia. BUN, blood urea nitrogen; CRI, chronic renal insufficiency; iPTH, intact parathyroid hormone; VDR, vitamin D receptor.

- *Low intact PTH*: primary hypoparathyroidism
- *Medication history*: anticonvulsants, loop diuretics, massive blood transfusions
- *Thyroid or parathyroid surgery*

Treatment of Hypocalcemia

Treatment depends on the severity and symptoms. Mild hypocalcemia may require only oral Ca^{2+} supplements (250–500 mg of elemental Ca^{2+} every 6–8 hours). Symptomatic hypocalcemia requires parenteral calcium gluconate (9 mg of Ca^{2+}/10-cc ampule) given in 10 cc of 5% dextrose over 10 minutes and repeated as necessary. Ca^{2+} gluconate can be infused with 10 ampules in 1 L of 5% dextrose at 50 cc/hr (45 mg/hr). A dose of 15 mg/kg of calcium over 4–6 hours usually raises the S_{Ca} 2–3 mg/dl.

II. **Phosphorus.** The normal serum concentration of phosphorus (S_P) is 3.0–4.5 mg/dl. Approximately 80% of P is contained in bone and 9% in skeletal muscle. S_P depends on P intake (800–1,600 mg/day), vitamin D, and PTH. Jejunal P absorption is stimulated by calcitriol. Approximately 80% of P is filtered at the glomerulus. It is reabsorbed in the proximal tubule with Na^+ that is stimulated by calcitriol. P stimulates PTH release, which inhibits its renal reabsorption.

A. **Hypophosphatemia.** Common presentations and findings are shown in Table 18.4.

Etiology and Differential Diagnosis of Hypophosphatemia

- *Decreased gastrointestinal (GI) absorption*: (a) starvation (combined with vitamin D deficiency, alcoholism); (b) corticosteroids; (c) aluminum, Mg, and Ca^{2+}-containing antacids.
- *Increased renal excretion* in hyperparathyroidism (including renal transplant).
- *Malignancies* can produce PTH-related protein.
- *Fanconi's syndrome* complicating multiple myeloma and proximal tubule dysfunction.
- *Diuresis* complicating (a) diuretics, mainly acetazolamide; (b) postobstruction; (c) recovery from acute tubular necrosis or diabetic ketoacidosis.
- *Cellular shifts* in respiratory alkalosis.

TABLE 18.4.   Presentation of hypophosphatemia

Asymptomatic (serum phosphorus, 1.0–2.5 mg/dl)
Muscle weakness (respiratory failure and left ventricular dysfunction)
Encephalopathy
Hemolysis, rhabdomyolysis
Decreased oxygen delivery by red blood cells (depletion of 2,3-diphosphoglycerate)
Impaired leukocyte chemotaxis
Reduced platelet survival
Defective bone mineralization

Treatment of Hypophosphatemia
Oral P providing 1–2 g of elemental P daily usually repletes body stores in 7–10 days. Skim milk is a good source. Intravenous infusion can provide 2 mg/kg over 6 hours.

B. Hyperphosphatemia. Hyperphosphatemia is S_P >4.5 mg/dl. It is common in secondary hyperparathyroidism (renal failure). It causes metastatic calcification if Ca^{2+} × P is >70.

Etiology and Differential Diagnosis

- *Pseudohyperphosphatemia* occurs with hemolysis or P binding by globulins.
- *Increased P intake or absorption*: (a) in vitamin D intoxication or (b) iatrogenic (phosphorus repletion or fleet enemas). This is a problem in renal insufficiency.
- *Release of P from tissues* in tumor lysis syndrome and rhabdomyolysis.
- *Transcellular shifts of P* in acidosis.
- *Decreased renal excretion of P* in renal insufficiency or when tubular reabsorption of P is increased in hypoparathyroidism, acromegaly, or thyrotoxicosis.

Treatment of Hyperphosphatemia
P absorption in the GI tract is prevented with oral P binders. $CaCO_3$ or Ca^{2+} acetate is given with meals unless the P level exceeds 6.5 mg/dl or the Ca^{2+} × P product exceeds 70 mg/dl, when non–calcium-containing binders, such as sevelamer hydrochloride, are preferable. Saline infusion increases renal P clearance, but dialysis is required in patients with renal failure.

III. Magnesium. Total body Mg is concentrated in intracellular fluid and bone. The average daily Mg intake is 300–360 mg, of which 25–60% is absorbed primarily in the small intestine. The majority of filtered Mg is reabsorbed in the cortical thick ascending limb and distal convoluted tubule. Less than 20% is reabsorbed in the proximal tubule.

A. Hypermagnesemia. This usually results from excess Mg intake (e.g., $MgSO_4$) in patients with reduced renal function. Common clinical findings are shown in Table 18.5.

Treatment of Hypermagnesemia
Intravenous Ca^{2+} (100–200 mg) antagonizes the effects of the Mg. A saline diuresis or hemodialysis enhances Mg^{2+} elimination.

TABLE 18.5.   Presentation of hypermagnesemia

Asymptomatic (serum magnesium, ≤5 mg/dl)
Nausea, vomiting, lethargy
Depressed neuromuscular function (decreased reflexes, muscle weakness, paralysis, hypoventilation)
Bradycardia, heart block, cardiac arrest
Effects exacerbated by hypocalcemia

TABLE 18.6. Presentation of hypomagnesemia

Asymptomatic, apathy, depression
Confusion, psychosis, brain stem signs
Hypocalcemia
Ventricular tachycardia, fibrillation, asystole, prolonged PR and QT
  intervals, flat T waves
Hypokalemia and hypophosphatemia

B. Hypomagnesemia. Common presentations and findings are listed in Table 18.6.

Etiology and Differential Diagnosis of Hypomagnesemia

- *Decreased intake* due to alcoholism, malnutrition, malabsorption, and GI losses.
- *Increased renal excretion*: diuresis from loop diuretics, hyperglycemia, or the diuretic phases of acute tubular necrosis; or postobstruction and in renal transplant recipients.
- *Drugs*: cisplatin, aminoglycosides, cyclosporine, amphotericin B, foscarnet, and ethanol.
- *Congenital defects of Mg absorption*: Bartter's and Gitelman's syndromes.
- *Hungry bone syndrome* after parathyroidectomy.

Evaluation of Hypomagnesemia

A Mg^{2+} excretion >24 mg/24 hr with low S_{Mg} indicates renal Mg^{2+} wasting (Fig. 18.4).

Treatment of Hypomagnesemia

Oral MgO provides 600 mg of elemental Mg^{2+} in 1 g in divided doses. Patients with hypomagnesemia and seizures or an acute arrhythmia require intravenous Mg^{2+} 8–16 mEq (1–2 g $MgSO_4$) over 15 minutes, followed by 48 mEq/day. Caution is required in renal failure, in which the dose should be halved and S_{Mg} monitored.

IV. Suggested Readings

Broadus AE. Mineral balance and homeostasis. In: Favus MJ, ed. *Primer on the metabolic bone diseases and disorders of mineral metabolism*. Philadelphia: Lippincott–Raven, 2003:105–110.

Bushinsky DA. Calcium, magnesium, and phosphorus: renal handling and urinary excretion. In: Favus MJ, ed. *Primer on the metabolic bone diseases and disorders of mineral metabolism*. Philadelphia: Lippincott–Raven, 2003:97–104.

Coe FL, Favus MJ. *Disorders of bone and mineral metabolism*. Philadelphia: Lippincott Williams & Wilkins, 2002.

Holick MF. Vitamin D: photobiology, metabolism, mechanism of action and clinical applications. In: Favus MJ, ed. *Primer on the metabolic bone diseases and disorders of mineral metabolism*. Philadelphia: Lippincott–Raven, 2003:129–136.

Hruska KA, Lederer ED. Hyperphosphatemia and hypophosphatemia. In: Favus MJ, ed. *Primer on the metabolic bone diseases and disorders of mineral metabolism*. Philadelphia: Lippincott–Raven, 2003:296–306.

LeBoff MS, Mikulec KH. Hypercalcemia: clinical manifestations, pathogenesis, diagnosis, and management. In: Favus MJ, ed. *Primer on the metabolic bone diseases and disorders of mineral metabolism*. Philadelphia: Lippincott–Raven, 2003:225–229.

Lemann J Jr., Favus MJ. Intestinal absorption of calcium, magnesium, and phosphate. In: Favus MJ, ed. *Primer on the metabolic bone diseases and disorders of mineral metabolism*. Philadelphia: Lippincott–Raven, 2003:93–96.

Rude RK. Magnesium depletion and hypermagnesemia. In: Favus MJ, ed. *Primer on the metabolic bone diseases and disorders of mineral metabolism*. Philadelphia: Lippincott–Raven, 2003:292–295.

Thakker RV. Hypocalcemia: pathogenesis, differential diagnosis, and management. In: Favus MJ, ed. *Primer on the metabolic bone diseases and disorders of mineral metabolism*. Philadelphia: Lippincott–Raven, 2003:271–273.

Ziegler R. Hypercalcemic crisis. *J Am Soc Nephrol* 2001;[Suppl 17]:S3–S9.

IV

Disease of the Urinary Collecting System and Bladder

Renal Stone Disease

I. David Weiner

Renal stone disease is a common condition that affects wide ranges of the population and causes significant morbidity. Therapeutic interventions, including extracorporeal shock wave lithotripsy (ESWL), percutaneous lithotripsy, and ureteroscopic laser treatment, simplify the treatment of acute manifestations of renal stone disease. However, renal stone disease recurs, often multiple times, in many individuals.

I. **Epidemiology.** Renal stone disease affects approximately one in every 500 individuals in the United States each year. Over a lifetime, approximately 3–5% of the population experiences symptoms. Men are approximately three times more likely than women to develop this disease. Asians, African Americans, and individuals of American Indian descent are relatively less likely to develop renal stone disease than are whites. Renal stone disease typically first occurs in individuals between the ages of 20 and 50 years. The prevalence of renal stone disease is greatest in a "stone belt" that encompasses Virginia, North Carolina, Georgia, Tennessee, and Kentucky, but it can occur in individuals in any state or country. The cause of the increased occurrence in this stone belt is incompletely understood. Individuals who have experienced an initial episode of renal stone disease are likely to experience further episodes. In the absence of preventive treatment, recurrence rates are approximately 10% at 1 year and 50% after 10 years.

II. **Physiology and Pathophysiology.** Most renal stones contain calcium in the form of calcium oxalate (35–70% of all stones), calcium phosphate (6–20%), or a mixture of both (10–30%). Pure uric acid stones account for 10% of all stones. Struvite stones, composed of magnesium ammonium phosphate, account for 15–20% of stones; rarely do stones consist primarily of cystine. Figure 19.1 summarizes the typical distribution of renal stones.

Kidney stones form when stone-forming crystalloids normally present in urine come out of solution. The most common stone-forming crystalloids are calcium phosphate, calcium oxalate, uric acid, magnesium ammonium phosphate, and cystine.

Several factors interact to cause these stone-forming crystalloids to come out of solution. The most important factors are (a) supersaturation of the crystalloids in the urine, (b) the presence of physical or chemical stimuli that promote stone formation, and (c) inadequate amounts of inhibitors of stone formation. Therefore, stone formation can result from any combination of the following:

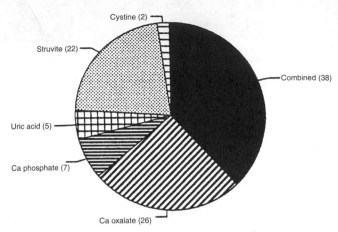

FIG. 19.1. The typical distribution of renal stones.

- Low urinary volume (e.g., hot climates)
- High urinary excretion of calcium, uric acid, or oxalate (the most common components of renal stones)
- Abnormal urinary pH (e.g., uric acid and cystine are less soluble in acid urine, whereas struvite and calcium phosphate are less soluble in alkaline urine)
- A nidus for crystal precipitation (e.g., sodium urate crystallization promotes calcium oxalate deposition on the sodium urate crystals and speeds the rate of stone formation)
- A deficiency of inhibitors of stone formation, such as citrate and Mg^{2+}

Most patients with renal stones have one or more identifiable causes of stone formation. The most common causes include hypercalciuria, hyperoxaluria, hypocitraturia, hyperuricosuria, and infection.

Hypercalciuria is the most commonly identified cause of renal stone disease. Excessive urinary calcium excretion leads to supersaturation of urine with calcium and the subsequent development of calcium oxalate (acid urine) or calcium phosphate (alkaline urine) stones. Hypercalciuria has several causes. Primary absorptive hypercalciuria leads to subclinical increases in serum calcium, mild suppression of parathyroid hormone, increased renal calcium filtration, and decreased calcium reabsorption, leading to an increase in urinary calcium excretion. A second cause is a primary renal calcium "leak," whereby a primary decrease in renal calcium reabsorption leads to increased urinary calcium excretion. A less common, but easily treatable, cause is a primary renal phosphate "leak" that leads to hypophosphatemia, with resultant stimulation of parathyroid hormone release, a secondary increase in gastrointestinal calcium absorption, a subclinical increase in the serum calcium, and a subsequent increase in urinary calcium excretion. Finally, excessive dietary sodium or protein intake increases urinary calcium excretion.

Most patients with calcium oxalate stones excrete normal amounts of urinary oxalate. However, increased gastrointestinal oxalate absorption can occur either from a primary increase in gastrointestinal uptake or from enhanced endogenous production. Gastrointestinal oxalate absorption can be increased by conditions that cause fat malabsorption, such as Crohn's disease, celiac sprue, or gastrointestinal bypass surgery. Increased endogenous production occurs from either increased intake of foods rich in oxalate such as spinach, peanuts, and cocoa, or excessive intake of vitamin C, which is metabolized to oxalate.

Citrate plays an important role in the defense against stone development because of its ability to complex urinary calcium, thereby preventing calcium incorporation into either calcium oxalate or calcium phosphate stones. Hypocitraturia may result from primary renal tubular acidosis or from conditions that increase endogenous acid production, such as excessive dietary protein intake, or that increase base loss, as in chronic diarrhea.

Hyperuricosuria can cause renal stone formation in either of two ways. First, uric acid crystals may serve as a nidus on which calcium oxalate crystals deposit, leading to increased rates of calcium oxalate stone growth. Second, pure uric acid stones can form in persistently acid urine. The solubility of uric acid is strongly pH dependent with markedly lower solubility at acid pH. For example, at pH 5, the normal rate of uric acid excretion for men, 800 mg/day, can lead to uric acid supersaturation and stone formation if urine volume is 1 L/day or less.

Infection with urea-splitting bacteria, such as *Proteus* and some *Klebsiella pneumoniae* species, can lead to increased formation of specific stones. A bacterial urease hydrolyzes urinary urea to ammonia in a reaction that consumes a proton, thereby increasing both urinary ammonia and pH. At high urine pH, magnesium, phosphate, and ammonium form struvite, which is insoluble and can rapidly grow in size until it fills the collecting system, forming the classic "staghorn" calculi. Bacteria are frequently incorporated into the growing struvite stone, leading to difficulty in sterilizing the urine.

III. Clinical Presentation. There are several clinical presentations of stone disease:

- *Severe, intense pain.* Severe pain is the most common presentation of renal stone disease. It typically has a sudden onset, although it slowly increases over a period of a few hours to a peak in some individuals. It may be either steady or colicky. An obstructing or partially obstructing stone in the renal pelvis or upper ureter is generally associated with flank and abdominal pain. Stones in the middle and lower thirds of the ureter typically cause pain that radiates downward to the inguinal ligament and into the urethra or testicle and penis. When stones are present in the portion of the ureter within the bladder wall, they may cause dysuria and frequency. Nausea and vomiting frequently accompany the pain and may contribute to the development of dehydration. Many affected individuals characterize the pain as the worst they have ever experienced. For unclear reasons, recurrent stones are typically less painful than on initial presentation.

- *Hematuria*. Hematuria may occur as a result of local trauma to the renal pelvis or bladder from the stones.
- *Infection*. Infection either of the stone or of the urinary tract, particularly if proximal to an obstructing renal stone, commonly occurs. Treating the infection is important in preventing recurrence. Infection proximal to an obstructing stone may require emergency admission and stone removal. If the stone is infected, a prolonged 6-week (or longer) course of antibiotics may be necessary to sterilize the stone because of poor penetration of antibiotics into the stone matrix.
- *Obstruction*. The stone may obstruct the renal pelvis or the ureter. Untreated obstruction, even if partial, can lead to irreversible loss of renal function.
- *Asymptomatic* stones may be discovered on an abdominal radiograph or ultrasound obtained for other reasons.

IV. Diagnosis. *History* should emphasize diet, drug ingestion, familial disorders, and the presence or absence of previous renal stones. If the afflicted individual is younger than 15 years or older than 50 years, then intensive evaluation of other possible etiologies of the presenting symptoms should be considered. In particular, appendicitis should be considered in the young, and an abdominal aortic aneurysm with possible rupture or dissection should be considered in those older than 50 years.

Urinalysis usually reveals either gross or microscopic hematuria. If pyuria is present, then infection should be excluded by urine culture. Crystalluria may permit a presumptive identification of stone type (Fig. 19.2). However, only freshly voided, warm urine should be used for examination; when urine is cooled, the solubility of dissolved crystalloids decreases, possibly leading to their precipitation and an incorrect diagnosis.

Radiologic studies play an important role in the evaluation of renal stone disease. A plain abdominal radiograph may show radiodense stones (85–90% of all stones) containing calcium, struvite, or cystine but may miss radiolucent uric acid stones. An ultrasound or an intravenous urogram is needed to identify radiolucent stones or to confirm that a radiodensity seen on plain radiograph is, in fact, within the renal pelvis or the ureter and to determine whether partial or complete ureteral obstruction is present. A helical computed tomography scan is very effective in diagnosing renal stone disease and assists in evaluating other causes of the presenting symptoms.

Crystallographic stone analysis is critical for establishing the chemical nature of a stone and guiding therapy.

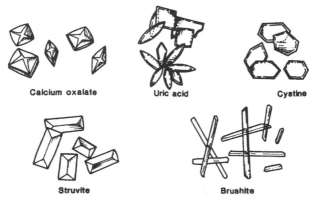

FIG. 19.2. Urinary crystal morphology.

Patients should strain their urine through a filter until the stone is passed to obtain the stone for crystallographic analysis of its composition.

V. **Management.** The management of renal stone disease should be divided into two components: the acute presentation, in the patient with acute renal colic, and the chronic management, after the pain, obstruction, or infection is treated.

A. **Acute Management.** Patients presenting with acute renal colic caused by renal stone disease are frequently in great discomfort and require aggressive treatment. Once other conditions such as appendicitis, cholecystitis, or pyelonephritis are shown not to be the cause of the patient's symptoms, pain control is essential. Most pain can be controlled with intravenous ketorolac or parenteral narcotics. Ketorolac has the benefit of combining analgesia with antiinflammatory effects and possible effects to promote ureteral relaxation. Oral analgesics should be avoided, in general, in the acute setting because of the nausea and vomiting that are frequently present. In addition, rapid pain control is generally desired and is best accomplished with parenteral analgesics.

Patients also frequently have intravascular volume depletion that is due to the associated nausea and vomiting. Intravenous rehydration assists in decreasing symptoms related to dehydration and increasing urine output, which may aid in the passage of the renal stone.

If infection is suspected, either because of the presence of fever and leukocytosis or pyuria and bacteriuria on urinalysis, empirical antibiotics should be started. In general, all patients should have their urine cultured for bacteria.

Most patients can be managed in an outpatient setting. An exception to this rule is the patient in whom

TABLE 19.1. Systemic diseases causing renal stone disease

Disease	Screening tests
Primary hyperparathyroidism	Serum calcium
Distal renal tubular acidosis	Serum electrolytes
Inflammatory bowel disease	History
Gout	History, uric acid
Inborn error of metabolism	History onset in childhood

nausea and vomiting cannot be controlled, requiring hospitalization for continued hydration. A second exception is the patient with a fever or urinary tract infection and ureteral obstruction, who is at high risk for severe, rapidly progressive urosepsis and should have emergent relief of the obstruction. Ureteral obstruction in the absence of infection is not an indication for emergent hospitalization unless the patient has a solitary functional kidney. Otherwise, the stone can be observed for spontaneous passage over a period of days.

Most renal stones pass spontaneously. The patient with acute renal colic should filter his or her urine until the stone passes to retrieve the stone for accurate identification of the composition, which will provide insight into the factors that caused the problem. However, stones >7 mm are less likely to pass spontaneously.

Stones that do not pass spontaneously or require urgent intervention for the reasons detailed above can be approached with a variety of techniques, including basket extraction, cystoscopy with laser lithotripsy, ESWL, and percutaneous extraction or shock wave lithotripsy. Usually, stones in the distal third of the ureter can be treated with cystoscopic techniques. Stones in other locations can be treated with ESWL, leading to the formation of multiple small fragments that usually pass with few symptoms.

B. **Chronic Management.** The chronic management of renal stone disease is based on two observations. First, renal stone disease may be the initial presentation of an underlying, systemic disease. Second, approximately 50% of patients develop one or more recurrences.

The first goal of the chronic management of renal stone disease is to exclude an underlying systemic disease that caused the renal stone disease. Table 19.1 lists the likely systemic diseases and their recommended screening tests. Patients with hypercalcemia, whether overt or borderline, should have an ionized calcium and a parathyroid hormone level measured to identify whether they have primary hyperparathyroidism. Patients with hypokalemic, non–anion gap metabolic acidosis should have the urine pH and urine anion gap measured to determine whether they have distal renal tubular acidosis. Inflammatory bowel disease and gout are generally suspected based on a typical history, although the presence of hyperuricemia may be helpful in the diagnosis of gout. Inborn errors of metabolism that cause renal stones are frequent causes of renal stones in children. These include cystine stones in cystinosis, glycine stones in hyperglycinuria, uric acid stones in Lesch-Nyhan syndrome, and oxalate stones in oxalosis. Congenital distal renal tubular acidosis may also present in children; it is frequently associated with impaired growth or failure to thrive, or both.

The second component of the chronic management of renal stone disease is prevention of recurrence. The simplest measure to prevent recurrence is to increase the urine volume to decrease the concentration of crystalloids, leading to a decreased rate of stone formation and even, in some patients, to dissolution of existing stones. Increasing urine volume by 1 L/day can decrease the risk of recurrence by 50%. In general, one should recommend an oral fluid intake of 2 L/day. Tea, coffee, and grapefruit juice should be used in limited amounts. Tea can contain substantial amounts of oxalate. Caffeine in coffee can lead to diuresis, intravascular volume depletion, and resulting urine concentration. Grapefruit juice ingestion has been associated with increased risk of recurrent stone disease; the mechanism is currently unknown.

Finally, some medications increase the risk of renal stone disease. In particular, the antiretroviral agent indinavir is associated with a substantial risk of stone disease. Approximately 8% of those receiving indinavir develop symptomatic renal stone disease. Increased oral hydration should be recommended to all patients receiving indinavir therapy. In some cases, indinavir withdrawal may be necessary. Other medications associated with renal stone formation include triamterene, sulfonamides, and oral carbonic anhydrase inhibitors.

Other measures to decrease recurrence are based on treating the common causes of stone formation. Automated analysis of calcium, oxalate, uric acid, citrate, pH, total volume, and sodium in a 24-hour urine specimen (e.g., StoneRisk Diagnostic Profile, Mission Pharmacal, San Antonio, TX) can be helpful. Any abnormalities that are found can be treated as described below.

Hypercalciuria should be treated by measures that decrease urinary calcium excretion. First, primary hyperparathyroidism or other causes of hypercalcemia should be investigated and treated if present. If hypercalcemia is not present, then thiazide diuretics are effective at decreasing urinary calcium excretion. Because thiazide diuretics decrease urinary citrate excretion, they should be combined with administration of potassium citrate. Sodium citrate should be avoided because the sodium content can increase urinary calcium excretion. Finally, dietary sodium and protein restriction decrease urinary calcium excretion. Dietary calcium restriction should not be used, as it can increase urinary oxalate excretion. This may lead, paradoxically, to an increased risk of recurrent stone formation.

Hyperoxaluria is treated by addressing the underlying cause whenever possible. Fat malabsorption should be treated aggressively. If marked hyperoxaluria more than five to ten times the upper limit of normal is present, then evaluation for primary hyperoxaluria related to genetic defects in oxalate metabolism should be initiated.

Hyperuricosuria can be treated by measures that either increase the solubility of uric acid or decrease the production of uric acid. Alkalinizing the urine markedly increases the solubility of uric acid. Potassium citrate is effective because oral citrate intake can cause mild metabolic alkalosis and subsequent alkalinization of the urine. Allopurinol, 300 mg/day, decreases the production of uric acid and is also beneficial in patients with documented hyperuricosuria, particularly if uric acid stones have been documented.

Hypocitraturia is easily treated with oral potassium citrate. As noted above, citrate ingestion leads to mild metabolic alkalosis, which increases urinary citrate excretion. Potassium citrate, 40–60 mEq/day in divided doses, should be used; sodium citrate should be avoided as noted previously.

Struvite stones require treatment of the underlying infection. Appropriate antibiotics should be administered based on the results of urine culture and sensitivity and should be continued for 4–6 months. Because the offending bacteria can become incorporated into the stone matrix, prolonged antibiotic treatment, even in the presence of apparently negative urine cultures, is necessary. Acetohydroxamic acid, a urease inhibitor, may be helpful.

VI. Suggested Readings

Borghi L, Meschi T, Schianchi T, et al. Medical treatment of nephrolithiasis. *Endocrinol Metab Clin North Am* 2002;31:1051–1064.

Borghi L, Schianchi T, Meschi T, et al. Comparison of two diets for the prevention of recurrent stones in idiopathic hypercalciuria. *N Engl J Med* 2002;346:77–84.

Delvecchio FC, Preminger GM. Medical management of stone disease. *Curr Opin Urol* 2003;13:229–233.

Manthey DE, Teichman J. Nephrolithiasis. *Emerg Med Clin North Am* 2001;19:633–654.

Monk RD, Bushinsky DA. Nephrolithiasis and nephrocalcinosis. In: Johnson RJ, Feehally J, eds. *Comprehensive clinical nephrology*, 2nd ed. St Louis: Mosby, 2003:731–744.

Pearle MS. Prevention of nephrolithiasis. *Curr Opin Nephrol Hypertens* 2001;10:203–209.

Urinary Tract Infections

Shakil Aslam

Urinary tract infections (UTIs) are among the most common bacterial infections. A UTI is called *complicated* if it is associated with an increased risk of serious complications or treatment failure (e.g., congenital malformations, obstruction, stones, presence of a foreign body, or immune deficiency states). This determines the therapy and the follow-up.

I. **Epidemiology.** In the United States, at least 250,000 episodes of acute pyelonephritis occur annually. The incidence of cystitis in young, sexually active women is approximately 0.5 per person-year and recurs in 27–44% of healthy women with normal urinary tracts. The incidence of symptomatic UTI in adult men <50 years of age is much lower and ranges from 5 to 8 per 10,000 person-years. Complicated UTI occurs in approximately 5 per 1,000 admissions. Catheter-associated infections account for 88% of these. More than 1 million nosocomial UTIs occur annually in the United States.

II. **Risk Factors.** UTIs are more common in women. The exceptions are those associated with congenital malformation in early childhood and obstruction, which occurs more frequently in men >50 years of age. This lower prevalence in men may relate to the greater distance between the anus and the male urethral meatus, its greater length, the drier environment, and the antibacterial activity of prostatic fluid. An increased risk of UTI in men is associated with lack of circumcision, homosexual activity, and intercourse with a woman colonized with an uropathogen.

III. **Pathogenesis**
   A. **Bacterial Factors.** More than 95% of UTIs result from ascension of uropathogens from the external genitalia. The remainder are due to hematogenous dissemination of organisms such as *Staphylococcus aureus*, *Pseudomonas aeruginosa*, and *Salmonella typhi* (Table 20.1). UTIs in women are often due to *Escherichia coli* that colonize the vaginal introitus and the periurethral area. Once within the bladder, bacteria may multiply and ascend to the ureters, especially if there is vesicoureteral reflux to the renal pelvis and parenchyma. Most UTIs are due to *E. coli*, especially serogroups (called *uropathogenic strains*) 01, 02, 04, 06, 07, 075, and 0150, which possess virulence factors that include adhesins that facilitate their adhesion to uroepithelium.
   B. **Host Factors.** The presence of lactobacilli in the normal vaginal flora prevents colonization. The use of spermicides for contraception and the hormonal changes of menopause inhibit the normal vaginal flora, thereby

TABLE 20.1.   Bacterial etiology of urinary tract infections (UTIs)

	Frequency in UTIs (%)	
Organisms	Uncomplicated	Complicated
Gram-negative organisms		
Escherichia coli	70–95	21–54
Proteus mirabilis	1–2	1–10
Klebsiella spp.	1–2	2–17
Citrobacter spp.	<1	5
Enterobacter spp.	<1	2–10
Pseudomonas aeruginosa	<1	2–19
Other	<1	6–20
Gram-positive organisms		
Coagulase-negative staphylococci	5–20	1–4
(*Staphylococcus saprophyticus*)		
Enterococci	1–2	1–23
Group B streptococci	<1	1–4
Staphylococcus aureus	<1	1–2
Other	<1	2

increasing the risk of recurrent UTIs. Sexual activity introduces pathogens into the bladder where they adhere to uroepithelial cells and cause infection. A normal bladder can eliminate these uropathogens, whereas incomplete bladder emptying severely attenuates this defense.

Within the kidney, the medulla is most susceptible to infection. This may relate to the high concentration of ammonia, which inactivates complement, and to poor chemotaxis in an area of high osmolality, low pH, low blood flow, and low PO_2.

IV. **Clinical Presentation and Diagnosis.** UTI syndromes range from asymptomatic bacteriuria to life-threatening, tissue-invasive infections associated with shock and multiple organ failure. Symptoms are not closely related either to the presence of bacteriuria or to the site of infection. Pyuria is suggestive of UTI. Urinary leukocyte esterase activity may be used as a screening test, but >10 leukocytes/mm^3 in unspun urine correlates better with true infection. In contrast, the examination of spun urine for leukocytes has high false-positive and -negative results. A Gram stain of unspun urine showing one or more organisms per oil immersion field correlates with the presence of $\geq 10^5$ bacteria/ml.

The cornerstone of diagnosis is a quantitative urine culture. Significant bacteriuria is $>10^5$ colony-forming units (CFUs)/ml of a single uropathogen. However, 20–30% of true, symptomatic bacterial UTIs in women that respond to appropriate treatment have lesser counts. Therefore, in a symptomatic woman, a lower cutoff improves the test sensitivity.

V. Major Urinary Tract Infection Syndromes

A. Asymptomatic Bacteriuria. *Asymptomatic bacteriuria* is defined as a positive urine culture in an asymptomatic patient. This is a common and generally benign condition. In elderly patients, it may be associated with pyuria. Treatment is generally not warranted except in high-risk patient groups that include pregnant patients, renal transplant recipients, those undergoing genitourinary surgery, and neutropenic patients.

B. Acute, Uncomplicated Cystitis or Urinary Tract Infection in Women. Acute, uncomplicated cystitis or UTI in women is characterized by burning on urination, dysuria, frequency, and/or suprapubic pain. Acute dysuria in a young, sexually active woman is usually caused by acute cystitis; acute urethritis from *Chlamydia trachomatis*, *Neisseria gonorrhoeae*, or *Herpes simplex*; or vaginitis caused by *Candida* spp. or *Trichomonas vaginalis*. The presence of pyuria favors acute cystitis and urethritis. However, definitive diagnosis requires the finding of significant bacteriuria in a midstream urine. In these circumstances, $>10^3$ CFU/ml should be used, because this increases the sensitivity from 50% to 80% and retains a specificity of 90%. Urine cultures are generally not necessary in uncomplicated acute cystitis.

Three-day regimens (Table 20.2) are preferred for the treatment of acute, uncomplicated cystitis. Single-dose regimens are somewhat less effective. Nitrofurantoin must be given for at least 7 days. The best cure rates are observed with trimethoprim-sulfamethoxazole (TMP-SMX) and fluoroquinolones (FQs). A 3-day oral regimen with TMP-SMX is the first-line therapy if tolerated. FQs are alternatives in those who are intolerant or in areas where resistance to this agent is $>10\%$. Routine follow-up cultures should be undertaken only when infection

TABLE 20.2. Commonly used oral regimens for acute, uncomplicated cystitis

Drug and dose	Interval	Duration (d)
Trimethoprim-sulfamethoxazole, 160/800 mg	q12h	3
Fluoroquinolone		
Ciprofloxacin, 250 mg	q12h	3
Ciprofloxacin, 500 mg extended release	q24h	3
Gatifloxacin, 200 mg	q24h	3
Levofloxacin, 250 mg	q24h	3
Nitrofurantoin (Macrobid), 100 mg	q12h	7
Nitrofurantoin macrocrystals, 50 mg	q6h	7
Amoxicillin, 500 mg	q12h	7
Amoxicillin-clavulanate, 500/125 mg	q12h	7
Cefpodoxime proxetil, 100 mg	q12h	7
Cefixime, 400 mg	q24h	7

persists or recurs within 2 weeks, when a longer course (10–14 days) with an agent based on sensitivities should be prescribed. A recurrence after 2 weeks should be treated as a new episode of UTI.

C. **Recurrent, Acute, Uncomplicated Cystitis in Women.** Most recurrent, acute, uncomplicated cystitis in women is due to reinfection with the same uropathogen. The first step should be postcoital voiding, avoiding spermicides, and local or systemic estrogen replacement in postmenopausal women. The next step should be imaging studies to detect sequestered focus of infection or a complicating structural or functional disorder. These may respond to an extended course (4–6 weeks) of TMP-SMX or an FQ. Prophylaxis should be considered for women who experience three or more infections annually. Effective strategies include

- Low-dose, long-term prophylaxis with either TMP-SMX (one or two tablets) or an FQ (e.g., ciprofloxacin, 250 mg, or ofloxacin, 200 mg) at bedtime
- A single dose of the above agents given after coitus
- A single dose at the onset of symptoms of UTI

D. **Acute Urethral Syndrome in Women.** Acute urethral syndrome in women is similar to acute, uncomplicated UTI but has a smaller number (10^2–10^4 CFU/ml) of usual uropathogens or infection with *C. trachomatis*. Pyuria is almost always present. Because vaginitis may present similarly, vaginal examination and cultures should be performed and appropriate treatment provided. Those with dysuria who lack pyuria or do not respond to antimicrobials should be managed symptomatically.

E. **Acute, Uncomplicated Pyelonephritis in Women.** Symptoms of acute, uncomplicated pyelonephritis in women range from a mild illness to septic shock and renal failure. These patients can have fever, chills, flank pain, nausea and vomiting, and costovertebral tenderness. Symptoms of cystitis are variable. A Gram stain of the urine sediment should guide empiric therapy. A urine culture of $\geq 10^4$ CFU/ml uropathogens is positive in >95% of patients.

Outpatient therapy (Fig. 20.1) with oral agents is safe and effective in selected patients. It can be instituted after initial stabilization in the emergency department (Table 20.3). Indications for hospitalization include inability to maintain oral hydration or to take medications, severe illness with high fevers, severe pain and debility, noncompliance, and uncertainty about the diagnosis. For Gram-positive organisms, therapy with ampicillin or amoxicillin/clavulanic acid, or vancomycin in patients with penicillin allergy, is appropriate. However, these infections are usually caused by Gram-negative bacilli. An FQ, a β-lactam/aminoglycoside combination, or a broad-spectrum β-lactam (e.g., imipenem, ceftazi-

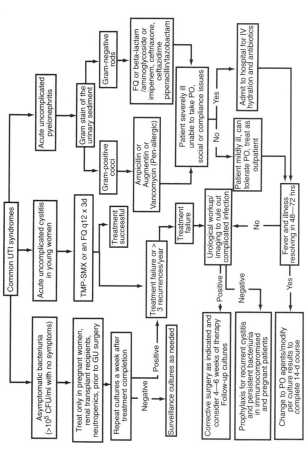

FIG. 20.1. Therapeutic approaches to urinary tract infection (UTI). CFU, colony-forming unit; C/S, culture and sensitivity; dx, diagnosis; FQ, fluoroquinolone; GU, genitourinary; TMP-SMX, trimethoprim-sulfamethoxazole.

TABLE 20.3. Commonly used oral agents for uncomplicated pyelonephritis

Drug and dose	Interval	Duration (d)
Fluoroquinolones	q12h	7–10
Ciprofloxacin, 500 mg	q12h	7–10
Gatifloxacin, 400 mg	q12h	7–10
Levofloxacin, 500 mg	q12h	7–10
Trimethoprim-sulfamethoxazole, 160/800 mg	q12h	10–14
Amoxicillin-clavulanate, 875/125 mg	q12h	10–14
Amoxicillin, 875 mg	q12h	10–14
Amoxicillin, 500 mg	q8h	10–14

dime, ceftriaxone, or piperacillin/tazobactam) are all appropriate (Table 20.4). Once sepsis is controlled and the patient is afebrile, oral therapy with an FQ or TMP-SMX should be given for 14 days. Failure to obtain response within 72 hours should trigger a search for a complicating problem, such as a stone, obstruction, or poor bladder emptying. Nitrofurantoin should not be used to treat pyelonephritis, as it does not achieve therapeutic tissue levels. Follow-up cultures should be done only if symptoms recur.

F. **Urinary Tract Infection in Pregnancy.** UTI in pregnancy is associated with premature labor and delivery, increased fetal loss, and prematurity. Routine screening and treatment of asymptomatic bacteriuria are standard practice at the first prenatal visit. Further screening is needed in women at high risk for infection (e.g., presence of urinary tract anomalies, hemoglobin S, or preterm labor). Treatment is similar to that for nonpregnant

TABLE 20.4. Commonly used parenteral regimens for acute, uncomplicated pyelonephritis

Drug and dose	Interval
Ceftriaxone, 1–2 g	q24h
Cefepime, 1 g	q12h
Ciprofloxacin, 200–400 mg	q12h
Gatifloxacin, 400 mg	q24h
Levofloxacin, 250–500 mg	q24h
Gentamicin, 3–5 mg/kg (± ampicillin)	q24h
Gentamicin, 1 mg/kg (± ampicillin)	q8h
Ampicillin, 1 g (+ gentamicin)	q6h
Trimethoprim-sulfamethoxazole, 160/800 mg	q12h
Aztreonam, 1 g	q8–12h
Ampicillin/sulbactam, 1.5 g	q6h
Piperacillin/tazobactam, 3.375 g	q6–8h

Note: See text for duration.

women with acute, uncomplicated UTI with a short-term course. However, sulfonamides should be avoided near term because of risk of kernicterus in the newborn, and FQs affect fetal cartilage development. Ampicillin and cephalexin are safe. Pregnant women with overt pyelonephritis should be admitted for parenteral therapy with β-lactams and aminoglycosides. Suppressive therapy is recommended for women with persistent bacteriuria (≥2 positive urine cultures). Nitrofurantoin (50–100 mg orally at bedtime) for the duration of the pregnancy or cephalexin (250–500 mg orally at bedtime) may be used. A culture should be obtained 1 week after completion of therapy and repeated monthly.

G. **Urinary Tract Infection in Men.** UTIs in men are usually associated with obstruction from congenital disorders in the young and acquired disorders in the old. In men <50 years of age, anal intercourse, intercourse with a woman colonized with uropathogens, and acquired immunodeficiency syndrome with CD4 count of <200/mm^3 are important risk factors. Men without one of these risk factors, and especially those who have recurrent infections, should undergo a urologic evaluation and an intensive treatment course (minimum of 4–6 weeks). UTI in men usually represents tissue invasion of the prostate or kidney, or both, and should be treated for at least 14 days. Recurrent infection often indicates a sequestered focus within the prostate that is difficult to eradicate due to poor antimicrobial penetration, presence of prostatic calculi, or prostatic enlargement causing bladder neck obstruction.

H. **Complicated Urinary Tract Infections.** Complicated UTIs involve a wide variety of structural and functional defects of the urinary system. There is a wide range of organisms. Resistance is common and mandates an individualized approach to therapy. Acutely septic patients should receive broad-spectrum antibiotic combinations until definitive bacteriologic data are available. If it is possible to correct an underlying structural defect, a shorter course of antibiotics (7–14 days) should be used to control the symptoms, and a prolonged 4- to 6-week course should be used if such correction is not possible. Catheter-related bacteriuria is a common source of Gram-negative bacteremia. Prevention should include avoidance of a catheter when possible, sterile insertion, prompt removal, and use of a closed collecting system. Prophylactic systemic antimicrobials are not indicated except in pregnant women or patients undergoing urologic surgery who require short-term catheterization.

Patients with spinal cord injuries who require catheter bladder drainage are predisposed to recurrent UTIs. Pyuria and significant bacteriuria (>10^5 CFU/ml) are usually present. Multi-drug resistance is common and may require parenteral antibiotics. Intermittent catheterization is preferred. Treatment of asymptomatic bacteriuria with prophylactic antibiotics is usually not successful.

Emphysematous pyelonephritis is necrotizing pyelonephritis with gas-forming *E. coli*, *Klebsiella pneumoniae*, *P. aeruginosa*, or *Proteus mirabilis*. Most cases occur in patients with diabetes and are associated with obstruction. Computed tomography shows gas within the renal parenchyma. Emergency nephrectomy and broad-spectrum antibiotics lower the mortality from 75% to 20%.

I. Candidal Infections of the Urinary Tract. Candidal infections of the urinary tract are increasingly common in patients with diabetes, those with indwelling catheters, or in patients receiving corticosteroids or broad-spectrum antibiotics. The first step is to reverse these factors. If candiduria persists, systemic antifungal therapy is recommended. Fluconazole (200–400 mg/day) is effective against *Candida albicans* and *Candida tropicalis* but not against *Candida krusei* or *Candida glabrata*, which should be treated with low-dose amphotericin (10 mg/day) plus flucytosine (100 mg/kg/day) in divided doses for 14 days. Patients who require an indwelling catheter may receive amphotericin or nystatin bladder rinses via a three-way catheter. However, this has an efficacy of only approximately 50%.

VI. Suggested Readings

Foxman B, Brown P. Epidemiology of urinary tract infections: transmission and risk factors, incidence, and costs. *Infect Dis Clin North Am* 2003;17:227–241.

Gilstrap LC III, Ramin SM. Urinary tract infections during pregnancy. *Obstet Gynecol Clin* 2001;28:581–591.

Hooton TM. The current management strategies for community-acquired urinary tract infection. *Infect Dis Clin North Am* 2003;17:303–332.

Nicolle LE. Urinary tract infection: traditional pharmacologic therapies. *Dis Mon* 2002;49:111–128.

Tolkoff-Rubin NE, Rubin RH. Therapy of urinary tract infection. In: Brady HR, Wilcox CS, eds. *Therapy in hypertension and nephrology*, 2nd ed. Philadelphia: WB Saunders, 2003:415–423.

V

Hypertension

Approach to the Hypertensive Patient

Christopher S. Wilcox

Hypertension is a level of blood pressure (BP) sufficient to increase the risk of stroke or renal or cardiovascular system disease. BP above 140/90 mm Hg in an adult is considered abnormal, and values of 130–139/80–89 mm Hg are considered borderline.

I. **Incidence.** The incidence of hypertension is approximately 5% in young adults, 50% by age 50 years, and 80% by age 80. It increases in diabetes mellitus or chronic renal insufficiency.

II. **Risks.** Hypertension increases the risk of many common conditions (Table 21.1). It is one of several factors that increase the risk of cardiovascular disease (Table 21.2). Hypertension accelerates the decline in renal function in azotemic patients with diabetic nephropathy and those with proteinuria >1 g daily. In these patients, the target BP should be 125/75 mm Hg. Hypertension accelerates the decline in cognitive function in patients with dementia and the decline in cardiac function in those with congestive heart failure, but optimum BP targets are not yet established for these conditions.

III. **Classification.** Each patient with hypertension should be classified according to the severity (Table 21.3), the pathologic type (Table 21.4), and the cause (see Chapter 22).

Treatment of borderline hypertension is generally nonpharmacologic. Treatment of stage 1 normally can be delayed during evaluation, but stage 2 requires treatment within days.

Isolated systolic hypertension in the young implies a high cardiac output and rapid left ventricular ejection. This responds well to β-adrenoceptor blockade. Isolated systolic hypertension is common in the elderly, in whom it results from the loss of elasticity in the large arteries or from aortic atherosclerosis. It carries an unfavorable prognosis for stroke and myocardial infarction. It responds well to diuretics.

A. **Pathologic Type.** Benign hypertension is usually asymptomatic and progresses slowly (Table 21.4). Malignant hypertension accounts for <1% of all hypertension. The hallmarks are grade II hypertension with grade IV funduscopic changes of papilledema, retinal hemorrhages, and exudates (Table 21.5) accompanied by headache and often by fluctuating neurologic signs caused by increased intracranial pressure and patchy cerebral ischemia. Untreated, malignant hypertension can progress to seizures, fixed neurologic deficits, coma, and death. Patients have proteinuria, hematuria, and an

TABLE 21.1.   Conditions associated with hypertension

Aortic aneurysm
Cerebrovascular accident
Chronic renal insufficiency (notably nephrosclerosis)
Congestive cardiac failure
Dementia
Myocardial infarction
Peripheral vascular disease

TABLE 21.2.   Factors that increase the cardiovascular risk of hypertension

African American ethnicity
Age
Chronic renal insufficiency
Coincident arterial disease
Dyslipidemia
Family history of myocardial infarction below age 50 y
Hyperhomocysteinemia
Left ventricular hypertrophy
Microalbuminuria
Obesity/underactivity
Previous organ injury
Smoking

TABLE 21.3.   Severity of hypertension

Normal: <130/<80 mm Hg
Prehypertensive: 130–139/80–89 mm Hg
Stage 1: 140–159/90–99 mm Hg
Stage 2: >160/>100 mm Hg

TABLE 21.4.   Pathologic type of hypertension

	Benign	Malignant
Onset	Gradual, ages 20–55	Sudden
Progression	Slow over years	Rapid over weeks
Vascular pathology	Medial hypertrophy	Myointimal proliferation and fibrinoid necrosis
Kidney pathology	Nephrosclerosis and atrophy	Ischemia and hemorrhagic microinfarction
Funduscopic changes	Arterial narrowing and tortuosity	Hemorrhages and exudates; usually papilledema
Renal failure	Absent or slowly progressive	Rapidly progressive with active urinary sediment

TABLE 21.5.   Classification of hypertensive retinopathy

Class	Arterial to venous ratio[a]	Focal arteriolar spasm[b]	Hemorrhages and exudates	Papilledema	Arteriolar light reflex
Normal	3:4	1:1	0	0	Fine yellow line; blood column
Grade I	1:2	1:1	0	0	Broad yellow line; blood column
Grade II	1:3	2:3	0	0	Broad "copper wiring" line; no blood
Grade III	1:4	1:3+	+	0	Broad "silver wire" line; no blood
Grade IV	Fine	Obliteration	+	+	Fibrous cords; no blood

[a]Ratio of arterial to venous diameters.
[b]Ratio of diameter of regions of spasm to more proximal segments.

active urinary sediment. They may progress over weeks or months to renal failure. Some have a microangiopathic hemolytic anemia and dysfunction of other organs. Further details appear in Chapter 28.

B. **Cause.** Essential hypertension encompasses 85–95% of patients who otherwise have no discernible cause. Most (70%) have a family history of hypertension, which usually presents between age 20 and 55 years. Secondary hypertension is described in Chapter 22.

IV. **Etiologic Factors in Essential Hypertension**

A. **Genetic Factors.** The probability of hypertension is increased if one parent is hypertensive. The genes responsible are not yet established.

B. **Diet.** Excessive intake of the following dietary constituents is associated with increased BP: sodium chloride, caffeine, and alcohol (more than two drinks per day). Lower BP is associated with high intakes of calcium and potassium. A DASH diet (Dietary Approaches to Stop Hypertension) lowers BP. It has a high content of calcium and potassium. It is based on fruits, vegetables, low-fat dairy products, white meat, and fish.

C. **Renin–Angiotensin–Aldosterone Axis.** Approximately 40% of hypertensive patients have low renin values. This includes many African Americans, the elderly, and those with chronic renal insufficiency. They often have salt-sensitive hypertension. Approximately 10% are high renin. They are often young, white patients.

D. **Sympathetic Nervous System.** Plasma levels of norepinephrine and epinephrine are normal or mildly elevated in most hypertensive patients. However, a subgroup has increased sympathetic tone (hyperdynamic circulation, raised heart rate, elevated catecholamines). Baroreceptor function is impaired in the elderly and those with extensive atherosclerosis who have elevated catecholamines and wider BP fluctuations.

E. **Renal Function.** Early in hypertension, the renal blood flow is reduced while the glomerular filtration rate is maintained. The ensuing rise in the filtration fraction promotes renal salt retention. Renal function deteriorates in a minority of hypertensive patients and creates a vicious cycle whereby a decline in renal function impairs salt excretion, which raises BP and perpetuates further renal damage. African Americans have more organ damage for a given level of hypertension. They are much more likely to develop nephrosclerosis and renal insufficiency.

F. **Lifestyle.** BP is increased by pain, emotion, anxiety, obesity, and smoking, but is reduced by exercise.

V. **Clinical Presentation of Hypertension.** There are no specific symptoms associated with hypertension. Headache occurs in severe or malignant hypertension. It is usually occipital, throbbing, and present on awakening. Initial examination of all hypertensive patients should include measurements of BP and pulse by the physician while the patient is lying down and after 2 minutes of standing. An orthostatic

**TABLE 21.6.   Questions to answer in each
hypertensive patient**

Does the patient have hypertension?
What is the severity of hypertension?
Is hypertension benign or malignant?
Is there a secondary cause?
Has there been organ damage?
Are there modifiable dietary or lifestyle factors?
What are the coincident risk factors for cardiovascular disease?
Are there specific drug indications or contraindications?

Note: These questions will not identify renovascular hypertension or pheochromocytoma.

fall in BP implies blocked cardiovascular reflexes (e.g., drugs,
such as α-receptor blockers, autonomic neuropathy, pheochromocytoma) and/or volume depletion. Initially, the BP
should be measured in both arms and the timing of femoral
and radial pulses correlated (marked differences in pulse
pressure or a delayed femoral pulse suggests severe aortic
atherosclerosis or coarctation). The BP of children or adoles-
cents should be measured in the leg to exclude coarctation of
the aorta. The fundi should be examined (Table 21.5) for
hypertensive or atherosclerotic changes. More severe changes
imply prolonged duration and a worse prognosis.

VI. **Questions to Answer in Each Hypertensive Patient.**
Key questions should be addressed in each patient suspected of hypertension (Table 21.6).

1. Does the patient have hypertension? Several measurements
   of BP are necessary because patients are often anxious at
   the first visit. They should take their BP regularly at home
   with an automated device. The BP records should be
   brought to clinic visits or transmitted via a computer link
   and e-mail to a central monitoring system. The self-recorded
   BP should be checked against a clinic measurement to
   ensure accuracy. "White coat" or "office" hypertension is an
   elevated BP in the clinic but not in the home setting. It is
   seen in 30% of hypertensive patients. It is associated with a
   higher probability of subsequent hypertension and a moderate increase in left ventricular hypertrophy. It does not need
   urgent treatment but should prompt arrangement for regular BP checks. A more precise diagnosis of white coat hypertension, and a more accurate definition of the true BP
   burden and response to treatment, require an ambulatory
   24-hour BP monitor. The following can overestimate BP:
   fear, pain, anxiety, a rigid arterial wall (checked by palpa-
   tion at wrist during BP measurement), or a large arm (use
   a large cuff).
2. What is the severity of hypertension? See Table 21.1.
3. Is hypertension benign or malignant? See Table 21.4.
4. Is there a secondary cause? See Chapter 22.
5. Has there been organ damage? Assess the impact on the

TABLE 21.7.   Tests for patients diagnosed as hypertensive

Urinalysis (protein, glucose, and blood; microscopy if dip is abnormal)
Electrolytes, calcium, blood urea nitrogen, and serum creatinine
Blood sugar and lipid profile (repeat fasting if abnormal)
Electrocardiogram (echocardiogram if abnormal)
Twenty-four–hour urine for sodium excretion, creatinine clearance, and
   microalbumin excretion.
For more severe hypertension or those with a family history of early car-
   diovascular disease:
   Plasma renin activity and serum aldosterone concentration.
   Plasma metanephrines
   Echocardiogram.
   Plasma homocysteine. If abnormal, plasma folate and vitamin B_{12}.
   Lipoprotein(a).

   heart (heart failure, hypertrophy, extra heart sounds,
   pulmonary rales, a raised jugular venous pressure), kidney
   (proteinuria, microalbuminuria, hematuria, azotemia,
   reduced creatinine clearance), vessels (peripheral pulses and
   bruits, abdominal aneurysms), and fundi (see Table 21.5).
6. Are there modifiable dietary or lifestyle factors contributing
   to hypertension? Assess the level of salt intake from measurements of 24-hour renal sodium excretion. (Measure creatinine excretion to assess the adequacy of collection, which
   should be 15–25 mg/kg.) Patients on a "no added salt" diet
   should achieve a daily sodium excretion of 120 mmol (equals
   120 mEq) or less. More than two alcoholic drinks daily raises
   BP. Aerobic, moderate exercise >30 minutes, three times
   weekly reduces BP and cardiovascular risk. A DASH diet
   reduces BP independent of weight reduction.
7. What are the coincident risk factors for cardiovascular disease? See Table 21.2.
8. Are there specific drug indications or contraindications?

VII. Routine Laboratory Tests. See Chapter 4.
   Tests to assess end-organ function and to screen for
   some secondary causes are detailed in Table 21.7.
VIII. Special Investigations. The following have value in
   selected patients.
   **A. Intravenous Pyelogram, Computed Tomography,
      or Renal Ultrasound.** An intravenous pyelogram, com-
      puted tomography, or renal ultrasound is indicated when
      the kidneys are palpated on examination (suggesting poly-
      cystic kidney disease or tumor) or anatomic abnormalities
      of the collecting system are suspected (patients with recur-
      rent urinary tract infection, unexplained pyuria or hema-
      turia, symptoms of prostatism, or previous renal stone
      disease). Renal ultrasound assesses renal size (decreased
      in unilateral renal artery stenosis, or parenchymal dis-
      ease) and is sensitive to detect renal cysts.
   B. Radionuclide Scanning. Radionuclide   scanning   is
      described in Chapters 3 and 22.

C. **Renal Arteriography.** Aortography and selective renal arteriography are the definitive procedures for visualizing renal artery stenosis (see Chapter 22). They are also valuable in the workup of classic-type polyarteritis nodosa (for demonstration of renal aneurysms) and in the diagnosis of renal infarction or tumor. A digital-subtraction arteriogram decreases the dye load and the risk of contrast-induced nephropathy in patients with impaired renal function or diabetes mellitus.

IX. Suggested Readings

DASH diet: http://www.nhlbi.nih.gov/health/public/heart/hbp/dash/.

Joint National Committee on Detection, Evaluation, and Treatment of High Blood Pressure. Seventh report. Bethesda, MD: National Institutes of Health, 2003.

Krakoff LR. Treatment decision for hypertension. In: Brady HR, Wilcox CS, eds. *Therapy in nephrology and hypertension*, 2nd ed. Philadelphia: WB Saunders, 2003:523–529.

Secondary Forms of Hypertension

Christopher S. Wilcox

Estimates of the percentage of hypertensive patients with a secondary cause vary widely (Table 22.1). The prevalence of secondary hypertension increases substantially among patients with severe and drug-resistant hypertension and in those with a suggestive clinical history or physical findings. Secondary causes should be considered in all whose blood pressure is not controlled while taking three or more medications (see Chapter 29). The low prevalence of many causes mandates a selective screening program to limit expensive testing. Suggestive clinical and laboratory findings should prompt appropriate screening tests. These must be highly sensitive (few false negatives) to avoid failing to diagnose a form of hypertension that may be curable or require specific therapy.

I. **Renal Parenchymal Disease.** Any decrease in renal function may cause hypertension. Conversely, hypertension itself may cause nephrosclerosis, especially in African Americans. Hypertension accounts for approximately one-fourth of patients with end-stage renal disease. It accelerates the progression of renal injury in patients with diabetes mellitus or those with proteinuria >1 g daily. Renal parenchymal hypertension is caused predominantly by excessive salt and water retention, but inappropriate secretion of renin and angiotensin and activation of the sympathetic nervous system contribute. Consequently, therapy with salt restriction plus a diuretic and an angiotensin-converting enzyme (ACE) inhibitor (ACEI) and/or an angiotensin receptor blocker are appropriate choices. Some patients require the addition of a sympatholytic agent. Calcium channel blockers are effective in most patients. For details of drug treatment, see Chapters 24–29.

II. **Renovascular Hypertension**

   A. **Definition and Causes.** Renal artery stenosis (RAS) is a narrowing (usually >80% to be functionally significant) of one or both renal arteries or their branches. Renovascular hypertension is that which is improved or cured by correction of an RAS. Renovascular disease encompasses both diagnoses. Ischemic nephropathy is chronic renal insufficiency caused by RAS that is often bilateral. If unilateral, it is accompanied by renal functional impairment, such as nephrosclerosis, in the contralateral kidney.

   The most common cause of renovascular hypertension is an atherosclerotic plaque that is often in the aorta overlaying the origin of the renal artery or in the proximal 1 cm (osteal lesion) (Table 22.2). Of the remainder,

TABLE 22.1. **Secondary causes of hypertension**

Cause	Prevalence (%)
Renal parenchymal disease	5
Renovascular disease	0.5–35.0
Primary aldosteronism	1–20
Thyroid disease	0.5
Pheochromocytoma	<0.2
Cushing's syndrome	<0.2
Drug-related	0.1–1.0

most are due to fibromuscular dysplasia of the renal arteries. Fibromuscular disease does not usually progress or cause renal arterial thrombosis, and, therefore, rarely causes ischemic nephropathy (Table 22.3).

B. **Pathophysiology.** Renal hypoperfusion releases renin from the myoepithelial cells of the afferent arteriole (see Fig. 26.1). Renin catalyzes the transformation of angiotensinogen, which is produced mainly in the liver, to angiotensin I (Ang I), which is inert until two amino acids are cleaved by ACE. ACE is located predominantly on the vascular endothelium. If only one kidney is hypoperfused, the effects of the reduced renal perfusion pressure and the increased Ang II and aldosterone secretion to enhance salt and water reabsorption are counterbalanced by a pressure natriuresis in the contralateral kidney. Therefore, there is little salt and water retention. However, in patients with bilateral RAS or stenosis of a transplanted, solitary, or dominant kidney, there is no normal kidney to allow pressure natriuresis. These patients can experience episodes of "flash" pulmonary edema caused by overfilling of the bloodstream. Acute or recurrent pulmonary edema in a hypertensive and azotemic patient, especially any with a preserved left ventricular ejection fraction, suggests this diagnosis. The natural history of untreated atherosclerotic renovascular diseases is a progressive decrease in renal blood flow, which ultimately results in ischemic nephropathy.

C. **Clinical Features.** Clinical features are outlined in Table 22.4.

TABLE 22.2. **Causes of renovascular hypertension**

Lesions intrinsic to kidney or its blood vessels	Extrinsic lesions
Atherosclerosis	Urinary tract obstruction
Fibromuscular dysplasia	Abdominal aortic aneurysm
Vasculitis	Emboli
Renal cysts	Renal capsular hematoma

TABLE 22.3.   Comparison of atherosclerotic and fibromuscular renal artery stenosis

Feature	Atherosclerosis	Fibromuscular dysplasia
Proportion of cases (%)	80	20
Age of onset	After 55 yr	Adolescence onward
Gender	Both	Female to male, 10:1
Site of lesion	Usually osteal	Distal renal artery or branch
Radiologic appearance	Single lesion	Often multiple, short lesions
Progression	Usual	Rare
Arterial occlusion/ thrombosis	Over time	Rare
Atherosclerosis elsewhere	Common	Less common
Renal failure	Over time	Rare

D. Screening Tests for Renovascular Hypertension.
Rapid-sequence intravenous pyelogram, simple renogram, unstimulated plasma renin activity (PRA), intravenous digital subtraction angiogram, and renal vein renins are not sufficiently accurate for routine use. Currently, three tests shown in clinical trials to have sensitivities >90% are available for screening.

1. The captopril-PRA or captopril challenge test is detailed in Table 22.5.
2. The ACEI renogram. This frequently uses technetium-99m mercaptotriglycine (MAG_3), which is filtered at the glomerulus and is secreted by the proximal tubule. The glomerular filtration rate (GFR) of a hypoperfused, post-stenotic kidney is maintained by the contractile effects of Ang II on the efferent arterioles. Thus, an ACEI reduces

TABLE 22.4.   Clinical features suggestive of renovascular hypertension

Hypertension resistant to two or more drugs and a diuretic
Onset of hypertension before age 20 yr in women or after age 55 yr
Accelerated or malignant hypertension
Arteriosclerotic disease elsewhere
Smoking history
Azotemia (especially that developing with angiotensin-converting enzyme inhibitors or angiotensin receptor blockers)
Abdominal bruit (especially diastolic or flank)
Recurrent pulmonary edema (especially if left ventricular ejection fraction is preserved)
Kidney size difference >1.5 cm (in the absence of cysts)
Unexplained hypokalemic alkalosis (suggesting hyperaldosteronism)

TABLE 22.5. Captopril challenge or captopril-plasma renin activity (PRA) test

Patients must have a moderate or high probability of renovascular hypertension.

Those with serum creatinine >3 mg/dl, cardiovascular system instability, or edema are excluded.

Antihypertensives and diuretics are discontinued over 10 days or replaced with alpha/beta blocker and/or calcium channel blocker.

Antihypertensives are withheld on the test day.

Administer 50 mg of crushed captopril with water while the patient is seated.

Monitor BP.

Blood for PRA is drawn 60 min after captopril.

Check standing BP to ensure patient is not orthostatic before discharge.

A postcaptopril PRA >5.7 ng/ml/h is a positive test.

Test sensitivity is 90–95%, and specificity is 80–90%.

BP, blood pressure.

the renal vascular resistance and the GFR. The ACEI maintains the renal blood flow of the post-stenotic kidney and, therefore, maintains the delivery of MAG_3 to the nephron, yet retards the elimination of MAG_3 because of the fall in GFR that reduces the rate of transit of the tracer through the nephron. This is detected as a reduced clearance of MAG_3 from the kidney. One hour after 50 mg of captopril is given, MAG_3 is injected, and the kidneys are scanned for 20–30 minutes. Diagnostic criteria for renovascular hypertension include an ACEI-induced delay in the time to peak or in the washout. In extreme cases, there is a progressive renal accumulation of the tracer after ACEI. If the test is abnormal, it is repeated without captopril to detect an ACEI-induced change in the renogram. A change implies functional renovascular hypertension, whereas a fixed abnormality implies renal parenchymal disease or outflow obstruction. Functional tests are used for screening and to predict the response to intervention.

3. Renal ultrasound with duplex Doppler velocimetry. This is a test of RAS. The lengths of the kidneys are measured with ultrasound. In the absence of renal cysts, a length difference >1.5 cm implies predominantly unilateral renal disease, and, in the context of hypertension, this is usually RAS. The peak systolic blood flow velocity is measured in the aorta and along the renal arteries. A threefold step up in velocity in a renal artery suggests RAS. The resistive index of the intrarenal vessels is calculated from the peak minus trough factored by the peak velocity. A resistive index >80% suggests fixed intrarenal vascular disease and predicts a poor response to correction of RAS. This noninvasive test is used for screening to predict response to intervention and for follow-up of patients after intervention. Its accuracy depends on the skill, experience, and time taken by the operator.

E. Diagnostic Tests for Renal Artery Stenosis.

1. Angiography is the gold standard for diagnosing RAS. Imaging must be undertaken in two planes. The quantity of dye injected is reduced to approximately 20–40 ml by computer enhancement (digital subtraction). To cause functionally significant renal ischemia, a stenosis must usually occlude >80% of the arterial lumen. However, the demonstration of an anatomic stenosis does not prove that it is the cause of the hypertension. Therefore, arteriography is performed only on selected patients. The complications include contrast-associated nephropathy, which is a particular risk in those with chronic renal failure, especially diabetic patients; cholesterol atheroembolism; dissection or puncture of the renal artery; spasm or thrombosis of the artery; or bleeding or pseudoaneurysm at the puncture site. Because of the risks and expense, the test is not suitable for screening. It is reserved for screened patients who have a high probability of an RAS.
2. Spiral computed tomography (CT). This is noninvasive and accurate but requires >100 ml of contrast. Therefore, it is best avoided in those with renal insufficiency.
3. Magnetic resonance angiography. This is noninvasive and does not use nephrotoxic agents. It is less expensive than angiography. Clinical trials have shown that it has a sensitivity >95% and a specificity >90% for detecting RAS that is proven by angiography. It is the test of choice to detect RAS, especially in azotemic or high-risk patients.

F. Intervention.
The goal is to improve or cure hypertension or to delay the progression to ischemic nephropathy. Percutaneous transluminal renal angioplasty (PTRA) is combined with stenting (S) for osteal lesions. PTRA(S) can cause arterial rupture or dissection, atheroemboli to the kidney or lower limbs, acute renal failure from contrast-associated nephropathy, or bleeding at the puncture site. The technical success rate is >90%, and at 1 year >75% of those arteries treated with stenting remain patent. Surgical revascularization is reserved for those who have failed PTRA(S) and for those with concomitant disease of the abdominal aorta requiring surgery.

G. Management.
Three controlled trials have failed to show a clear benefit over 6–12 months for patients with RAS randomized to PTRA compared to medical theory. Therefore, the finding of RAS does not necessarily imply that the patient should be offered intervention. Only those with renal artery narrowing of >80% should be considered for intervention. Clinical criteria favoring intervention are outlined in Table 22.6. All patients with atherosclerotic RAS require cardiovascular risk factor management and careful control of hypertension. ACEIs and angiotensin receptor blockers should be avoided when possible because of the associated risk of azotemia. Patients should be evaluated carefully at 3–4

TABLE 22.6. Criteria for intervention in renal artery stenosis (RAS)

Progressive or advanced azotemia
Recurrent flash pulmonary edema
Tight bilateral RAS
Angiotensin-converting enzyme inhibitor–induced renal failure
Uncontrolled hypertension or congestive heart failure
Stenosis of a single functioning kidney

months then every 6 months to determine whether their condition is stable (Table 22.7). Those with documented progression and no contraindications should be offered intervention.

III. **Pheochromocytoma.** Hypertension is caused by a tumor (pheochromocytoma) that secretes catecholamines. More than 90% are benign.

A. **Pathophysiology, Associated Conditions, and Clinical Features.** Some 90% of pheochromocytomas are in the adrenal medulla, but neural crest cells that can harbor a pheochromocytoma are found in autonomic ganglia, organs of Zuckerkandl (lying anterior to the aortic bifurcation), carotid bodies, and bladder. Tumors are bilateral in 10–20%.

Pheochromocytoma may be inherited as an autosomal-dominant trait either alone or as part of the syndromes of multiple endocrine neoplasia type 2 (medullary thyroid carcinoma, pheochromocytoma, and parathyroid hyperplasia), von Hippel-Lindau syndrome (retinal and cerebellar hemangioblastomas, renal cysts, and renal cell carcinomas), von Recklinghausen's syndrome (neurofibromatosis and café-au-lait skin pigmentation), or tuberous sclerosis (mental deficiency, renal cysts, and tumors). Hypertension is sustained in approximately 60% of patients but may be paroxysmal when catecholamines are released and cause severe hypertension, headache, sweating, and palpitations. Paroxysms may be precipitated by exercise, urination, defecation, sexual intercourse, anesthesia, contrast agents, or certain drugs, including vasodilators. Other clinical features

TABLE 22.7. Noninvasive tests to evaluate progression of renovascular disease

Blood pressure (ideally ambulatory blood pressure monitoring)
Creatinine clearance and microalbuminuria
Renal size by ultrasound
Renal artery stenosis by duplex Doppler velocimetry
Plasma renin activity
Individual renal function by angiotensin-converting enzyme inhibitor renography

include weight loss, fever, anxiety, tremors, psychotic illness, and glucose intolerance. Orthostatic hypotension is secondary to diminished plasma volume from pressure natriuresis and blunted sympathetic reflexes.

B. **Screening Tests.** The features that suggest the need to screen for pheochromocytoma are

- Hypertension accompanied by headache, palpitations, and sweating
- Paroxysmal hypertension
- Sustained diastolic blood pressure >120 mm Hg
- Hypertension and unexplained orthostatic hypotension

The most sensitive and specific screening test is plasma metanephrines. An increase in plasma catecholamines >3- to 5-fold while the patient is hypertensive is highly suggestive of pheochromocytoma, whereas less severe elevations accompany anxiety, pain, hypoglycemia, hypoxemia, old age, and tricyclic antidepressant or vasodilator therapy.

C. **Diagnostic Tests.** Clonidine inhibits the sympathetic outflow from the brain. It thereby reduces plasma catecholamines in healthy individuals and patients in whom elevated levels are caused by physiologic stimulation from anxiety but not from an autonomous pheochromocytoma (Table 22.8).

D. **Localization Tests.** A CT scan, magnetic resonance imaging, or selective adrenal venous sampling for catecholamines is used for localization. Magnetic resonance imaging is preferred because it is noninvasive and accurate in localizing tumors larger than 0.5 cm. It can discriminate between pheochromocytomas and adrenal adenomas or cysts. Imaging slices of 0.3 cm should be taken through the regions of the adrenals and the anterior aspect of the aortic bifurcation, bladder, chest, and neck.

E. **Management.** Surgical excision is curative. Preoperative stabilization with α-blockade and volume expansion is essential. Acute pheochromocytoma crisis responds to intravenous α-blockade with phentolamine. Prolonged, predictable α-blockade is achieved with phenoxybenzamine, which is a noncompetitive α-antagonist. After hypertension is controlled, a β-antagonist can be admin-

TABLE 22.8.   Clonidine suppression test

Withhold beta blockers and diuretics for 2 wk before testing.
Hold antihypertensives on the day of the test.
Patient is recumbent with an IV cannula 30 min before and during the test.
Administer 0.3 mg of clonidine orally.
Obtain plasma for catecholamines before and 3 h after the clonidine.
A positive test is total catecholamines >500 pg/ml or failure to fall by >50%.
The sensitivity for detecting pheochromocytoma is >90%.

istered to control tachycardia. A shorter-acting combined alpha and beta blocker, such as labetalol or carvetalol, is useful for less hypertensive subjects.

IV. **Primary Hyperaldosteronism.** In primary hyperaldosteronism, hypertension is caused by excess aldosterone and is accompanied by suppression of renin.

A. **Pathophysiology and Clinical Features.** Aldosterone-producing adenomas (APAs) of the adrenal zona glomerulosa cells, also called *Conn's syndrome*, previously accounted for 60% of cases of primary hyperaldosteronism. Currently, many more patients are being diagnosed with primary hyperaldosteronism. Most now have bilateral adrenal hyperplasia, also called *idiopathic hyperaldosteronism* (IHA). Multiple adenomas occur in <10% of patients. Rare causes include glucocorticoid-remediable hyperaldosteronism, also called *dexamethasone-suppressible hyperaldosteronism*. This is caused by a chimeric mutation in the promoter for aldosterone synthase that leads to its activation by adrenocorticotrophic hormone (ACTH). Glucocorticoid-remediable hyperaldosteronism is inherited as a dominant condition. It is diagnosed by DNA analysis and from the reversal of hyperaldosteronism and hypertension after suppression of ACTH secretion with dexamethasone. The excessive producuction of aldosterone results in renal salt retention, causing extracellular fluid volume expansion, hypertension, and enhanced secretion of K^+ and H^+ in the collecting ducts, causing hypokalemic metabolic alkalosis. Aldosterone activates a cytoplasmic mineralocorticosteroid receptor (MC-R). The MC-R is also activated by glucocorticosteroids, which are present in much higher concentrations than aldosterone. However, the MC-R normally is protected from glucocorticosteriods by 11-β hydroxysteroid dehydrogenase (11-β HSD) that is coexpressed at sites of MC-R expression. 11-β HSD metabolizes glucocorticosteriods such as cortisol to inactive cortisone. The 11-β HSD can be inhibited by glycoyrrhine acid present in licorice or chewing tobacco or may be defective due to a dominant mutation. These conditions give rise to pseudohyperaldosteronism.

Primary aldosteronism should be differentiated from secondary aldosteronism caused by excess renin secretion, as occurs in renovascular hypertension or edematous states, and from pseudohyperaldosteronism and Liddle's syndrome that is caused by excessive reabsorption of Na^+ via the epithelial sodium channel in the collecting ducts. Patients with pseudohyperaldosteronism have the clinical and biochemical changes of primary hyperaldosteronism but have suppressed levels of serum aldosterone concentration (SAC).

The hallmarks of hyperaldosteronism are hypertension, hypokalemic metabolic alkalosis, and suppressed PRA, but elevated SAC.

TABLE 22.9.   Screening test for primary hyperaldosteronism

24-h urine potassium >40 mEq despite hypokalemia
Low basal or frusemide-stimulated PRA
SAC >15 ng · dl^{-1}; SAC to PRA ratio >25 ng · ml^{-1}/ng · ml^{-1} · h^{-1}
Excessive aldosterone or tetrahydroaldosterone excretion after 3 days
   with Na$^+$ intake >200 mmol/day (check 24-h urine) or with 9α-
   fludrocortisone (0.1 mg t.i.d.)

PRA, plasma renin activity; SAC, serum aldosterone concentration.

B. Screening Tests. Screening should be undertaken in selected patients. The features that should prompt screening are

- Unprovoked or diuretic-induced hypokalemia with alkalosis
- Resistance to therapy with two or more drugs
- Suppression of PRA and/or elevation of SAC

Screening should follow correction of potassium deficits, because hypokalemia suppresses aldosterone secretion even from adenomas (Table 22.9). Blood for serum potassium must be taken without stasis or fist clenching.

C. Diagnostic Tests. The following tests confirm the diagnosis and distinguish between APAs and IHAs.

1. The saline suppression test assesses the dependency of aldosterone secretion on Ang II. Two liters of 0.9% NaCl are infused intravenously over 2 hours to suppress PRA and Ang II. Blood is drawn before and after the infusion for plasma cortisol and aldosterone. Patients with APAs continue to secrete aldosterone independent of Ang II. Therefore, these patients have an elevated post-saline SAC (above 10 ng · dl^{-1} or <50% reduction) and an aldosterone: cortisol ratio >2.2, whereas those with normal adrenals or IHAs show a >50% reduction in these measurements.

2. The postural stimulation test assesses the relative response of adrenal aldosterone secretion to Ang II and ACTH. The test is conducted while ACTH and cortisol normally are declining during the morning. After 1 hour of recumbency at 8 a.m., a blood sample is obtained for SAC, 18-hydroxycorticosterone, PRA, and cortisol and repeated after 4 hours of upright ambulation to stimulate renin and angiotensin secretion. A decrease in cortisol confirms that ACTH has fallen. The diagnosis of APA is suggested by an elevated SAC and 18-hydroxycorticosterone that fail to increase further with standing. Healthy individuals and those with IHA show an orthostatic increase in SAC.

3. CT scan with 0.3 mm imaging cuts through the adrenals detects tumors >0.5 cm.

4. Adrenal venous sampling is required when functional tests suggest an APA but no mass is seen on CT scan. It is techni-

TABLE 22.10. Additional causes of secondary hypertension

Cause	Clinical features
Preeclampsia	Third-trimester pregnancy, proteinuria, and edema
Cushing's syndrome	Central obesity, hirsutism, glycosuria
Coarctation of the aorta	Delayed pulses in legs
Hyperparathyroidism	Increased calcium and parathyroid hormone levels
Congenital adrenal hyperplasia	
11-Hydroxylase deficiency	Virilization
17-Hydroxylase deficiency	Abnormal sexual development
Sleep apnea	Obesity, snoring, somnolence
Hypothyroidism	Bradycardia, hair loss, amenorrhea
Acromegaly	Excessive growth, glycosuria

cally difficult. An SAC to cortisol ratio that is >4-fold higher on one side compared to the other suggests a unilateral source for aldosterone secretion from a microadenoma that will respond to adrenalectomy. Patients with IHA have elevated SAC in both adrenal veins.

D. Treatment. APAs should be removed laparoscopically. Blood pressure is normalized in 50–75% of patients, and the biochemical abnormalities are corrected in almost all. IHA is managed with a mineralocorticosteroid antagonist such as spironolactone or eplerenone (see Chapter 26). In those who develop adverse effects, high doses of amiloride

TABLE 22.11. Drug-induced hypertension

Adrenergic agonists
    Methylphenidate
    Neo-Synephrine
    Phenylephrine
    Phenylpropanolamine
    Pseudoephedrine
Hypertension after abrupt withdrawal
    Clonidine
    Barbiturates
Catecholamine-releasing drugs
    Amphetamines
    Cocaine
    Caffeine
    Monoamine oxidase inhibitors (plus tyramine or cheese)
Other agents
    Alcohol (>2 drinks)
    Smoking
    Cyclosporine
    Disulfiram (plus alcohol)
    Ergotamine
    Estrogen and birth control pills (high doses)

usually control hypokalemia, after which incremental doses of a thiazide diuretic are usually effective.

V. Other Causes of Secondary Hypertension. Additional causes of hypertension are presented in Table 22.10, and drug-induced causes in Table 22.11.

VI. Suggested Readings

Brady HR, Wilcox CS. *Therapy in nephrology and hypertension*, 2nd ed. Philadelphia: WB Saunders, 2003.

Wilcox CS. *Atlas of diseases of the kidney*, Vol 3. Schrier RW, ed. Philadelphia: Current Medicine, 1998.

Wilcox CS, ed. Renal vascular disease. *Semin Nephrol* 2000;20: 387–502.

Hypertension and Renal Disease in Pregnancy

Lillian J. Borrego Conde and Jason G. Umans

Renal physiology and blood pressure (BP) control change dramatically with normal pregnancy. This makes diagnosis more difficult and may alter the course and severity of renal disease. Likewise, renal disease and hypertension each increase the risk to the mother and the fetus. There are causes of hypertension and renal failure that are unique to pregnancy. Table 23.1 outlines some physiologic changes in normal pregnancy.

I. Specific Renal Problems in Pregnancy

A. Urinary Infection. Asymptomatic bacteriuria is apparent in 40% of pregnancies, with pyelonephritis occurring in 1–2% of all pregnancies. The clinical diagnosis of cystitis is unreliable in pregnancy. Standard obstetric practice includes screening cultures by the sixteenth week of gestation, with treatment of those who test positive for 7–10 days (see Chapter 20). Single-dose or 3-day antibiotic regimens are inadequate in pregnancy. Several antibiotics present specific risks to the fetus. Sulfonamides should be avoided for several weeks before delivery. Fluoroquinolones can result in an arthropathy. Tetracyclines cause dental problems. Aminoglycosides entail a 2–3% risk of ototoxicity. Relapse requires an additional 2–3 weeks of antibiotics, followed by suppressive therapy until delivery. Pyelonephritis in pregnancy requires hospitalization and intravenous antibiotics.

B. Nephrolithiasis. Despite a doubling of urinary calcium excretion and urinary supersaturation, stone frequency is not increased in pregnancy. Collecting system dilation might favor stone passage. However, even when clinically silent, stone disease may lead to recurrent urinary infection. Suppressive therapy with thiazide diuretics or allopurinol should be discontinued during pregnancy and urine output maintained >2.5 L/day. Ultrasound only visualizes ~60% of symptomatic stones. Single-shot, intravenous pyelography may be required if clinical suspicion is high. Most symptomatic women respond to intravenous fluids and analgesics. The remainder require urologic intervention.

C. Acute Renal Failure. Acute renal failure was a common, and often fatal, accompaniment of septic illegal abortion but is now rare. Acute tubular necrosis may complicate the concealed hemorrhage of placental abruption. It occurs in 1–2% of women with preeclampsia and in 7% of those with the *h*emolysis, *e*levated *l*iver function

TABLE 23.1.   Physiologic changes in normal pregnancy

Adaptations in pregnancy	Consequences
Increased renal perfusion and glomerular filtration rate (30–50%)	Serum creatinine >0.8 or blood urea nitrogen >13 is suspicious
Respiratory alkalosis with renal compensation	Normal P_{CO_2} ~30; normal HCO_3^- ~19–20
Retention of 8 L water, ~900 mEq Na^+, plasma volume increased ~42%	Some edema is expected; volume sensed as normal
Reset of osmotic regulation with osmolality decreased by 10 mOsm/L	Normal serum sodium ~135
Circulating renin, angiotensin, aldosterone increased, but angiotensin and aldosterone effects decreased	Difficult to diagnose secondary hypertension
Decreased blood pressure by ~10 mm Hg in healthy individuals and by 20–40 mm Hg in women with hypertension	Easy to miss underlying hypertension
Altered tubular function; increased urinary protein, glucose, uric acid, and amino acids	Proteinuria worsens with underlying glomerular disease; normal uric acid, 2.8–3.0

tests, *l*ow *p*latelets (HELLP) variant. Recognition of the normal gestational dilatation of the collecting system and ureters is key to avoiding misdiagnosis of obstructive uropathy.

D. **Chronic Renal Insufficiency.** Subtle renal insufficiency often goes unrecognized in pregnancy, as the glomerular filtration rate (GFR) is increased 30–50% even in women with advanced chronic renal insufficiency. The degree of renal insufficiency before conception and the presence of hypertension predict pregnancy outcome. More than 95% of pregnancies succeed in a live birth without adverse impact on renal disease progression in those women whose renal function is stable and well preserved (serum creatinine, 1.4 mg/dl) and in whom hypertension is absent or well controlled. Risk remains high, with preeclampsia in up to 30% of cases and worsened proteinuria in women with glomerular disease. Lower preconception GFR (serum creatinine up to 2.8) or more severe hypertension predicts severe maternal hypertension, prematurity, and fetal growth restriction and a 40% chance of more rapid progression to renal failure. Women with more severe chronic renal failure should avoid pregnancy.

Disease flares of lupus nephropathy may be difficult to differentiate from superimposed preeclampsia except by biopsy. Antiphospholipid antibodies lead to recurrent, usually mid-trimester, pregnancy loss and require low-molecular-weight heparin and aspirin.

Women with diabetic nephropathy or proteinuric renal disease should remain on angiotensin-converting enzyme inhibitors or angiotensin receptor blockers until pregnancy is confirmed, as these drugs are only contraindicated in the second and third trimesters.

Nephrotic syndrome and pregnancy are each hypercoagulable states. Prophylaxis with low-molecular-weight heparin is common. Warfarin is contraindicated during pregnancy. Hyperlipidemia is rarely treated during pregnancy because hepatic 3-hydroxy-3-methylglutaryl coenzyme A reductase inhibitors are contraindicated. Risk of bacteriuria is increased in women with nephrotic proteinuria.

When renal disease presents during pregnancy and treatment depends on a specific pathologic diagnosis, it is reasonable to perform a renal biopsy.

E. **Transplantation.** Renal transplantation restores fertility. More than 12% of women of childbearing age with renal allografts become pregnant. Pregnancy does not impair graft survival or promote rejection, although these pregnancies are often complicated by hypertension, preeclampsia, and prematurity. Outcome is predicted by renal function and hypertension. Immunosuppression with prednisone, azathioprine, and calcineurin inhibitors is acceptable. There is little experience with mycophenolate, and sirolimus is ill advised. It is difficult to distinguish preeclampsia from acute rejection or calcineurin inhibitor toxicity. Calcineurin inhibitors require dose adjustment during pregnancy. In the absence of graft dysfunction, new or worsened hypertension or proteinuria should be considered as superimposed preeclampsia. Patients should be hospitalized, observed closely, and have their BP controlled.

II. **Hypertensive Disorders in Pregnancy.** Systemic vasodilation decreases BP in normal pregnancy by ~10 mm Hg. Falls of 20–40 mm Hg are common in women with underlying hypertension and obscure the diagnosis of unsuspected hypertension. Hypertension increases the risk of maternal and neonatal morbidity and mortality. BP measurement during pregnancy depends on auscultation, as most automated devices are unreliable.

Hypertension in pregnancy is classified as gestational hypertension, preeclampsia, chronic hypertension, or preeclampsia superimposed on chronic hypertension. Gestational hypertension is a new onset of hypertension without proteinuria in the latter half of pregnancy that resolves with delivery. It often recurs in subsequent pregnancies and predicts essential hypertension later in life. The diagnosis of chronic hypertension depends on its recognition before or early in pregnancy. Gestational vasodilation usually allows discontinuation of antihypertensives early in pregnancy. Treatment is usually reinstituted if systolic BP rises to >150 or diastolic to >100, or at lower values with underlying renal disease.

Preeclampsia is a hypertensive disorder unique to pregnancy, occurring in its latter half, and accompanied by proteinuria (>300 mg/day). The onset of proteinuria may be delayed relative to the hypertension. The hypertension is due to intense systemic vasoconstriction. Preeclampsia is most common in nulliparas, at extremes of maternal age, or with multifetal gestations. Risk is genetic and is increased by maternal microvascular disease, diabetes mellitus, collagen vascular disease, underlying renal disease, and hypertension. Diagnosis is often surprisingly difficult, but, because of its risks, one should always err in favor of diagnosing preeclampsia. Target organ damage is common. Subtle laboratory evidence of multisystem involvement may aid in diagnosis. Preeclampsia is the most common cause of nephrotic syndrome in pregnancy. It is associated with decreased GFR and often with hyperuricemia. Any evidence of microangiopathy should suggest the HELLP syndrome. Epigastric or right upper quadrant tenderness, especially with liver function test abnormalities, is an ominous finding that suggests the possibility of incipient hepatic hemorrhage or rupture. Also ominous are progressive renal dysfunction or neurologic findings (including headache or blurred vision), no matter how mild. Any of these ominous findings should prompt urgent delivery.

When preeclampsia is complicated by grand mal seizures, it is termed *eclampsia*, and mortality is increased. Eclamptic seizures may be prevented or treated with magnesium sulfate, but not with classic anticonvulsants. Women are usually loaded with 4–6 g of $MgSO_4$ (over 10 minutes, not as a bolus) followed by infusion at 1–2 g/hr to achieve plasma Mg^{2+} levels of 5–9 mg/dl. Dosing is decreased in women with renal insufficiency. Toxicity can manifest as areflexia or hypoventilation and is treated with calcium gluconate.

Delivery is the definitive treatment for preeclampsia. This may be delayed in women with milder disease to gain added fetal maturation, but this should only be contemplated in a tertiary setting with close observation in the absence of ominous findings or disease progression and with careful BP control.

A. **Treatment of Hypertension during Pregnancy.** Goals of BP control are not well defined by clinical trials. The most commonly used oral antihypertensives include methyldopa, β-receptor blockers (especially labetalol), and calcium channel blockers (especially sustained-release nifedipine). Hydralazine is a second-line agent (in combination with a drug to block reflex tachycardia). Diuretics are usually avoided. Both angiotensin-converting enzyme inhibitors and angiotensin receptor blockers are contraindicated after early pregnancy due to drug-induced fetopathy and potentially lethal fetal and neonatal acute renal failure.

TABLE 24.2. Antihypertensive drugs used commonly in pregnancy

Drug	Dose	Concerns and comments
Most commonly used oral agents		
Methyl-dopa	0.5–3.0 g/day in 2–3 divided doses	Preferred agent of the NHB-PEP working group; longest experience, including study of offspring.
Labetalol	200–1,200 mg/day in 2–3 divided doses	Labetalol is preferred by NHBPEP working group as alternative to methyldopa. Beta blockers, especially atenolol, may impair fetal growth in first trimester; no specific problems noted later in pregnancy.
Nifedipine	30–120 mg/day of a slow-release preparation	Less experience with other calcium entry blockers.
Adjunctive agents		
Hydrala-zine	20–300 mg/day in 2–4 divided doses	Useful only in combination with sympatholytic agent. May cause neonatal thrombocytopenia.
Thiazide diuretics	Depends on specific agents	Few studies in hypertensive pregnancy. Can cause volume depletion and electrolyte disorders.
Agents for severe hypertension		
Hydrala-zine	5 mg IV or IM, then 5–10 mg q20–40 min or infuse 0.5–10.0 mg/h	Long experience. Higher doses or more frequent administration often precipitates fetal distress.
Labetalol	20 mg IV, then 20–80 mg q20–30 min up to 300 mg; or infusion 1–2 mg/min	Fewer adverse effects, and less blood pressure control than with hydralazine.
Nifedipine	5–10 mg PO repeat q30 min as needed, then 10–20 mg q2–4 h	Immediate-release nifedipine not approved by U.S. Food and Drug Administration for treatment of hypertension, though seems equivalent to parenteral hydralazine or labetalol.

NHBPEP, National High Blood Pressure Education Project.

Severe hypertension warrants hospitalization and often parenteral antihypertensives, including hydralazine or labetalol. Table 23.2 summarizes antihypertensives most commonly used in pregnancy.

III. Suggested Readings

Duley L, the Magpie Trial Collaborative Group. Do women with pre-eclampsia, and their babies benefit from magnesium sulphate. The Magpie Trial. A randomized placebo controlled trial. *Lancet* 2002;359:1877–1890.

Lindheimer MD, Roberts JM, Cunningham FG, eds. *Chesley's hypertensive disorders in pregnancy*. Connecticut: Appleton & Lange, 1999.

Report of the National High Blood Pressure Education Project (NHBPEP) Working Group on High Blood Pressure in Pregnancy. NIH Publication No. 00-3029. July 2000 (available in pdf format at www.nhlbi.nih.gov/health/prof/heart/hbp/hbp_preg.htm).

Umans JG. Hypertension in pregnancy. In: Brady HR, Wilcox CS, eds. *Therapy in nephrology and hypertension: companion to Brenner and Rector's the kidney*, 2nd ed. Philadelphia: WB Saunders, 2003:445–452.

Umans JG. Renal disease in pregnancy. In: Brady HR, Wilcox CS, eds. *Therapy in nephrology and hypertension: companion to Brenner and Rector's the kidney*, 2nd ed. Philadelphia: WB Saunders, 2003:453–457.

VI

Drug Use in Hypertension and Renal Disease

Diuretics

Paul S. Modlinger and Christopher S. Wilcox

Diuretics and beta blockers have been proven in placebo-controlled trials to reduce cardiovascular mortality in hypertensive patients. They have long been recommended by the Joint National Committee on Prevention, Detection, Evaluation, and Treatment of High Blood Pressure as first-line therapy for uncomplicated essential hypertension. They are inexpensive and well tolerated. Diuretics abolish all of the increased risk of stroke and more than half of the increased risk of myocardial infarction associated with hypertension. In the randomized controlled Antihypertensive and Lipid Lowering Treatment to Prevent Heart Attack Trial (ALLHAT), diuretics were as effective as or more effective than angiotensin-converting enzyme (ACE) inhibitors, calcium channel blockers, and alpha blockers at decreasing blood pressure, cardiovascular events, strokes, and congestive heart failure.

I. **Classes of Diuretics**
   A. **Proximal Tubule Diuretics.** Proximal tubule diuretics inhibit luminal and cytosolic carbonic anhydrase. This enzyme provides intracellular H^+ for luminal exchange with Na^+ that accounts for reabsorption of >65% of Na^+, bicarbonate, and water in the proximal tubule. Although 60–70% of filtered Na^+ is normally absorbed in the proximal tubule, carbonic anhydrase inhibitors (CAIs) do not induce a large loss of bodily fluids because the accompanying metabolic acidosis reduces the filtered load of bicarbonate to a level at which it can be reabsorbed by other mechanisms. Moreover, increased delivery of NaCl to the macula densa activates tubuloglomerular feedback to decrease the glomerular filtration rate (GFR).

   CAIs are used to treat diuretic resistance and metabolic alkalosis. Escalating doses of loop diuretics exacerbate metabolic alkalosis, which can cause hypoventilation, CO_2 retention, and cardiac arrhythmias. Chloride merely exacerbates the edema. Therefore, CAIs are a rational choice to add to loop diuretics in these circumstances.

   CAIs are also used to prevent high-altitude sickness and glaucoma. Monitoring is necessary to avoid volume depletion and severe metabolic acidosis. Other uncommon side effects are allergic reactions, hepatitis, blood dyscrasias, and erectile dysfunction.

   Three CAIs are in clinical practice (Table 24.1). Methazolamide is lipid soluble and is preferred for the treatment of glaucoma.

TABLE 24.1. Carbonic anhydrase inhibitors

Agent	Dose range (mg)	Dose interval	Difference between agents
Acetazolamide	250–500	b.i.d.	—
Dichlorphenamide	25–200	qd	—
Methazolamide	100–300	qd	Lipid soluble

B. Loop Diuretics

Mechanism of Action

Loop diuretics inhibit the $Na^+/K^+/2Cl^-$ cotransporter on the luminal membrane of the thick ascending limb, where 20–30% of filtered sodium is reabsorbed. They are the most powerful natriuretics and aquaretics. The $Na^+/K^+/2Cl^-$ cotransporter is also located on the macula densa cells. Therefore, loop diuretics block the tubuloglomerular feedback and are less likely than other diuretics to reduce the GFR.

Pharmacokinetics

Loop diuretics are strongly bound to albumin and are not filtered by the glomerulus. They are transported into the lumen via an organic anion transporter (OAT) located on the basolateral membrane of proximal tubule cells. A reduction in renal blood flow, or an increase in organic acids, as occurs in chronic renal insufficiency (CRI), diminishes the potency of loop diuretics, necessitating increased dosage. Protein binding is required for secretion by an OAT. Therefore, hypoalbuminemia is a cause of diuretic resistance (see Diuretic Resistance).

Clinical Uses

Loop diuretics are the drugs of choice for edema and refractory hypertension in patients with CRI. They increase the renal excretion of free water, potassium, calcium, magnesium, and hydrogen ions. Therefore, they are useful for the treatment of several commonly encountered metabolic disturbances (Table 24.2).

The four available loop diuretics differ in oral bioavailability, half-life, and metabolism (Table 24.3). None has been shown to be superior, although bumetanide and torsemide may be preferred in renal failure because they are metabolized mainly by the liver and, therefore, do not accumulate. Ethacrynic acid lacks a sulfhydryl moiety. It is a good choice for patients who become allergic to loop or thiazide diuretics. Ceiling doses are the maximal effective doses and should not normally be exceeded.

Adverse Effects

Prerenal azotemia is more common when loop diuretics are used in combination with thiazides (Table 24.4). Hypokalemia and alkalosis can be avoided by the addition of a potassium-sparing diuretic. Ototoxicity is a

TABLE 24.2. Conditions that may be treated with diuretics

Carbonic anhydrase inhibitors
  High-altitude sickness
  Glaucoma
  Metabolic alkalosis complicating diuretic resistance
Loop diuretics and thiazides
  Edematous disorders (congestive heart failure, cirrhosis, and neph-
    rotic syndrome)
  Hypertension with GFR >35 ml/min
  Hyperkalemia
  Hypermagnesemia
  Renal tubular acidosis type IV
Loop diuretics only
  Hypertension with GFR <35 ml/min
  Hypercalcemia
  Hyponatremia/syndrome of inappropriate secretion of antidiuretic
    hormone
Thiazides only
  Diabetes insipidus
  Loop diuretic resistance
  Recurrent calcium-containing nephrolithiasis
Potassium-sparing diuretics
  Diuretic-induced hypokalemic metabolic alkalosis
  Lithium-induced polyuria
Aldosterone antagonists
  Primary hyperaldosteronism
  Congestive heart failure and cirrhosis with ascites
Osmotic diuretics
  Cerebral edema

GFR, glomerular filtration rate.

risk in patients with CRI, in whom it correlates with diuretic blood levels, which relate to the dose and the rate of administration.

A randomized placebo-controlled trial in patients with ARF showed that loop diuretics increase urine output but do not affect renal recovery, death, or the need for dialysis. The authors recommend that loop diuretics be reserved for patients with oliguric or nonoliguric ARF who have volume overload.

C. **Thiazide Diuretics.** Thiazide diuretics act in the early distal convoluted tubule by blocking the luminal Na^+/Cl^- cotransporter, where 3–5% of filtered Na^+ and a significant fraction of free water are absorbed. Consequently, unlike loop diuretics, thiazides inhibit free water excretion and can cause hyponatremia, which is most commonly observed in elderly women. They also cause hypokalemia, hypomagnesemia, and metabolic alkalosis. Blockade of luminal Na^+ entry by thiazides reduces the intracellular $[Na^+]$ and thereby stimulates Na^+/Ca^{2+} counterexchange at the basolateral membrane. This increases tubular Ca^{2+} reabsorption. Thus, unlike loop diuretics, thiazide reduces Ca^{2+} excretion and may exacerbate hypercalcemia.

TABLE 24.3. Loop diuretics

Agent	Duration (h)	Equivalent oral dose (mg)	Equivalent IV dose (mg)	Metabolism	Ceiling IV dose (mg)	Infusion dose (mg/h)
Bumetanide	2–4	0.5–1.0	1	L>>K	10	0.5–1.0
Furosemide	3–6	20–40	40	K>>L	200	5–40
Ethacrynic acid	3–6	50	50	L>K	100	5–20
Torsemide	8–12	5–10	20	L>>K	100	5–20

>, is greater than; >>, is much greater than; K, kidney; L, liver.
Note: Equivalent doses are compared to 1 mg of oral bumetanide.

TABLE 24.4. Adverse effects of loop diuretics

Adverse effect	Prevention or treatment
Hypokalemia	Potassium-sparing diuretic or MCA
Hypomagnesemia	Potassium-sparing diuretic or MCA
Metabolic alkalosis	KCl, potassium-sparing diuretic, MCA, or carbonic anhydrase inhibitor
Hyperuricemia	Avoid therapy if possible; allopurinol
Impotence	Avoid therapy if possible; sildenafil
Ototoxicity	Reduce dose, avoid furosemide in chronic renal insufficiency
Prerenal azotemia	Hold diuretic, volume repletion
Hyperglycemia	Potassium-sparing diuretic or MCA
Hyperlipidemia	Statins
Allergy	Switch to ethacrynic acid
Hyponatremia	Restrict free water intake

MCA, mineralocorticosteroid antagonist.

Thiazides are drugs of first choice for uncomplicated essential hypertension. They are useful for treatment of mild edema and as adjuvants for refractory edema (see Diuretic Resistance and Table 24.2). Thiazides used alone are relatively ineffective in advanced renal insufficiency with a GFR <35 ml/min. Adverse effects include glucose intolerance (related to potassium depletion) and hyperuricemia. Commonly used thiazides are shown in Table 24.5.

D. **Potassium-Sparing Diuretics.** The cortical collecting duct reabsorbs only 3% of filtered Na^+, but it is the primary site for secretion of the positively charged ions, K^+ and H^+. Diuretics that inhibit Na^+ entry at this site reduce the negative charge in the tubular lumen and thereby inhibit the secretion of K^+ and H^+ from the cell into the tubular fluid. Amiloride and triamterene block epithelial Na^+ channels, whereas spironolactone and eplerenone are mineralocorticosteroid antagonists. Potassium-sparing diuretics are most often used to prevent or treat hypokalemic metabolic alkalosis provoked by loop or thiazide diuretics. Spironolactone is used for primary hyperaldosteronism or decompensated cirrho-

TABLE 24.5. Thiazide diuretics

Agent	Dose range (mg)	Dose interval	Duration of action (h)
Hydrochlorothiazide	12.5–50.0	qd	6–12
Chlorothiazide	500–1,000	b.i.d.	6–12
Metolazone	5–20	qd	Up to 24
Chlorthalidone	25–100	qd	Up to 72

TABLE 24.6. Distal potassium-sparing diuretics and mineralocorticosteroid antagonists (MCAs)

Agent	Dose range (mg)	Dose interval	Duration of action (h)	Other info
Amiloride	5–20	qd	Up to 24	—
Triamterene	50–100	b.i.d.	7–9	—
Spironolactone	50–100	qd	24–72	MCA
Eplerenone	50–100	qd	12–24	MCA

sis with ascites. Recent clinical trials have shown that spironolactone or eplerenone given in addition to an ACE inhibitor reduces the morbidity and mortality in patients with severe left ventricular failure.

Amiloride is excreted by the kidney in active form, whereas triamterene is partly metabolized by the liver and accumulates in patients with cirrhosis. Spironolactone is metabolized to canrenoates that are fully active over 72 hours. Side effects include hyperkalemia and metabolic acidosis, which is a special risk in patients with renal insufficiency or when spironolactone is used with other drugs that predispose to these conditions (see Chapters 16 and 17). Spironolactone has considerable antiandrogenic and pro-progestogenic actions that cause impotence, loss of libido, and painful gynecomastia in men and postmenopausal bleeding in women. These effects limit the use of spironolactone in doses >25 mg daily. Eplerenone is a new agent that does not have these adverse effects (see Chapter 26). Available agents are listed in Table 24.6.

E. **Osmotic Diuretics.** Mannitol is an osmotic diuretic that is freely filtered by the glomerulus but not reabsorbed. This provides an osmotic gradient that causes a rapid and substantial increase in the excretion of fluid, Na^+, K^+, and other ions. Mannitol is used to treat cerebral edema because it does not penetrate the blood–brain barrier. It prevents ARF in some high-risk settings, such as contrast nephropathy and rhabdomyolysis, but some trials indicate that it is no more effective than hydration alone (see Chapter 30). Side effects include hypernatremia, hyperkalemia, acidosis, and intravascular volume expansion in patients with renal failure.

II. **Diuretic Resistance.** Diuretic resistance is the inability to cause negative salt balance with conventional doses of loop diuretics. Figure 24.1 shows an algorithm for managing diuretic resistance. Causes include the following:

• *Noncompliance.* Patients must take the diuretic and adhere to a low-sodium diet (<2–3 g or 80–120 mmol/ day). Sodium intake can be quantified with a 24-hour urine even in patients on regular diuretic therapy.

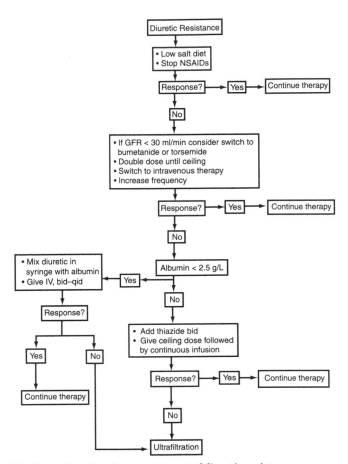

FIG. 24.1. Algorithm for management of diuretic resistance.

- *Nonsteroidal antiinflammatory drugs.* Nonsteroidal anti-inflammatory drugs block the actions of loop diuretics.
- *Inadequate absorption.* Some patients with bowel edema from decompensated congestive heart failure respond to the more bioavailable torsemide or bumetanide or to intravenous administration of a loop diuretic.
- *"Braking phenomenon."* Braking phenomenon refers to the observation that, after a day to a few weeks (depending on the degree of edema), there is a brake on progressive loss of NaCl and fluid. A new steady state is achieved when losses match intake and body weight stabilizes. Consequently, patients frequently cannot achieve an adequate loss of NaCl and fluid with a single diuretic. Diure-

sis can be increased by dosing the drug more frequently, switching to the longer-acting torsemide, adding a diuretic that acts at another site, or using a continuous intravenous infusion.

- *Tachyphylaxis.* Patients receiving loop diuretics may have decreased natriuresis due to increased tubular absorption in the distal nephron and collecting duct. This is best treated with the addition of a thiazide or a potassium-sparing diuretic.

- *Renal insufficiency.* The efficacy of diuretics is reduced in proportion to the GFR in renal insufficiency because of decreased renal blood flow, decreased functional nephron mass, and accumulation of organic anions that compete for proximal diuretic secretion via OAT. Thiazide diuretics are relatively inactive alone once the GFR is <35 ml/min. However, diuresis can be achieved with a loop diuretic even with severe renal insufficiency by doubling the dosage until the ceiling is achieved (Table 24.2), administering it several times per day, using a continuous infusion after a ceiling dose, and/or by adding a thiazide diuretic, preferably metolazone.

- *Hypoalbuminemia.* Severe hypoalbuminemia causes diuretic resistance by increasing the volume of distribution of the drug (decreased plasma protein binding), inhibiting the uptake of the drug by the proximal tubule, and promoting its metabolism within the tubular cells. Patients with the nephrotic syndrome have decreased levels of free drug in the tubular fluid because of extensive binding to albumin within the glomerular filtrate. Some have reported an increased natriuresis by premixing a loop diuretic in the syringe with salt-poor albumin, but this has not been confirmed. Cirrhotic patients respond well to a mineralocorticosteroid antagonists. Nephrotic patients should receive an ACE inhibitor or an angiotensin receptor blocker to minimize proteinuria. Extra caution is required when using diuretics in severely hypoalbuminemic patients because of the increased risk of prerenal azotemia. Albumin infusion in hypoalbuminemic patients is expensive, increases the blood volume, and very rarely promotes negative salt balance.

III. Suggested Readings

Ellison DR, Wilcox CS. Therapeutic use of diuretics. In: Brady HR, Wilcox CS, eds. *Therapy in nephrology and hypertension*, 2nd ed. Philadelphia: WB Saunders, 2003:537–545.

Wilcox CS. New insights into diuretic use in patients with chronic renal disease. *J Am Soc Nephrol* 2002;13:798–805.

Wilcox CS. Diuretics. In: Brenner BM, ed. *The kidney*, 7th ed. WB Saunders, 2004:2345–2380.

Beta Blockers, Alpha Blockers, and Sympatholytics

Paul S. Modlinger and Christopher S. Wilcox

Beta blockers and diuretics are the classes of antihypertensive agents that have been proven in placebo-controlled trials to reduce cardiovascular mortality and death in patients with hypertension. Clinical trials also demonstrate that beta blockers decrease mortality and recurrence of myocardial infarction in survivors. They are recognized as first-line pharmacologic therapy for patients with established coronary artery disease. Alpha blockers inhibit vasoconstriction of the peripheral vasculature and are considered third- or fourth-line antihypertensive agents. Central sympatholytics are among the oldest blood pressure medications. α-Methyldopa is especially useful for the treatment of hypertension in pregnancy.

I. Beta Blockers

A. Mechanism of Action.
Beta blockers antagonize the effects of the sympathetic nervous system by competing with epinephrine and norepinephrine for β_2-receptors on target organs. β_1-Receptors predominate in the heart and in the renin-containing cells of the renal afferent arteriole, whereas β_2-receptors are located primarily in bronchioles, skeletal muscle, and vascular smooth muscle. Beta blockers are nonselective when they block both subtypes and selective when they block only β_1-receptors. Both classes of beta blockers lower blood pressure by decreasing cardiac output, decreasing sympathetic outflow from the brain, and inhibiting renin release by the juxtaglomerular apparatus in the kidney. Nonselective blockers may also potentiate sympathetic-induced vasoconstriction of resistance vessels. Selective beta blockers also offer the advantage of decreased bronchospasm, which is occasionally associated with beta blockade. Some beta blockers have intrinsic sympathomimetic activity, which may help prevent bradycardia, congestive heart failure (CHF), or metabolic disturbances. Table 25.1 provides details of individual agents. Table 25.2 lists side effects commonly associated with beta blocker use. Carvedilol and labetalol are two nonselective beta blockers that also have α_1-receptor–blocking properties. Carvedilol has significant antioxidant effects. Both are often effective in African Americans and in patients with low renin hypertension. In addition, carvedilol was the first beta blocking agent to be shown to improve mortality in patients with moderate to severe CHF. These drugs are also useful in treating hypertension associated

TABLE 25.1.   Beta blockers

Agent	ISA	Half-life	IV use	Metabolism	Usual dosage GFR >50 (mg)	Maximal daily dose (mg)	Dose for GFR[a] 10–50 (mg)	<10 (mg)	Comments and special indications
Nonselective									
Nadolol	0	20–24 h	No	K	40–240 qd	320	50%	25%	Hydrophilic
Propranolol	0	3–4 h	Yes	L	40–120 b.i.d.	640	No change	No change	Lipophilic; thyrotoxicosis
Propranolol LA	0	10 h	No	L	80–240 qd	640	No change	No change	Lipophilic
Timolol	0	3–4 h	No	L>>K	10–30 b.i.d.	60	No change	No change	Lipophilic
Carteolol	++	5–6 h	No	K>L	2.5–10 qd	10	50%	25%	Hydrophilic
Penbutolol	+	5 h	No	L>>K	10–20 qd	80	No change	No change	Lipophilic
Pindolol	+++	4–5 h	No	L>K	10–30 b.i.d.	60	No change	50%	Lipophilic
Selective									
Atenolol	0	6–7 h	Yes	K	20–100 qd	100	50%	30–50%	Hydrophilic
Betaxolol	0	14–22 h	No	L>K	10–20 qd	20	No change	50%	Lipophilic
Bisoprolol	0	9–12 h	No	K = L	5–20 qd	20	75%	50%	Lipophilic = hydrophilic; CHF
Metoprolol	0	3–7 h	Yes	L	50–150 b.i.d.	450	No change	No change	Lipophilic; CHF
Acebutolol	+	7–9 h	No	K>L	400–800 qd	1,200	50%	30–50%	Lipophilic
Esmolol	0	9 min	Yes	RBCs	50–200 μg/kg/min	7.2 mg/kg	No change	No change	Hydrophilic; hypertensive emergencies

Beta/alpha								
Labetalol	0	3–4 h	Yes	L	100–600 qd	2,400	No change	No change	Lipophilic; cocaine intoxication
Carvedilol	0	7–10 h	No	L	6.25–25 b.i.d.	50	No change	No change	Lipophilic; CHF, antioxidant

CHF, congestive heart failure; ISA, intrinsic sympathomimetic activity; K, kidney; L, liver; RBCs, red blood cells.
[a]Dose for GFR indicates percentage of usual dose for patients with these levels of GFR (ml/min).

TABLE 25.2.   Adverse effects of beta blockers

Bradycardia
Hypotension
Depression
Malaise
Decreased exercise capacity
Bronchospasm
Hyperkalemia
Sexual dysfunction
Increase risk of diabetes
Increased triglycerides
Claudication
Raynaud's phenomenon

with catecholamine excess, such as cocaine intoxication or pheochromocytoma.

B. Pharmacokinetics. The various beta blockers differ widely in oral bioavailability, hepatic first-pass metabolism, and route of elimination. Agents that have significant elimination in the urine require a dose reduction in renal failure. Beta blockers that are hydrophilic may have less blood–brain barrier penetrance and, therefore, fewer central nervous system side effects. See Table 25.1 for dosage suggestions for individual agents.

C. Indications and Contraindications. Beta blockers are indicated for the treatment of hypertension, especially in patients with coronary artery disease. Table 25.3 lists the most recent prospective, randomized controlled trials comparing beta blockers to other antihypertensive agents. Beta blockers decrease perioperative myocardial infarction and mortality in patients at risk for coronary artery disease and reinfarction in those with a prior myocardial infarction. To date, three beta blocking drugs—carvedilol, bisoprolol, and metoprolol—have been shown to improve mortality in patients with moderate CHF and systolic dysfunction with an ejection fraction <40%. The protective mechanism is most likely due to a decrease in ventricular arrhythmias and protection from cardiac remodeling by the sympathetic nervous system. Carvedilol was more beneficial than metoprolol in a recent trial, which may be due to the intrinsic antioxidant properties of carvedilol. For additional diseases that may be treated with beta blockers, see Table 25.4. Nonselective beta blockers are contraindicated in patients with asthma, although patients with chronic obstructive pulmonary disease are usually tolerant of these drugs. Relative contraindications include mild conduction abnormalities, asymptomatic hypotension and/or bradycardia, decompensated CHF, and severe peripheral vascular disease.

II. Alpha Blockers. Alpha blockers antagonize the effects of the sympathetic nervous system by competing with epinephrine and norepinephrine for postsynaptic α_1-receptors on

TABLE 25.3. Major long-term trials of beta blockers for cardiovascular or renal protection

Name	Category	Number studied	Duration (yr)	Beta blocker vs. comparator	Outcome
AASK	HTN and CRI in African Americans	1,094	7	Metoprolol vs. amlodipine or ramipril	Increased incidence of composite end point (ESRD, death, or decreased GFR) with metoprolol vs. ramipril. No difference metoprolol vs. amlodipine.
CONVINCE	HTN + CV risk factors	16,602	3	Atenolol vs. verapamil or hydrochlorothiazide	No difference in first occurrence of stroke, MI, or CV-related death.
ELSA	HTN + carotid atherosclerosis	2,334	4	Atenolol vs. lacidipine	Lacidipine more effective in reversing carotid intima-media thickness. No difference in CV events.
UKPDS 39	HTN + DM	1,148	9	Atenolol vs. captopril	No difference in CV events, retinopathy, or nephropathy.
NORDIL	HTN	10,881	4.5	Beta blocker ± diuretic vs. diltiazem	Diltiazem more effective in reducing stroke.
CAPPP	HTN	10,985	6.1	Beta blocker vs. diuretic or captopril	No difference in MI, stroke, or CV-related death.
STOP-2	HTN + age >70	6,614	4.9	Beta blocker vs. diuretic, ACE-1 or calcium channel blocker	No difference in MI, stroke, or CV-related death.

AASK, African American Study of Kidney Disease and Hypertension; ACE, angiotensin-converting enzyme; CAPPP, Captopril Prevention Project; CONVINCE, Controlled Onset Verapamil Investigation of Cardiovascular Endpoints; CRI, chronic renal insufficiency; CV, cardiovascular; DM, diabetes mellitus; ELSA, European Lacidipine Study on Atherosclerosis; ESRD, end-stage renal disease; GFR, glomerular filtration rate; HTN, hypertension; MI, myocardial infarction; NORDIL, Nordic Diltiazem; STOP-2, Swedish Trial in Old Patients with Hypertension-2; UKPDS, U.K. Prospective Diabetes Study Group.

TABLE 25.4.   Diseases that may be treated with beta blockers

Migraine prophylaxis
Supraventricular tachycardia
Angina
Essential tremor
Preoperative cardiovascular protection
Congestive heart failure
Thyrotoxicosis
Vasovagal syncope
Palpitations
Hypertension

resistance vessels. The net effect is a decrease in peripheral vascular resistance. Selective α_1-blockers have no affinity for presynaptic α_2-receptors. They do not cause reflex tachycardia or increase cardiac output. Older-generation (moderately selective) alpha blockers have some affinity for the presynaptic α_1-receptors, which results in an increase in local norepinephrine release by sympathetic nerve endings. This leads to a decrease in peripheral vascular resistance but an increase in heart rate and cardiac output. Table 25.5 lists the various agents.

The selective alpha blockers are considered third- or fourth-line agents for the treatment of hypertension. The doxazosin arm of the Antihypertensive and Lipid Lowering Treatment to Prevent Heart Attack Trial (ALLHAT) was terminated prematurely due to a doubling of episodes of CHF compared with chlorthalidone. These agents are widely used to improve the obstructive symptoms of benign prostatic hypertrophy. Selective alpha blockers are associated with a profound hypotensive effect when the first dose is

TABLE 25.5.   Alpha blockers

Agent	Half-life	Metabolism	Initial dosage (mg)	Usual dosage (mg)	Dose range (mg/d)
Selective					
Doxazosin	22 h	Liver	1 qd	2–4 qd	1–16
Prazosin	2–4 h	Liver	1 b.i.d.	2–6 b.i.d.	2–30
Terazosin	12 h	Liver	1 qd	2–5 qd	1–20
Moderately selective					
Phenoxy-ben-zamine	24 h	Liver	10 b.i.d.	20–40 b.i.d. –t.i.d.	20–120
Phentola-mine	19 min	Liver	5 IV PRN	Same	—

TABLE 25.6. Alpha agonists

Agent	Half-life (h)	Metabolism	Initial dosage (mg)	Usual dosage (mg)	Daily dose range (mg)
α-Methyl-dopa	2	L>K	250 b.i.d.	250–1,000 b.i.d.	500–3,000
Cloni-dine (Cat-apres)	12	L = K	0.1 b.i.d.	0.1–0.6 b.i.d.	0.2–2.4
Catapres-TTS	12	L = K	TTS-1 is equiva-lent to 0.1 mg t.i.d.	TTS-3 is equiva-lent to 0.3 mg t.i.d.	TTS-3 qwk
Guana-benz	4–6	L	4 b.i.d.	4–16 b.i.d.	8–64
Guanfa-cine	12–24	L = K	1 qd	1–3 qd	1–3

K, kidney; L, liver.

taken. Administration of a low initial dose at nighttime while sitting or lying is recommended. All of the selective alpha blockers are associated with a decrease in triglycerides, total cholesterol, and low-density lipoprotein, with a concomitant increase in high-density lipoprotein. Moderately selective alpha blockers are used mainly for the treatment or perioperative management of pheochromocytoma in which alpha blockade precedes beta blockade to prevent paradoxical hypertension. This use may be extended to treat the hypertension associated with cocaine intoxication.

III. **Alpha Agonists**

A. **Central Sympatholytic Agents.** Alpha agonists reduce sympathetic outflow from the brain by binding to pre- and postsynaptic α_2-receptors in the midbrain and medulla. Consequently, they reduce plasma catecholamines. Alpha agonists reduce peripheral vascular resistance and heart rate without changing cardiac output. Orthostatic hypotension is unusual. Table 25.6 lists the various agents.

Common side effects of the α_2-receptor agonists include sedation, dry mouth, and depression. α-Methyldopa can cause hypersensitivity reactions, hepatitis, and a Coombs'-positive hemolytic anemia. Abrupt withdrawal from clonidine can cause a severe rebound hypertension that is accentuated by beta blockers. Clonidine is available as a skin patch (Catapres-TTS) that provides a steady drug delivery over a 1-week period. The patch is useful in noncompliant patients and in patients who cannot take medication orally. α-Methyldopa has been the most widely studied agent in pregnancy and is considered the first-line agent for pregnancy-associated hypertensive disorders. Both α-methyldopa and guanfacine carry a pregnancy category B rating from the U.S. Food and Drug Administration, whereas all other antihypertensives are considered category C or D.

B. Peripheral Sympatholytic Agents. Peripheral sympatholytic agents reduce blood pressure by depleting sympathetic nerves of catecholamines. This class includes the drugs reserpine, guanethidine, and guanadrel. They are associated with a variety of potentially severe side effects, including depression, peptic ulcer disease, fluid retention, asthma, and syncope. Reserpine may precipitate a hypertensive crisis in patients receiving monoamine oxidase inhibitors. Other effects include diarrhea and retrograde ejaculation. These agents are not frequently prescribed.

IV. Suggested Readings

Cleland JGF. Beta blockers for heart failure: why, which, when and where. *Med Clin North Am* 2003;87:339–371.

Dobbie H, Capasso G, Unwin R. Diuretics and beta-blockers. In: Brady HR, Wilcox CS, eds. *Theory in nephrology and hypertension*, 2nd ed. Philadelphia: WB Saunders, 2003:537–546.

Weir MR, Hanes DS, Klassen DK. Antihypertensive drugs. In: Brenner BM, ed. *The kidney*, 7th ed. Philadelphia: WB Saunders, 2004:2381–2452.

Angiotensin-Converting Enzyme Inhibitors, Angiotensin II Receptor Blockers, and Mineralocorticosteroid Antagonists

Wen-Ting Ouyang and Christopher S. Wilcox

I. **Renin–Angiotensin–Aldosterone System.** The renin–angiotensin–aldosterone system (RAAS) has a unique role in hypertension because angiotensin II (Ang II), acting on its type I receptors (AT_1-Rs), not only contracts blood vessels but also enhances renal salt retention. Ang II increases renal vascular resistance and the filtration fraction and increases NaCl reabsorption in the proximal tubule, loop segment, and distal nephron. Moreover, Ang II stimulates aldosterone, whose action in the collection ducts enhances Na^+ reabsorption. Ang II coordinates the body's response to salt depletion and hypotension. Accordingly, renin secretion is enhanced by salt restriction, diuretic therapy, or a decrease in blood pressure (BP) during antihypertensive therapy. An exception is beta blockers, which lower BP and inhibit renin secretion. Ang II itself inhibits renin secretion (Fig. 26.1).

Prolonged effects of Ang II on AT_1-R cause hypertrophy of the left ventricle, remodeling of blood vessels, sclerosis of glomeruli, and fibrosis of the renal interstitium. Ang II type 2 receptors (AT_2-Rs) enhance bradykinin (Bk) release that activates its type 2 receptors to generate nitric oxide and cyclic guanosine monophosphate. The actions of AT_2-Rs generally offset those of AT_1-Rs (Fig. 26.1). Ang II receptor blockers (ARBs) stimulate renin secretion and Ang II generation and thereby active AT_2-Rs.

Renin cleaves angiotensinogen to produce Ang I. Angiotensin-converting enzyme (ACE) is a carboxypeptidase that not only cleaves two amino acids from the inert Ang I to form the active Ang II, but also inactivates Bk. Therefore, ACE inhibitors diminish Ang II and enhance Bk. It is presently unclear whether there are special clinical benefits of ACE inhibitors mediated via Bk or of ARBs mediated via AT_2-R. ACE inhibitors and ARBs are equally effective antihypertensive agents.

The circulating RAAS is complemented by a tissue RAAS expressed in the heart, kidney, brain, and adrenal glands, where Ang II acts as a local autocoid.

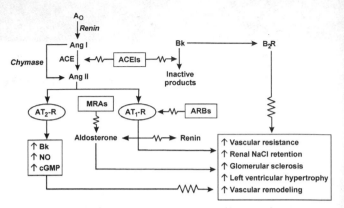

FIG. 26.1. Diagrammatic representation of the renin–angiotensin–aldosterone system and the sites of action of angiotensin-converting enzyme (ACE) inhibitors (ACEIs), angiotensin receptor blockers (ARBs), and mineralocorticosteroid receptor antagonists (MRAs). Ang, angiotensin; A_O, angiotensinogen; AT_1-R, angiotensin II type 1 receptor; AT_2-R, angiotensin II type 2 receptor; Bk, bradykinin; B_2R, bradykinin type 2 receptor; cGMP, cyclic guanosine monophosphate; NO, nitric oxide.

II. Angiotensin-Converting Enzyme Inhibitors

A. Mechanism of Action. ACE inhibitors are potent antihypertensive agents that reduce BP by peripheral vasodilation and natriuresis. Unlike some other vasodilators, such as hydralazine or minoxidil, they reset the baroreflex and do not cause tachycardia or stimulate the sympathetic nervous system. Their natriuretic actions prevent compensatory renal fluid retention. Peripheral vasodilation involves a reduction in vascular smooth muscle contraction, sympathetic tone, and aldosterone secretion. ACE inhibitors also are venodilators, which benefits patients with congestive heart failure (CHF).

B. Adverse Effects. ACE inhibitors can induce functional renal insufficiency in patients with renal artery stenosis that is bilateral or affects a single functioning kidney, or in some patients with CHF, especially those receiving excessive diuretic therapy. In these circumstances, there is an activated RAS and a compromised glomerular ultrafiltration pressure that falls further after prevention of the effects of Ang II to maintain the BP and constrict the efferent arterioles. The glomerular filtration rate (GFR) normally returns promptly after withdrawal of ACE inhibitors. ACE inhibitors do not affect the GFR of normal subjects or those with essential hypertension. The kidneys of patients with chronic renal insufficiency (CRI) generally have lost the ability to autoregulate. Therefore, any abrupt decrease in BP can reduce the GFR in the short term.

Hyperkalemia occurs in predisposed patients. CRI is not a contraindication to the use of ACE inhibitors, but the serum potassium concentration (S_K) must be monitored before and within 1 week of initiation of therapy and after an increase in ACE inhibitor dose. Concurrent use of loop diuretics and avoidance of foods with high K^+ content may obviate hyperkalemia and allow continuance of ACE inhibitor therapy.

A dry cough occurs in 10–20% and angioedema in <1%. These adverse effects likely represent kinin action. Neutropenia is a rare complication. ACE inhibitors are contraindicated in pregnancy, where they can affect fetal survival during the third trimester. ACE inhibitors do not perturb lipids and may improve carbohydrate tolerance. Indeed, they can reduce the incidence of new-onset diabetes mellitus. They do not provoke erectile dysfunction or depression and are generally well tolerated.

C. **Differences between Agents.** ACE inhibitors are structurally heterogeneous. All ACE inhibitors except captopril and lisinopril are prodrugs, which prolongs their action. Some agents are highly lipophilic and provide superior ACE inhibition in tissues, but the clinical consequences of this are not yet clear (Table 26.1). Benazepril, fosinopril, quinapril, and other lipid-soluble agents are preferred in patients on hemodialysis or with CRI, because only a small fraction of the dose is removed during dialysis, and the normal route of elimination by hepatic metabolism is preserved.

D. **Patient Selection and Drug Interactions.** Patient groups with low-renin hypertension are less responsive to monotherapy with ACE inhibitors. These include African Americans, elderly, individuals with diabetes, obese patients, and those consuming a high-salt diet. However, the addition of a diuretic stimulates the RAAS, thereby potentiating the antihypertensive effect of ACE inhibitors and permitting these patient groups to respond fully. Moreover, thiazide diuretics counteract ACE inhibitor–induced hyperkalemia, whereas ACE inhibitors counteract diuretic-induced glucose intolerance. Thus, ACE inhibitors and thiazide diuretics make an ideal, and even synergistic, combination.

Nonsteroidal antiinflammatory drugs blunt the effects of ACE inhibitors. Close biochemical monitoring is required when ACE inhibitors are used with other drugs that cause hyperkalemia, such as KCl supplements, mineralocorticosteroid receptor antagonists (MRAs), distal diuretics, trimethoprim-sulfamethoxazole, pentamidine, or heparin. Certain ACE inhibitors should not be taken with food (Table 26.1).

E. **Clinical Trials.** The results of the major controlled clinical trials with ACE inhibitors for hypertension and cardiovascular disease are shown in Table 26.2 and for progression of chronic renal failure in Table 26.3. ACE inhibitors are generally similar to diuretics in preventing

TABLE 26.1.   Angiotensin-converting enzyme inhibitors

Agent	Half-life (h)	Initial dose (mg/d)	Dosing frequency (per day)	Dose range (mg/d)	Lipophilicity	Interaction with food
Benazepril (Lotensin)	10–11	5	Once or twice	5–40	Mild	No
Captopril (Capoten)	2	25–20	Twice or three times	25–150	Little	Yes
Enalapril (Vasotec)	11	2.5–5	Once or twice	5–40	Mild	No
Fosinopril (Monopril)	12	10	Once	10–40	High	No
Lisinopril (Zestril, Prinivil)	12	5	Once	5–40	None	No
Moexipril (Univasc)	2–9	7.5	Twice	7.5–15	?Moderate	Yes
Perindopril (Aceon)	0.8–1.0	4	Once	4–16	Moderate	No
Quinapril (Accupril)	25	10	Once	5–80	Moderate	Yes
Ramipril (Altace)	13–17	2.5	Once	1.25–20	Moderate	Yes
Trandolapril (Mavik)	16–24	1	Once	1–4	Moderate	No

TABLE 26.2.   Summary of major recent controlled clinical trials in hypertension and cardiovascular disease using angiotensin-converting enzyme (ACE) inhibitors, angiotensin II receptor blockers, or mineralocorticosteroid antagonists

Study	Description, inclusion criteria, and drugs	Conclusion
ABCD (Appropriate Blood Pressure Control in Diabetes Trial) (hypertensive group + non-hypertensive subgroup)	N = 950 F/U, 5 yr Type II DM DBP <75 vs. DBP <90 Enalapril vs. nisoldipine	Enalapril was better than nisoldipine at reducing MI.
ALLHAT (Antihypertensive and Lipid Lowering Treatment to Prevent Heart Attack Trial)	N = 42,000 F/U, 5 yr Hypertension and 1 coronary risk factor Chlorthalidone vs. lisinopril vs. amlodipine vs. doxazosin	Diuretics were most effective in reducing CVA and CHF. Doxazosin had higher rate of CHF and complications.
ANBP2 (Second Australian National Blood Pressure Study)	N = 6,083 F/U, 5 yr Hypertensives and older patients Enalapril vs. diuretic	Compared to diuretics, ACE inhibitors reduced CV events or death by 17%. Biggest effect in men.
CAPP (Captopril Prevention Project)	N = 10,985 F/U, 6 yr Hypertension Captopril vs. beta blocker or diuretic	Captopril and conventional therapy did not differ in efficacy in preventing CV mortality. There was a slight increase in stroke risk in the captopril group, which is probably related to higher BP.
EPHASUS (Eplerenone Post-AMI Heart Failure Efficacy and Survival Study)	N = 6,632 F/U, 16 mo MI + CHF or systolic dysfunction	Eplerenone reduced mortality by 15% and CV mortality by 17%.

(continued)

TABLE 26.2. (continued)

Study	Description, inclusion criteria, and drugs	Conclusion
HOPE (Heart Outcomes Prevention Evaluation)	Eplerenone vs. placebo N = 9,297 F/U, 4 yr DM, 3,496 Hypertension and ≥1 CVD risk factors Ramipril vs. placebo	Ramipril reduced composite end point of MI, CVA, and CV mortality by 25% and development of diabetic nephropathy by 24%.
LIFE (Losartan Intervention for Endpoint Reduction in Hypertension)	N = 8,300 F/U, 4 yr Isolated systolic hypertension with LVH Losartan vs. atenolol	Compared to atenolol, losartan reduced composite end point of stroke and MI by 25%.
QUIET (Quinapril Ischemic Event Trial)	N = 6,175 F/U, 2 yr CAD Quinapril vs. placebo	No evidence that quinapril has antiatherosclerotic effect in CAD.
PROGRESS (Perindopril Protection Against Recurrent Stroke Study)	N = 6,105 F/U, 4 yr History of TIA or stroke in hypertensives and nonhypertensives Perindopril ± indapamide vs. placebo	Perindopril reduced stroke incidence and recurrence, even in nonhypertensives.
RALES (Randomized Aldactone Evaluation Study)	N = 1,663 F/U, 2 yr Classes III and VI heart failure Spironolactone vs. placebo	Spironolactone reduced nonfatal hospitalizations and total mortality by 22%.

STOP-2 (Swedish Trial in Older Patients with Hypertension-2)	N = 6,614 F/U, 5 yr Hypertension in elderly ACE inhibitor vs. CCB vs. beta blocker	Old and new antihypertensives had similar outcomes. CV events were related to BP lowering rather than to class.
UKPDS-HDS (U.K. Prospective Diabetes Study–Hypertension in Diabetic Study)	N = 1,148 F/U, 4 yr DM type II Captopril vs. atenolol	Complications of DM and new events related to achieved BP, not to class of agent used.

BP, blood pressure; CAD, coronary artery disease; CCB, calcium channel blocker; CHF, congestive heart failure; CV, cardiovascular; CVA, cerebrovascular accident; CVD, cardiovascular disease; DBP, diastolic blood pressure; DM, diabetes mellitus; F/U, follow-up period; LVH, left ventricular hypertrophy; MI, myocardial infarction; TIA, transient ischemic attack.

Note: For further details, see Brady HR, Wilcox CS, eds. *Therapy in nephrology and hypertension.* 2nd ed. Philadelphia: WB Saunders, 2003:415–422.

TABLE 26.3.   Summary of major recent controlled clinical trials in prevention of progressive kidney disease using angiotensin-converting enzyme inhibitors or angiotensin II receptor blockers

Study	Description, inclusion criteria, and drugs	Conclusion
AASK (African American Study of Kidney Disease and Hypertension)	N = 1,150 F/U, 5 years African Americans with hypertension and nephrosclerosis Ramipril vs. amlodipine vs. metoprolol vs. others	No benefit of lower BP goal. No difference between angiotensin-converting enzyme inhibitor and beta blocker, but CCB was less effective. Adequate BP goal can be achieved.
AI PRI (Angiotensin-Converting Enzyme Inhibition to Prevent Renal Insufficiency)	N = 583 F/U, 3 yr Chronic renal insufficiency Benazepril vs. placebo	Benazepril reduced the risk of doubling of S_{cr} or need for dialysis by 53%.
COOPERATE SCOPE (Combination Treatment of Angiotensin-II Receptor Blocker and Angiotensin-Converting Enzyme Inhibitor in Nondiabetic Renal Disease)	N = 263 F/U, 3 yr Nondiabetic proteinuric nephropathies Trandolapril vs. losartan vs. halved doses of both drugs in combination	Risk of doubling S_{cr} or ESRD reduced from 23% with losartan or 23% with trandolapril to 11% with combined treatment.
The Collaborative Study Group	N = 409 F/U, 3 yr DM type I with nephropathy Captopril vs. placebo	Captopril reduced the risk of doubling of S_{cr} by 48%.
IDNT (Irbesartan Diabetic Nephropathy Trial)	N = 1,715 F/U, 2.6 yr DM type II with nephropathy Irbesartan vs. amlodipine vs. placebo	Irbesartan reduced the risk of doubling S_{cr} by 23% and of ESRD by 37%.

Study	Details	Results
IRMA (Irbesartan in Type 2 Diabetes and Microalbuminuria Study)	N = 590 F/U, 2 yr Hypertension and DM type II with microalbuminuria Irbesartan vs. placebo	Progress from microalbuminuria to overt proteinuria reduced to 5% with irbesartan, 300 mg, compared to 10% with 150 mg, and to 15% in the placebo group.
RENAAL (Reduction of Endpoint in NIDDM with Angiotensin II Antagonist Losartan)	N = 1,513 F/U, 4.5 yr DM type II with nephropathy Losartan vs. placebo	Losartan reduced the risk of doubling of S_{cr} by 25% and of ESRD to 28%.
REIN (Ramipril Efficacy in Nephropathy)	N = 352 F/U, 2.6 yr Nondiabetic nephropathy with proteinuria of 1–2.9 g vs. >3 g/24-h and chronic renal insufficiency S_{cr} = 3 vs. 2 vs. 1.5 mg·dl^{-1} Ramipril vs. placebo + conventional antihypertensive therapy	GFR reduced to 0.53 ml/min/mo in ramipril group vs. 0.88 ml/min/mo in placebo. ESRD reduced by 33% in ramipril group.

BP, blood pressure; DM, diabetes mellitus; ESRD, end-stage renal disease; F/U, follow-up period; GFR, glomerular filtration rate; NIDDM, non-insulin-dependent diabetes mellitus; S_{cr}, serum creatinine.

Note: For further details, see Brady HR, Wilcox CS, eds. *Therapy in nephrology and hypertension*, 2nd ed. Philadelphia: WB Saunders, 2003:415–422.

cardiovascular disease in patients with essential or systolic hypertension [Antihypertensive and Lipid Lowering Treatment to Prevent Heart Attack Trial (ALLHAT), Second Australian National Blood Pressure Study (ANBP2), Captopril Prevention Project (CAPP), and Swedish Trial in Older Patients with Hypertension-2 (STOP-2)] but are more effective in those with associated risk factors [Heart Outcomes Prevention Evaluation (HOPE)]. ACE inhibitors reduce stroke incidence and recurrence, even in normotensives [Perindopril Protection Against Recurrent Stroke Study (PROGRESS)], and are as effective as other antihypertensives in preventing complications in patients with diabetes mellitus [U.K. Prospective Diabetes Study–Hypertension in Diabetic Study (UKPDS-HDS)]. ACE inhibitors are more effective than equivalent antihypertensive therapy in preventing progression of renal disease in patients with proteinuria >1 g/d [Effects of ACE Inhibitors in Diabetic Nephropathy, Ramipril Efficacy in Nephropathy (REIN)], but not in those with nephrosclerosis and low-grade proteinuria [African American Study of Kidney Disease and Hypertension (AASK)]: ACE inhibitors are of established benefit in preventing recurrent MI and prolonging life expectancy in moderate or severe CHF, even in the absence of hypertension. Therefore, ACE inhibitors are preferred agents for patients with CRI and proteinuria >1 g/d, and for those with a myocardial infarction or CHF, and they are also an excellent choice for patients with essential hypertension, especially those with associated cardiovascular risk factors.

III. **Angiotensin II Receptor Blockers.** ARBs bind selectively to AT_1-R, where they are competitive or insurmountable antagonists. They block all the primary action of Ang II.

    A. **Actions, Uses, Interactions, and Adverse Effects.** ARBs' major effects and uses are similar to those of ACE inhibitors. However, ARBs do not stimulate kinins and therefore do not cause a dry cough or angioedema. Consequently, they have an even lower profile of adverse effects. Some ARBs are prodrugs. They have variable bioavailability (Table 26.4). Losartan is the only uricosuric ARB.

    B. **Clinical Trials.** Results of controlled clinical trials have shown that ARBs are superior to beta blockers in the prevention of stroke in hypertensive patients [Losartan Intervention for Endpoint Reduction in Hypertension (LIFE)] (Table 26.2) and superior to equivalent antihypertensive therapy in reducing proteinuria and progression of nephropathy due to diabetes mellitus type 2 [Irbesartan Diabetic Nephropathy Trial (IDNT), Irbesartan in Type 2 Diabetes and Microalbuminuria Study (IRMA), and Reduction of Endpoint in NIDDM with Angiotensin II Antagonist Losartan (RENAAL)]. Therefore, they are excellent choices in those conditions.

IV. **Natriuretic Peptides.** Atrial natriuretic peptide and brain natriuretic peptide are secreted during volume expansion and

TABLE 26.4. Angiotensin receptor blockers

Agent	Half-life (h)	Initial daily dose (mg)	Dosing frequency (per day)	Dose range (mg/d)	Predominant elimination	Active metabolites	Interaction with food
Candesartan (Atacand)	7^a (4–11)	8–16	Once	8–32	B	Y	N
Eprosartan (Teveten)	7 (5–9)	600	Twice	400–800	B	N	N
Irbesartan (Avapro)	13 (11–15)	150	Once	150–300	B	N	N
Losartan (Cozaar)	2^a (6–9)	25	Once or twice	25–100	B	Y	Y
Olmesartan (Benicar)	13^a	20	Once	20–40	B & R	Y	?
Telmisartan (Micardis)	24	20–40	Once	40–80	B	Y	N
Valsartan (Diovan)	9	80	Once	80–320	B	N	Y

B, biliary; N, no; R, renal; Y, yes.
[a]Effective half-life prolonged by active metabolites.

cardiac pressure overload. These peptides are natriuretic, inhibit renin secretion, lower BP, and generally oppose the actions of Ang II and aldosterone. They are degraded by neutral endopeptidase. Omapatrilat inhibits both ACE and neutral endopeptidase. It reduces BP in both high- and low-renin hypertension and is a mild diuretic. It shares the adverse effects of ACE inhibitors.

V. **Mineralocorticosteroid Receptor Antagonists.** Aldosterone activates the cortical and medullary collecting duct epithelial Na^+ entry channels and the Na^+/K^+-ATPase on the basolateral cell membrane. The ensuing increase in cellular Na^+ uptake enhances the negative charge across the luminal cell membrane, thereby enhancing tubular secretion of the positively charged K^+ and H^+ ions. Aldosterone secretion is enhanced by activation of the AT_1-R. Therefore, it is increased in patients with salt restriction, renovascular hypertension, CHF, and advanced cirrhosis with ascites and in those taking diuretics, and is inhibited by ACE inhibitors and ARBs. Aldosterone secretion also is enhanced by hyperkalemia and metabolic acidosis, which account for elevated levels in patients with renal failure. The highest levels are found in patients with primary hyperaldosteronism (see Chapter 22).

MRAs enhance renal Na^+ loss, but the effect may take several days to become apparent. The blockade of distal K^+ and H^+ secretion increases S_K and causes a metabolic acidosis. These effects are used to advantage when MRAs are combined with loop or thiazide diuretics to prevent hypokalemic metabolic alkalosis and the associated magnesium depletion. Aldosterone also contributes to vasoconstriction, vascular inflammation, endothelial dysfunction, myocardial and renal fibrosis, and left ventricular hypertrophy.

MRAs added to conventional therapy, including ACE inhibitors, reduce hospitalization and prolong life in patients with CHF [Randomized Aldactone Evaluation Study (RALES), Eplerenone Post-AMI Heart Failure Efficacy and Survival Study (EPHASUS)]. Therefore, they should be added to ACE inhibitors in patients with CHF, unless there is a contraindication.

Spironolactone (Aldactone) blocks the nuclear (genomic) MR. It is the preferred drug for medical management of primary hyperaldosteronism (see Chapter 22). It is particularly useful in patients with uncompensated edema due to advanced cirrhosis and ascites, or CHF in which hypokalemia and alkalosis complicate diuretic therapy. It is also effective in essential hypertension, but this is limited by adverse effects.

Spironolactone is well absorbed. It is metabolized to canrenoates that are fully active and have a long half-life of 16.5 hours. It should be given only once daily.

Some side effects are predictable—for example, hyperkalemia and metabolic acidosis, which preclude its use in any patients with even a borderline elevation of S_K. Additionally, it has pronounced, dose-dependent antiandrogenic and pro-progestogenic effects that cause loss of libido, impotence, and painful gynecomastia in men, and menstrual irregularities and postmenopausal bleeding in women. Wherever possible, the dose should be limited to 12.5–25.0 mg daily to obviate these adverse effects.

Eplerenone (Inspra) is a novel MRA without antiandrogenic or pro-progestogenic actions. It is much better tolerated than spironolactone. It is cleared by hepatic metabolism with a half-life of 4–6 hours. The effective daily dose range is 25–100 mg. It is an effective antihypertensive agent.

VI. Renin Inhibitors. Renin inhibitors block the binding of renin substrate (angiotensinogen) to renin (Fig. 26.1). Zankiren, remikiren, ciprokiren, and A-74273 are currently under investigation.

VII. Suggested Readings

American Society of Hypertension. Completed and ongoing trials included within the BP Trialists' Collaboration. Available at: http://www.ash-us.org/about_hypertension/trialslist.htm. Accessed April 23, 2004.

Brady HR, Wilcox CS, eds. *Therapy in nephrology and hypertension*, 2nd ed. Philadelphia: WB Saunders, 2003:415–422.

Hostetter TH, Ibrahim HN. Aldosterone in chronic kidney and cardiac disease. *J Am Soc Nephrol* 2003;14:2395–2401.

Turnball F. Effects of different blood-pressure-lowering regimens on major cardiovascular events: results of prospectively designed overview of randomized trials. *Lancet* 2003;362:1527–1535.

Calcium Channel Blockers and Other Vasodilators

Oscar Adler and Christopher S. Wilcox

I. Calcium Channel Blockers

A. Mechanism of Action. Calcium channel blockers (CCBs) block the influx of Ca^{2+} into vascular smooth muscle cells (VSMCs) via voltage-gate, L-type calcium channels. The ensuing fall in intracellular $[Ca^{2+}]$ causes relaxation that dilates coronary arteries and decreases peripheral vascular resistance. CCBs release nitric oxide from the vascular endothelium, which augments the relaxation of VSMCs. They reduce basal vascular tone and the reactivity to adrenergic stimulation, angiotensin II, and endothelin. In the kidneys, they are weak inhibitors of distal NaCl reabsorption, but powerful dilators of the afferent arteriole. The efferent arteriole does not contain L-type Ca^{2+} channels and is unresponsive to CCBs.

B. Classification and Differences between Calcium Channel Blockers. CCBs can be divided into *nondihydropyridines* (verapamil and diltiazem) and *dihydropyridines* (the remainder). Dihydropyridines block L-type Ca^{2+} channels in VSMCs quite selectively, whereas nondihydropyridines also block L-type Ca^{2+} channels in cardiac tissue and therefore depress conduction through the atrioventricular node and reduce cardiac rate and contractility. All agents lower blood pressure similarly, and all except the relatively short-acting isradipine and nimodipine are available in a formulation that permits effective once-daily dosing for hypertension (Table 27.1).

C. Metabolism and Elimination. CCBs undergo oxidative biotransformation, predominantly via cytochrome P450 CYP 3A in the liver. The absence of significant renal clearance prevents accumulation, or the need for major dosage modifications, in renal insufficiency.

D. Drug Interactions. Verapamil and diltiazem inhibit the metabolic clearance of other drugs that are substrates for hepatic cytochrome P450 CYP 3A, whereas dihydropyridines generally do not (Table 27.2). Additionally, verapamil and diltiazem inhibit P-glycoprotein–mediated drug transport. This may delay the intestinal absorption of drugs and their distribution into the central nervous system.

Both verapamil and diltiazem delay the metabolic clearance of cyclosporine, necessitating a reduction in its dosage. Cimetidine, sulfinpyrazone, rifampin, phenytoin, and ketoconazole reduce the metabolic clearance

TABLE 27.1. Calcium channel blockers

Drug	Daily dose (mg)	Dosing frequency (per day)	Time to peak (h)	Elimination half-life (h)
Amlodipine	2.5–10.0	Daily	6–12	30–50
Diltiazem SR	180–480	Daily	6–11	2–5
Felodipine	2.5–10.0	Daily	2.5–5.0	11–16
Isradipine	2.5–10.0	Twice daily	1–5	8–12
Nicardipine SR	60–120	Daily	1–4	8
Nifedipine SR	30–120	Daily	6	2
Nimodipine	60	Each 4 h	1	1–2
Nisoldipine SR	20–40	Daily	6–12	7–12
Verapamil SR	120–480	Daily	4–6	4.5–12.0

of CCBs. They can thereby cause bradyarrhythmias when administered with verapamil or diltiazem.

E. Use for Hypertension, Renal Disease, and Cardiovascular Protection. Thiazide diuretics and long-acting CCBs are especially effective antihypertensives in low-renin hypertension, which is common in African Americans, the elderly, obese patients, diabetics, and those with renal insufficiency. Large, placebo-controlled trials of CCBs in hypertension are not available. However, when compared with standard diuretic or beta blocker therapy in primary hypertension, CCBs were as effective as standard therapy in preventing cardiovascular events or

TABLE 27.2. Interactions between calcium channel blockers and other drugs

Calcium channel blocker and drug affected	Clinical effect
Bepridil, verapamil:	
Digoxin	Digoxin toxicity
Diltiazem, verapamil:	
Carbamazepine	Neurotoxicity
Antihistamines:	
Astemizole	Prolonged QT interval
Terfenadine	Torsade de pointes
Cisapride	Torsade de pointes
Quinidine	Torsade de pointes
HMG-CoA reductase inhibitors:	
Atorvastatin, lovastatin, simvastatin	Myopathy, rhabdomyolysis
Immunosuppressive drugs:	
Cyclosporine, tacrolimus	Nephrotoxicity
Beta blockers	Bradyarrhythmias
Theophylline	Theophylline toxicity

HMG-CoA, hydroxymethylglutaryl-coenzyme A.

strokes, or both, in the Nordic Diltiazem (NORDIL), International Nifedipine GITS (INSIGHT), Systolic Hypertension in the Elderly Long-Term Lacidipine (SHELL), Swedish Trial in Old Patients with Hypertension-2 (STOP-2), and Controlled Onset Verapamil Investigation of Cardiovascular End Points (CONVINCE) trials but slightly less effective in the Antihypertensive and Lipid-Lowering Treatment to Prevent Heart Attack Trial (ALL-HAT) and Systolic Hypertension in Europe (Syst-Eur) trial in hypertension, or the Appropriate Blood Pressure Control in Diabetes (ABCD) trial in type II diabetes mellitus (Table 27.3). A CCB was more effective than a beta blocker or diuretic in reducing or reversing arterial remodeling in the European Lacidipine Study on Atherosclerosis (ELSA) and Verapamil in Hypertension and Atherosclerosis Study (VHAS) trials of hypertension compared to placebo. A CCB reduced hospitalizations in patients with congestive heart failure in the Prospective Randomized Evaluation of the Vascular Effects of Norvasc Trial (PREVENT) and reduced revascularizations after percutaneous transluminal coronary angioplasty in the Nisoldipine in Coronary Artery Disease in Leuven (NICOLE) trial. Metaanalysis suggests that there is little difference between classes of drugs in prevention of cardiovascular disease in patients with essential hypertension. Greater reduction in blood pressure is associated with greater reduction in cardiovascular risk. Subgroup analysis shows that CCBs may be somewhat less effective in preventing heart failure but somewhat more effective in preventing stroke.

Proteinuria is little changed by dihydropyridines but is reduced by nondihydropyridines. An angiotensin-converting enzyme inhibitor (ACEI) given with a non-dihydropyridine CCB reduces proteinuria more than either agent alone. The African American Study of Kidney Disease and Hypertension (AASK) reported that an ACEI or a beta blocker is more effective than amlodipine in preventing the slow but progressive fall in glomerular filtration rate in African Americans with hypertension and nephrosclerosis (Table 27.3). The Irbesartan Diabetic Nephropathy Trial (IDNT) reported that an angiotension receptor blocker is more effective than amlodipine in preventing the more rapid fall in glomerular filtration rate in patients with nephropathy from type II diabetes mellitus (Table 27.3). Therefore, dihydropyridine CCBs should not be used as primary therapy to prevent progression of chronic renal insufficiency.

A long-acting CCB and an ACEI are excellent first-line antihypertensives in renal transplant recipients because CCBs alleviate the renal afferent arteriolar vasoconstriction caused by cyclosporine. CCBs are indicated in hypertensives with angina pectoris or Raynaud's phenomenon. They are effective antihypertensives in patients with chronic renal insufficiency and are used frequently in

TABLE 27.3. Major long-term trials of calcium channel blockers (CCBs) for cardiovascular or renal protection

Name	Category	Number studied	Duration (yr)	CCB vs. comparator	Outcome
AASK	HTN + nephrosclerosis in African Americans	1,094	7	Amlodipine vs. metoprolol or ramipril	1.6-fold increased incidence with CCB vs. ACEI for composite end point of decreased glomerular filtration rate, ESRD, or death.
ABCD	HTN + DM type II	470	5	Nisoldipine vs. enalapril	CCB increased incidence of myocardial infarction.
ALLHAT	HTN + CVD risk factors	42,488	6	Amlodipine vs. chlorthalidone	Diuretic had better outcome for CHF.
CONVINCE	HTN + CVD risk factors	16,602	3	Verapamil vs. HCTZ or atenolol	CV events similar with all therapies.
ELSA	HTN + carotid atherosclerosis	2,334	4	Lacidipine vs. atenolol	CCB more effective in reversing carotid intima-media thickness.
IDNT	HTN + DM type II + chronic renal insufficiency	1,715	2.6	Amlodipine vs. irbesartan	Irbesartan 23% more effective in preventing composite end point of doubling of serum creatinine, ESRD, or death.
INSIGHT	HTN + CVD risk factor	6,321	3–5	Nifedipine SR vs. HCTZ + amiloride	Similar CV events and stroke.
JMIC-B	HTN + CHD	1,650	3	ACEI vs. nifedipine	Similar CV events.
NICOLE	CHD	826	3	Nisoldipine vs. placebo	CCB reduced number of revascularizations after PTCA.
NORDIL	Diastolic HTN in aged	10,881	4.5	Diltiazem SR vs. thiazide ± beta blocker	CCB reduced risk of stroke.

(continued)

TABLE 27.3. (continued)

Name	Category	Number studied	Duration (yr)	CCB vs. comparator	Outcome
PREVENT	CHD	825	3	Amlodipine vs. placebo	CCB had fewer hospitalizations.
SHELL	Systolic HTN in aged	1,882	3.6	Lacidipine vs. chlorthalidone	Both therapies had similar CV events.
STOP-2	HTN in aged	4,409	5	Felodipine or isradipine vs. atenolol or metoprolol	Therapies had similar CV mortality.
Syst-EUR	Systolic HTN in aged	4,695	5	Nitrendipine ± enalapril ± HCTZ vs. placebo	Reduction in stroke with active drugs. HCTZ slightly superior.
VHAS	HTN	1,414	2	Verapamil vs. chlorthalidone	CCB had better regression in carotid intima-media thickness.

AASK, African American Study of Kidney Disease and Hypertension; ABCD, Appropriate Blood Pressure Control in Diabetes; ACEI, angiotensin-converting enzyme inhibitor; ALLHAT, Antihypertensive and Lipid-Lowering Treatment to Prevent Heart Attack Trial; CHD, congestive heart disease; CHF, congestive heart failure; CONVINCE, Controlled Onset Verapamil Investigation of Cardiovascular End Points; CV, cardiovascular; DM, diabetes mellitus; ELSA, European Lacidipine Study on Atherosclerosis; ESRD, end-stage renal disease; HCTZ, hydrochlorothiazide; HTN, hypertension; IDNT, Irbesartan Diabetic Nephropathy Trial; INSIGHT, International Nifedipine GITS study; JMIC-B, Japan Multicenter Investigation for Cardiovascular Diseases-B; NICOLE, Nisoldipine in Coronary Artery Disease in Leuven; NORDIL, Nordic Diltiazem study; PREVENT, Prospective Randomized Evaluation of the Vascular Effects of Norvasc Trial; PTCA, percutaneous transluminal coronary angioplasty; SHELL, Systolic Hypertension in the Elderly Long-Term Lacidipine; SR, sustained release; STOP-2, Swedish Trial in Old Patients with Hypertension-2; Syst-Eur, Systolic Hypertension in Europe study; VHAS, Verapamil in Hypertension and Atherosclerosis Study.
For details of trials, see Dworkin LD, Shemin DG. Calcium channel blockers. In: Brady HR, Wilcox CS, eds. *Therapy in nephrology and hypertension*, 2nd ed. Philadelphia: WB Saunders, 2003:555–564.

those with end-stage renal disease. They are not removed by dialysis.

CCBs are very helpful as third-line antihypertensives in patients receiving a diuretic and an ACEI or an adrenergic receptor blocker to achieve the low-blood-pressure goal recommended to delay the progression of renal insufficiency in patients with diabetic nephropathy and other causes of high-grade proteinuria (see Chapter 32). Nondihydropyridines slow the ventricular rate in patients with atrial fibrillation.

F. **Adverse Effects.** CCBs are generally very well tolerated. Nondihydropyridines can cause bradyarrhythmias, and any CCBs may worsen congestive heart failure. They can cause constipation and headache. Dihydropyridines cause dose-dependent edema by redistribution of plasma fluid into the interstitium because of arteriolar vasodilatation. The edema is relatively resistant to diuretics but is reduced by ACEI therapy. Dihydropyridines activate the sympathetic nervous system. Therefore, they are best used in combination with beta blockers to treat patients with myocardial ischemia and angina.

II. **Other Vasodilators.** Hydralazine and minoxidil are direct-acting arteriolar vasodilators. Minoxidil opens potassium channels on VSMCs. The ensuing hyperpolarization closes voltage-gated Ca^{2+} channels, thereby reducing intracellular $[Ca^{2+}]$ and causing vasorelaxation.

These agents are effective antihypertensives. However, long-term therapy is limited by tachyphylaxis and a spectrum of adverse effects. Both agents lead to reflex activation of the sympathetic nervous system that can worsen angina pectoris and myocardial ischemia and cause tachyarrhythmias. They also cause renal salt and fluid retention, leading to edema or worsening of congestive heart failure. Headache is frequent. Hydralazine can cause a lupuslike syndrome. Minoxidil can cause carbohydrate intolerance, hirsutism, and pericardial effusions that occasionally cause cardiac tamponade.

Hydralazine is used in patients who are resistant to α-methyldopa to control pregnancy-associated hypertension (see Chapter 23). Minoxidil is used as a short-term treatment in severe, drug-resistant hypertension, especially in those with renal insufficiency (see Chapter 29). Both agents usually require coadministration of a beta blocker to prevent reflex tachycardia and a diuretic to prevent fluid retention. Neither agent should be used for long-term therapy.

III. **Suggested Readings**

Abernethy DR, Schwartz JB. Drug therapy: calcium-antagonist drugs. *N Engl J Med* 1999;341:1447–1457.

August P. Initial treatment of hypertension. *N Engl J Med* 2003;348:610–617.

Dworkin LD, Shemin DG. Calcium channel blockers. In: Brady HR, Wilcox CS, eds. *Therapy in nephrology and hypertension*, 2nd ed. Philadelphia: WB Saunders, 2003: 555–564.

Muntwyler J, Follath F. Calcium channel blockers in treatment of hypertension. *Prog Cardiovasc Dis* 2001;44:207–216.

Sica DA. Current concepts of pharmacotherapy in hypertension: combination calcium channel blocker therapy in the treatment of hypertension. *J Clin Hyperten* 2001;3:322–327.

White WB. Clinical trial experience around the globe: focus on calcium-channel blockers. *Clin Cardiol* 2003;26[Suppl 2]:II7–II11.

Urgent, Emergent, and Resistant Hypertension

Chagriya Kitiyakara and Christopher S. Wilcox

I. **Definitions.** A *hypertensive crisis* is the point at which the management of an acutely elevated blood pressure (BP) is decisive in the outcome. The level of BP is less important than the extent of end-organ damage. *Hypertensive urgency* denotes a sudden rise in BP without an acute deterioration in the function of a critical organ. Typically, the BP can be lowered in the ward or clinic with oral antihypertensive agents over a few hours or days. *Hypertensive emergency* denotes a sudden rise in BP with an acute deterioration in function of a critical target organ. The BP should be lowered (not necessarily to the normal range) in minutes under close monitoring in an intensive care unit. Clinical disorders that meet the criteria for hypertensive urgencies and emergencies are shown in Tables 28.1 and 28.2. *Severe hypertension* denotes a BP >160/110 mm Hg, but the patient is asymptomatic, the rise in BP is gradual, and there are no retinal hemorrhages or papilledema. Severe hypertension can be treated in the clinic under close supervision. *Resistant hypertension* denotes a failure to reach goal BP despite adhering to appropriate doses of a three-drug regimen that includes a diuretic.

II. **Hypertensive Emergencies and Urgencies**

   A. **Epidemiology, Etiology, and Pathogenesis.** A crisis occurs in less than 1% of all hypertensives. Smokers and African Americans are at increased risk. Essential hypertension and all secondary forms can give rise to a hypertensive crisis. Many patients have renal parenchymal or renovascular disease.

   The pathophysiology of a hypertensive emergency remains incompletely understood. An abrupt rise in vascular resistance and activation of the renin-angiotensin-aldosterone (RAA) system are key features. Other circulating factors and cytokines reinforce the vasoconstriction and vascular damage. Endothelial damage from a severe and abrupt elevation in BP decreases autoregulatory responses and promotes vasoconstriction. Renal ischemia, pressure-induced injury, and volume depletion due to pressure natriuresis further activate the RAA system. A vicious cycle can develop when hypertension causes endothelial damage, fibrinoid necrosis, vascular obstruction from platelets and fibrin deposition, and renal ischemia that activate the RAA system, which promotes further hypertension.

   Autoregulation of renal and cerebral vessels normally maintains a stable blood flow during variations of mean

TABLE 28.1.   Hypertensive emergencies and initial parenteral treatment with preferred drug(s)

Hypertensive emergency	Preferred drugs (alternatives)	Contraindication
Hypertensive encephalo-pathy	SNP, LAB, FEN	Clonidine
HTN with intracranial hemorrhage	SNP, LAB, FEN	Clonidine
HTN with ischemic stroke	LAB, SNP, FEN	—
HTN with myocardial ischemia	NTG, BB, LAB	HYD
HTN with pulmonary edema	NTG, loop diuretic	BB
Dissecting aortic aneurysm	BB, verapamil, SNP[a]	HYD
Eclampsia	HYD, LAB, nicardipine	Angiotensin-converting enzyme inhibitor, angiotensin II receptor blocker
Perioperative HTN	SNP, nicardipine, NTG, LAB, BB	—
Adrenergic crisis	Phentolamine, LAB, SNP, FEN	BB

BB, β-adrenergic blocker; FEN, fenoldopam; HTN, hypertension; HYD, hydralazine; LAB, labetalol; NTG, nitroglycerine; SNP, sodium nitroprusside.
[a]SNP should be added only after complete β-adrenergic blockade is achieved.

arterial pressure (MAP) within the physiologic range of approximately 70–120 mm Hg. If the MAP abruptly exceeds this limit of autoregulation, capillary pressures and flows increase. In the brain, this leads to capillary hypertension, hyperemia, disruption of the blood–brain barrier, cerebral swelling, necrosis, and microhemorrhage. In the kidney, there is patchy ischemia and necrosis in glomerular capillaries, leading to the escape of red blood cells into tubular fluid, the appearance of red blood cell casts, and generalized capillary hypertension leading to proteinuria. Patients with long-standing hypertension develop a compensatory vascular hypertrophy and a shift in the

TABLE 28.2.   Hypertensive urgencies

Malignant HTN
HTN with angina
HTN with left ventricular failure
Acute glomerulonephritis
Scleroderma renal crisis
Preeclampsia

HTN, hypertension.

autoregulation curve toward higher levels of MAP. This provides protection from hypertensive encephalopathy even when the BP exceeds 220/110 mm Hg. By contrast, cerebral autoregulation can be exceeded in a previously normotensive patient, even at a BP of 160/100 mm Hg. This is seen in acute glomerulonephritis or preeclampsia. Thus, the rate of rise of BP can be more important than the level of BP achieved.

B. Clinical Manifestations and Patient Evaluation. The manifestations of a hypertensive crisis are those of the end-organ dysfunction. *Malignant hypertension* is characterized by BP >160/100 mm Hg, retinal hemorrhages, and, usually, papilledema. Azotemia, proteinuria, and microangiopathic hemolytic anemia are frequent. *Hypertensive encephalopathy* is characterized by a reversible alteration in the level of consciousness, with headache, vision changes (including blindness), and seizures. If untreated, this can progress to cerebral hemorrhage, coma, and death.

Patients should be questioned concerning their use of medications, including monoamine oxidase inhibitors, cocaine, amphetamines, and recent clonidine withdrawal. Careful funduscopic examination is mandatory to detect the presence of arterial hemorrhages and papilledema (see Table 21.5). Investigations should include complete blood cell count, serum electrolytes, blood urea nitrogen, creatinine, urinalysis, electrocardiogram, and chest x-ray to assess end-organ damage. Hypokalemic metabolic alkalosis suggests hyperaldosteronism. A peripheral blood smear can detect schistocytes. Appropriate drug screening should be considered. Proteinuria and hematuria are common. Computed tomography or magnetic resonance imaging scans are required in those with an abrupt onset of focal neurologic signs or decreased consciousness. The magnetic resonance imaging scan of patients with hypertensive encephalopathy shows edema of the parieto-occipital white matter, which is termed *posterior leukoencephalopathy*. Investigations for secondary causes of hypertension are usually deferred until the crisis is resolved.

C. Management. The goal of treatment of a hypertensive emergency is to decrease the BP sufficiently to prevent or limit end-organ damage. This must be balanced against the danger of hypoperfusion and ischemia of vital organs. BP should be lowered within minutes in patients with hypertensive emergencies by using parenteral agents. However, the MAP normally should not be lowered by >20%, or the diastolic (DBP) reduced <100–110 mm Hg, within the first 2 hours. Special caution is necessary in patients with preexisting neurologic or cardiac dysfunction and in the elderly. The selection of a drug to reduce the BP in a controlled and predictable manner depends on the clinical condition and the end-organ damage (Table 28.1). Monitoring of arterial pressure and other parameters in the intensive care unit is required for patients with a hypertensive emergency. Sodium nitroprusside is reliable and safe in many settings. It provides optimal minute-to-minute control of BP but requires intraarterial monitoring. It carries a risk of thiocyanate toxicity when infused at high rates for >24–48 hours, especially in patients with renal or hepatic impairment. Other intravenous (IV) drugs that have slightly slower onset and offset times include labetalol (a combined α- and β-adrenergic receptor blocker) and fenoldopam (a selective dopamine D1 receptor agonist). Volume depletion should be anticipated in patients with malignant hypertension or adrenergic crisis, who may require saline infusion. Diuretics should be used cautiously, if at all, in patients with emergency hypertension, except in those with pulmonary edema or renal failure. The drugs used to treat hypertensive emergencies are outlined in Table 28.3.

The BP of patients with a hypertensive urgency may be lowered to target levels over several hours with oral agents, such as an angiotensin-converting enzyme inhibitor (ACEI), clonidine, labetalol, or a calcium channel blocker (CCB). However, short-acting dihydropyridines, such as nifedipine, have caused permanent neurologic damage in some patients with an abrupt or severe fall in BP. Moreover, they cause reflex activation of cardiac sympathetic nerves, which may worsen myocardial ischemia. Therefore, these drugs should be avoided. Patients should be monitored after achieving the target BP. Thereafter, they should be followed up in the clinic, where they may require evaluation for secondary causes of hypertension and a change of medication, usually including a diuretic, for maintenance therapy.

D. Management in Specific Settings
Hypertensive Encephalopathy
Sodium nitroprusside is the preferred agent because it allows rapid onset and offset for tight control of BP. Although it is a vasodilator, the sharp fall in BP with sodium nitroprusside is usually sufficient to reduce the cerebral capillary pressure and thereby improve cerebral edema. Loop diuretics activate the RAA and sympathetic nervous systems and can induce hypovolemia and hypotension. Therefore, they should be used cautiously. Intraarterial monitoring is required. The BP should be decreased during the first hour by a maximum of 20% or to a DBP of 100–110 mm Hg. A higher target is desirable in patients with preexisting or evolving fixed neurologic deficits. Any neurologic deterioration should prompt a search for alternative or additional causes, such as a new stroke. Clonidine should be avoided because of its central depressant action.

Hypertensive Cerebral Hemorrhage
The optimal treatment is uncertain. Reducing BP has been shown to reduce further bleeding but may result in ischemia, especially in patients with subarachnoid

TABLE 28.3. Selected parenteral drugs for hypertensive emergencies

Drug	Mechanism of action	Route (dose range)	Onset (min)	Duration	Adverse effects
Sodium nitroprusside	Dilates arterioles > veins	IVi (0.5–10.0 µg/kg/min)	<1	3–5 min	Thiocyanate toxicity[a]
Nitroglycerin	Dilates veins > arterioles	IVi (5–100 µg/min)	2–5	5–10 min	Headache, tachyphylaxis
Fenoldopam	Dopamine D1 agonist	IVi (0.1–1.6 µg/kg/min)	4–5	10–15 min	Tachyphylaxis, increased ocular pressure[b]
Labetalol	Beta/alpha blocker	IVi (0.5–3.0 mg/min) or IV (20 mg in 2 min; 40–80 mg per 10 min)	5	6–10 h	Bronchospasm, bradycardia
Esmolol	β_1-Blocker	IV 500 µg/kg + IVi 25–250 µg/kg/min	<1	10–20 min	Bronchospasm, bradycardia
Phentolamine	Nonselective alpha blocker	IV (1–15 mg/min)	1–2	3–5 min	Reflex tachycardia
Enalaprilat	Angiotensin-converting enzyme inhibitor	IV (1.25–5.00 mg/6 h)	15	4–6 h	Renal failure in bilateral renal artery stenosis or volume depletion
Hydralazine	Direct vasodilator	IV (10–20 mg)	10	2–6 h	Reflex tachycardia
Nicardipine	Calcium channel blocker	IVi (2–10 mg/h)	5–10	2–4 h	Reflex tachycardia, flushing

IV, intravenous bolus; IVi, intravenous infusion.
[a]Rare below 3 µg/kg/min for up to 72 h unless patient is in hepatic or renal failure.
[b]Avoid in patients with glaucoma.

hemorrhage complicated by vasospasm. Therapy with IV sodium nitroprusside or labetalol is almost always required for acute intracerebral hemorrhage with systolic BP >170 mm Hg. The target systolic BP is usually 140–160 mm Hg. In contrast, IV antihypertensive therapy is generally withheld in patients with subarachnoid hemorrhage, because of concern for worsening zonal cerebral ischemia, unless hypertension is severe (DBP >130 mm Hg). Nimodipine is a short-acting, parenteral CCB that decreases vasospasm and improves outcome in patients with subarachnoid hemorrhage. It should be used cautiously to obviate hypotension, especially in patients receiving diuretics.

Hypertension and Cerebral Ischemia

Many patients have a temporary increase in BP after an acute thrombotic stroke. Because cerebral autoregulation is impaired in the ischemic periumbra, antihypertensive therapy should not normally be instituted for 5–10 days after an ischemic stroke, unless the BP is particularly high. Some neurologists set a goal for the upper limit of BP at 185/110 mm Hg if thrombolytic therapy is given. Labetalol, nitroprusside, or fenoldopam can be used, but dihydropyridine CCBs should be avoided.

Acute Aortic Dissection

Acute aortic dissection requires complete initial blockade of cardiac (β_1) adrenergic receptors to reduce the cardiac rate and contractility and thereby to reduce the shear stress on the vessel wall. Esmolol given IV is a good choice. Verapamil is an alternative in patients with bronchospasm or other contraindications to beta blockade. Vasodilators, such as sodium nitroprusside or fenoldopam, should be used only after 24-hr/day beta blockade is fully achieved. Given alone, these drugs are dangerous, because a reflex increase in cardiac rate and contractility increases the shear force on the aortic wall and may extend the dissection.

Hypertension with Myocardial Ischemia

Nitroglycerine improves coronary perfusion, reduces myocardial stretch and energy metabolism, and reduces preload. Although not normally an effective antihypertensive agent, it frequently lowers BP in this setting. It is the initial drug of choice. Parenteral labetalol or beta blockers are useful. Sodium nitroprusside and direct vasodilators cause reflex tachycardia and may worsen ischemia. They should be avoided.

Hypertension with Left Ventricular Failure

Hypertension with left ventricular failure should be treated with IV nitroglycerin, usually combined with sodium nitroprusside. When given parenterally, loop diuretics can cause vasodilatation, which, together with the diuresis, reduces the effective blood volume and the cardiac preload. However, vasodilatation is not seen in patients who are established on oral loop diuretic therapy or in those receiving ACEIs or nonsteroidal antiinflammatory agents. ACEIs are often useful, but β-adrenergic blockers should be avoided in the acute phase because of the risk of worsening bronchospasm or reducing cardiac output.

Preeclampsia and Eclampsia

Parenteral therapy is reserved for patients with systolic BP >180 mm Hg or DBP >110 mm Hg. Timely delivery of the fetus is the only cure. Before this, the DBP should not be lowered excessively, or <90 mm Hg, because the uteroplacental blood flow is not autoregulated. Indeed, any reduction in maternal BP can induce fetal distress. Hydralazine is the traditional choice, but labetalol and nicardipine are alternatives. Magnesium sulfate is used as prophylaxis for seizures. Sodium nitroprusside may be toxic to the fetus, and ACEIs cause nephrotoxicity to the newborn. These agents should be avoided (see Chapter 23).

Perioperative Hypertension

Perioperative hypertension increases risks of bleeding, myocardial ischemia, and stroke. Sodium nitroprusside provides excellent BP control. Esmolol and labetalol are used to lower BP further and to limit reflex tachycardia. Nicardipine and fenoldopam are useful alternatives.

Sympathetic Crises

Pheochromocytoma, sympathomimetic drugs (e.g., cocaine, amphetamine, phencyclidine), a combination of a monoamine oxidase inhibitor with tyramine-containing foods, or abrupt discontinuation of treatment with a short-acting central sympatholytic agent (e.g., clonidine) all can cause severe, adrenergically-mediated hypertension. The first step is to reintroduce clonidine, if that is the culprit. An α-adrenergic antagonist, such as phentolamine, is rational, but nicardipine, sodium nitroprusside, or fenoldopam can control less severe episodes of hypertension. Monotherapy with β-adrenergic blockers evokes unopposed α-adrenergic vasoconstriction of blood vessels and may paradoxically worsen the hypertension.

Renal Insufficiency

Renal insufficiency can be a cause or a consequence of severe or malignant hypertension. Fenoldopam is valuable to preserve the glomerular filtration rate (GFR) and urine flow in patients with new-onset or worsening renal insufficiency. A CCB, labetalol, and sodium nitroprusside are alternatives. Diuretics should be used in patients with volume overload, pulmonary edema, or resistant hypertension. ACEIs are drugs of first choice for patients with scleroderma renal crisis and may be valuable in others with malignant hypertension. However, ACEIs should not be used in patients with bilateral renal artery stenosis or stenosis of a single (e.g., transplanted) functioning kidney, as they may precipitate acute renal failure. Because autoregulation is impaired or absent in patients with malignant hypertension or renal insufficiency, any drug that lowers the BP may reduce the GFR abruptly. Thus, an ini-

TABLE 28.4.   Causes of drug-resistant hypertension

Pseudoresistance
   "White coat" or "office" hypertension
   Inappropriate use of regular-sized cuff in obese subjects
   Nonadherence to drug therapy or diet
   Inadequate drug dose or inappropriate drug combination
Salt and fluid overload
   Absent or inadequate diuretic therapy
   Excess salt intake
   Kidney disease
   Compensation to vasodilator therapy
Drug induced
   Nonsteroidal antiinflammatory drugs, cyclooxygenase-2 inhibitors
   Cocaine, amphetamines, other illicit drugs
   Sympathomimetics (decongestants, anorectics)
   Oral contraceptives, adrenal steroids
   Cyclosporine and tacrolimus
   Erythropoietin
   Licorice and some chewing tobaccos
   Some over-the-counter supplements (e.g., ephedra, ma huang)
Associated conditions
   Obesity and sleep apnea
   Excessive alcohol intake
   Secondary hypertension

tial increase in serum creatinine concentration or blood urea nitrogen is not necessarily an indication to change therapy. With restoration of a normal BP, renal autoregulation and hemodynamics improve, and the elevated serum creatinine and blood urea nitrogen usually return to baseline over the subsequent few days or weeks. Ultrafiltration with hemodialysis may be required to control BP in oliguric patients. Ultrafiltration may improve the GFR over the next few months if the BP control is optimal, although most patients have residual renal impairment, and many remain dialysis dependent.

III. **Resistant Hypertension.** After confirming good compliance, the clinician should exclude secondary causes of hypertension (see Chapter 22). Causes of drug-resistant hypertension are shown in Table 28.4. Ambulatory BP monitoring may reveal patients with the "white coat" effect. Volume overload in patients with renal impairment or those receiving aggressive vasodilator therapy is an important cause. Dietary salt restriction and appropriate doses of furosemide given two or three times daily produce better diuresis than a thiazide alone in patients with a reduced GFR. The most common cause of drug-resistant hypertension is a failure to use a diuretic or use of a diuretic in inadequate dose.

IV. **Suggested Readings**
   Blumenfeld JD, Laragh JH. Management of hypertensive crises: the scientific basis for treatment decisions. *Am J Hypertens* 2001;11:1154–1167.

Joint National Committee on Detection, Evaluation, and Treatment of High Blood Pressure. *Seventh report*. Bethesda, MD: National Institutes of Health, 2003. Available at http://www.nhlbi.nih.gov/guidelines/hypertension/express.pdf.

Mann SJ. Hypertensive emergencies. In: Brady HR, Wilcox CS, eds. *Therapy in nephrology and hypertension*, 2nd ed. Philadelphia: WB Saunders, 2003:569–579.

Murphy MB, Murray C, Shorten GD. Fenoldopam: a selective peripheral dopamine-receptor agonist for the treatment of severe hypertension. *N Engl J Med* 2001;345:1548–1557.

Vaughan CJ, Delanty N. Hypertensive emergencies. *Lancet* 2000;356:411–417.

Use of Drugs in Renal Failure

Brendan J. Smyth and Jason G. Umans

The activity of a drug is related to the concentration of free drug in the tissue compartment in which the effect occurs (Fig. 29.1). The kidney is a major route of elimination for most drugs. Therefore, patients with renal disease, or with unsuspected renal insufficiency, as in the elderly, are more susceptible to adverse drug reactions and toxicity. Uremia may alter drug pharmacokinetics, including absorption, volume of distribution (V_D), degree of protein binding, and biotransformation. It also reduces the hepatic elimination of certain drugs, which can result in accumulation of the parent drug or its active metabolites to toxic levels (e.g., acyclovir, captopril, codeine, meperidine, and procainamide). The nephrotoxicity of commonly used drugs is discussed in Chapter 30.

I. **Drug Bioavailability and Absorption.** The bioavailability of a drug is the fraction of a dose absorbed into the circulation. It depends on the route of administration and on factors that could interfere with absorption, such as drug binding in the gut or *first-pass* biotransformation in the gut wall or liver. Gastrointestinal drug absorption can be impaired in uremia due to vomiting, delayed gastric emptying, diarrhea, or impaired gastric acidity. Likewise, phosphate binders may bind or chelate drugs in the gut, preventing their absorption.

II. **Drug Distribution.** Factors that affect the extent of drug distribution in the body include molecular size, plasma protein binding, and drug tissue binding. Edema and ascites can increase the V_D for hydrophilic and highly protein-bound agents. Decreased binding of acidic drugs to proteins in uremia increases the unbound drug levels and, consequently, their distribution and elimination. The alteration in protein binding may be caused by one of the following three mechanisms: (a) decreased serum albumin concentration, (b) accumulation of endogenous organic acids in uremic plasma that displace acidic drugs from albumin-binding sites, or (c) altered albumin drug-binding capacity. By contrast, binding of basic drugs to acidic glycoproteins can be increased in renal failure.

Reduced protein binding decreases the total plasma drug concentration while increasing the unbound fraction of that total concentration. For example, because of decreased phenytoin binding to albumin in chronic renal insufficiency, total plasma drug concentrations underestimate free drug levels and therapeutic responses. There is a transient rise in free drug levels, but these later return to steady state as the total drug level decreases. The finding of a low total drug

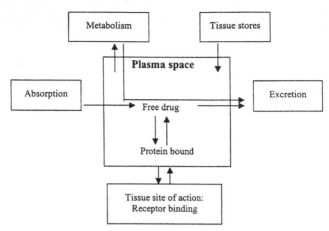

FIG. 29.1. The relationships among absorption, distribution, protein binding, and excretion of a drug and its concentration at its site of action.

level may prompt the physician to increase drug dosage to reestablish therapeutic total plasma drug levels, with the danger of drug toxicity. Specific measurement of plasma free drug concentrations avoids drug toxicity.

III. **Clearance.** The total plasma clearance of a drug depends on renal elimination and hepatic metabolism and conjugation. Renal elimination of drugs is determined by the glomerular filtration rate, tubular secretion, and tubular reabsorption. Glomerular filtration rate should be estimated from creatinine clearance or from a prediction formula such as the Cockcroft-Gault or Modification of Diet in Renal Disease equations (see Chapter 3). Protein-bound drugs are poorly filtered, but they may be efficiently secreted by the proximal tubule. Unbound drugs are usually freely filtered through the glomerulus. Drugs with primarily hepatic elimination are preferred in patients with renal insufficiency. However, renal insufficiency may alter hepatic drug metabolism.

IV. **Prescribing for the Patient with Renal Insufficiency**
   A. **Calculation of Initial Loading Dosage.** Because loading dose depends only on the V_D and not on drug clearance, patients with renal failure and normal extracellular volume are given a normal loading dose, whereas those with edema or ascites may require a larger loading dose. Loading dose is calculated as

   $$\text{desired plasma drug concentration} \times V_D$$

   B. **Calculation of Maintenance Dosage.** The fraction of the normal dose for a patient with renal insufficiency can be calculated from

dose in renal failure = dose in normal renal function
$$\times (t_{1/2} \text{ normal}/t_{1/2} \text{ renal failure})$$

where $t_{1/2}$ is the half-life for elimination and inversely proportional to clearance.

Alternatively, the dose can often be kept constant and the dosing interval increased:

Dose interval in renal failure = normal dose interval/
$$(t_{1/2} \text{ normal}/t_{1/2} \text{ renal failure})$$

V. Hemodialysis of Drugs. Drug removal by hemodialysis (HD) is directly proportional to the plasma concentration of free drug and to the clearance characteristics of the dialysis membrane. High drug molecular weight does not limit drug removal by HD with high-flux membranes (e.g., polysulfone, cellulose triacetate, polyacrylonitrile). It is only important with less "leaky" cellulosic (e.g., cuprophane or cellulose acetate) membranes. The most important variables limiting drug removal by HD are a large V_D and high protein binding. Drug removal during HD can be substantial—for instance, requiring replacement of approximately 50% of total body stores of an aminoglycoside. As in the case of urea kinetic modeling, there can be substantial postdialysis redistribution of drug from tissue to the central (plasma-containing) compartment. This phenomenon can limit drug removal during HD and lead to overestimates of drug removal if plasma levels are measured immediately after dialysis before equilibration is complete.

Whenever possible, drug dosing in HD patients should be estimated using aids such as Table 29.1, then the accuracy of these estimates should be confirmed by measurement of plasma drug levels. This strategy avoids the wide variation in drug levels that may result if drugs are only dosed when the plasma levels fall below the therapeutic target.

VI. Drug Therapy during Continuous Renal Replacement Therapy. Drug removal by continuous renal replacement therapy (CRRT), either venovenous hemofiltration or venovenous HD, differs from that in intermittent HD because dialytic clearance is usually much higher, and intercompartmental redistribution during and after dialysis is relatively unimportant. The dialyzer membranes do not differ from those used in high-flux HD, offering effective pore size larger than nearly all unbound drugs. Consequently, drug-dosing adjustments during CRRT are much more dependent on the relative contribution of CRRT to total body clearance of the drug than on the drug's V_D. One simple approach to drug-dosing adjustment during CRRT is to estimate mean 24-hour creatinine clearance from total dialysate or ultrafiltration volume (often in the range of 30–35 ml/min), then to look up dose adjustments in Table 29.1 or similar published references for patients with chronic renal insufficiency and residual function of 10–50 ml/min. More precise estimates can be made when protein-

TABLE 29.1. Details of drugs requiring dose adjustments in patients with renal insufficiency and those receiving dialysis

Drug	Excreted unchanged (%)	Protein bound (%)	t½ Normal/renal failure (h)	Dose or frequency adjustment for GFR (ml/min) GFR >50	GFR 10–50	GFR <10	Supplemental dose for HD	Peritoneal dialysis
Analgesics								
Narcotics								
Codeine	Hepatic	7	2.5–3.5/?	100%	75%	50%	?	?
Fentanyl	Hepatic	80–84	2–7/?	100%	75%	50%	Not applicable	Not applicable
Meperidine[a]	Hepatic	70	2–7/7–32	100%	Avoid	Avoid	Avoid	Avoid
Methadone	Hepatic	60–90	13–58/?	100%	75%	50–75%	None	None
Morphine[b]	Hepatic	20–30	1–4/unchanged	100%	75%	50%	None	?
Nonsteroidal antiinflammatory drugs and cyclooxygenase-2 enzyme inhibitors								
Acetamino-phen	Hepatic	20–30	2/2	q4h	q6h	q8h	None	None
Aspirin	Hepatic/renal	80–90	2–3/unchanged	q4h	q4–6h	Avoid	Dose after HD	None
Celecoxib	Hepatic	97	11/unchanged	?	Avoid	Avoid	?	?
Ibuprofen	<1	99	2/unchanged	100%	100%	100%	None	None
Rofecoxib	Hepatic	85	17/unchanged	25 mg qd	Avoid	Avoid	?	?
Antimicrobials								
Aminoglycosides[c,d] (traditional multiple daily doses; see alternative once-daily dosing at end of table)								

(continued)

TABLE 29.1. (continued)

Drug	Excreted unchanged (%)	Protein bound (%)	t½ Normal/renal failure (h)	Dose or frequency adjustment for GFR (ml/min) GFR >50	GFR 10–50	GFR <10	Supplemental dose for HD	Peritoneal dialysis
Amikacin	95	<5	1.4–2.3/17–150	60–90% q12h OR 100% q12–24h	30–70% q12–18h OR 100% q24–48h	20–30% q24–48h OR 100% q48–72 h	½ Full dose after HD	15–20 mg/L/d
Gentamicin	95	<5	1.8/20–60	60–90% q8–12h OR 100% q12–24h	30–70% q12h OR 100% q24–48h	20–30% q24–48h OR 100% q48–72h	½ Full dose after HD	3–4 mg/L/d
Streptomycin	70	35	2.5/100	q24h	q24–72h	q27–96h	½ Full dose	20–40 mg/L/d
Tobramycin	95	<5	2.5/27–60	60–90% q8–12h	30–70% q12h	20–30% q24–48h	⅔ Full dose	3–4 mg/L/d
Carbapenems Imipenem[e]	20–70	13–21	1.0/4.0	100%	50%	25%	Dose after HD	50%

Drug	Excreted Unchanged (%)	Protein Binding (%)	Half-Life Normal/ESRD (hr)	GFR >50	GFR 10–50	GFR <10	Supplement for Hemodialysis	Supplement for CAPD
Cephalosporins								
Cefaclor	70	25	1.0/3.0	100%	50–100%	50%	250 mg after HD	250 mg q8–12h
Cefazolin	75–95	80	2/40–70	q8h	q12h	q24–48h	0.5–1.0 g after HD	0.5 g q12h
Cefotaxime	60	37	1.0/15	q6h	q8–12h	q24h	1 g after HD	1 g/d
Ceftazidime	60–85	17	1.2/13–25	q8–12h	q24–48h	q24h	1 g after HD	0.5 g/d
Ceftriaxone	30–65	90	7–9/12–24	100%	100%	100%	Dose after HD	750 mg q12h
Cephalexin	98	20	0.7/16	q8h	q12h	q12h	Dose after HD	Dose for GFR <10
Macrolides								
Azithromycin	6–12	8.0–50.0	10–60/?	100%	100%	100%	None	None
Clarithromycin	15	70	2.3–6.0/?	100%	75%	50–70%	Dose after HD	None
Erythromycin	15	60–90	1.4/5–6	100%	100%	50–70%	None	None
Miscellaneous								
Clindamycin	10	60–95	2–4/3–5	100%	100%	100%	None	None
Metronidazole	20	20	6–14/7–21	100%	100%	50%	Dose after HD	Dose for GFR <10
Sulfamethoxazole	70	50	10/20–50	q12h	q18h	q24h	1 g after HD	1 g/d
Trimethoprim	40–70	30–70	9–13/20–49	q12h	q18h	q24h	Dose after HD	—
Vancomycin	90–100	10–50	6–8/200	500 mg q12h	500 mg q24–48h	500 mg q48–96h	Dose for GFR <10	Dose for GFR <10

(continued)

TABLE 29.1. (continued)

Drug	Excreted unchanged (%)	Protein bound (%)	t½ Normal/renal failure (h)	Dose or frequency adjustment for GFR (ml/min) GFR >50	GFR 10–50	GFR <10	Supplemental dose for HD	Peritoneal dialysis
Penicillins								
Amoxicillin	50–70	15–25	2.3/5–20	q8h	q8–12h	q24h	Dose after HD	250 mg q12h
Ampicillin	30–70	20	1.5/7–20	q6h	q6–12h	q12–24h	Dose after HD	250 mg q12h
Aztreonam	75	45–60	2.9/6–8	100%	50–75%	25%	0.5 g after HD	Dose for GFR <10
Nafcillin	36	85	0.5/1.2	100%	100%	100%	None	None
Penicillin G	60–85	<5	0.5/6–20	100%	75%	20–50%	Dose after HD	Dose for GFR <10
Piperacillin	75–90	30	0.8–2.0/3.0–5.1	q4–6h	q6–8h	q8h	Dose after HD	Dose for GFR <10
Ticarcillin	85	45–60	1.2/11–16	1–2 g q4h	1–2 g q8h	1–2 g q12h	3 g after HD	Dose for GFR <10
Quinolones								
Ciprofloxacin	50–70	20–40	3–6/6–9	100%	50–75%	50%	250 mg q12h	250 mg q12h
Gatifloxacin	74–84	20	7–14/36	400 mg q24h	200 mg q24h	200 mg q24h	200 mg q24h after HD	200 mg q24h
Levofloxacin	67–87	24–38	4–8/76	100%	500 mg initially then 250 mg q24–48h	500 mg initially then 250 mg q48h	Dose for GFR <10	Dose for GFR <10

Drug								
Ofloxacin	68–80	25	5–8/28–37	100%	50%	25–50%	100 mg q12h	Dose for GFR <10
Tetracyclines[g]								
Doxycycline	35–45	80–90	20/18–25	100%	100%	100%	None	?
Minocycline	6–10	70	16/12–18	100%	100%	100%	None	None
Antifungals								
Amphotericin B		90	24/unchanged	q24h	q24h	q24–36h	None	Dose for GFR <10
Fluconazole		12	22/?	100%	100%	100%	200 mg after HD	Dose for GFR <10
Caspofungin		97	β-Phase 9–11 h then 40–50 h/ no change	100%	100%	100%	None	?
Flucytosine		<10	3–6/75–200	q12h	q16h	q24h	Dose after HD	0.5–1.0 g/q24h
Itraconazole		99	21/25	100%	100%	50%	100 mg q12–24h	100 mg q12–24h
Antiparasitics								
Chloroquine	40	50–65	4/5–50 d	100%	100%	50%	None	None
Pentamidine	20	69	29/118	q24h	q24–36h	q48h	None	None
Dapsone	5–20	70–90	20–30/?	?	?	?	?	?
Antituberculosis								
Ethambutol	75–90	10–30	4–7/15	q24h	q24–36h	q48h	Dose after HD	Dose for GFR <10
Isoniazid	5–30	4–30	0.7–4.0/8–17	100%	100%	50%	Dose after HD	Dose for GFR <10
Pyrazinamide	1–3	0.5	54/?	100%	Avoid	Avoid	Avoid	Dose for GFR <10
Rifampin	15–30	60–90	1.5/1.8–11	100%	50–100%	50%	None	Dose for GFR <10

(continued)

TABLE 29.1. (continued)

| Drug | Excreted unchanged (%) | Protein bound (%) | t½ Normal/renal failure (h) | Dose or frequency adjustment for GFR (ml/min) | | | Supplemental dose for | |
				GFR >50	GFR 10–50	GFR <10	HD	Peritoneal dialysis
Antiviral[h]								
Abacavir	Hepatic 40–70	50	1.5–2.7/none	100%	100%	100%	None	?
Acyclovir (prodrug = valacyclovir)		15–30	2.1–3.5/19	5 mg/kg q8h	5 mg/kg q12h	5 mg/kg q24h	Dose after HD	Dose for GFR <10
Amantadine	90	60	12/500	q24–48h	q48–72h	q7d	None	None
Amprenavir	<3	90	7.6–10.1/?	100%	100%	100%	?	?
Cidofovir/probenecid	70–85%	<6%	2.6/not applicable	See note	Avoid	Avoid	Avoid	Avoid
Didanosine	60	<5	1.3–1.6/4.5	q12h	q24h	q48h	25% of daily dose	Dose for GFR <10
Efavirenz	Hepatic 50–65	>99	40–76/?	?	?	?	?	?
Famciclovir		<25	1.6–2.9/10–22	q8h	250 mg q12h	250 mg q48h	250 mg after HD	?
Foscarnet	85	17	3/prolonged	28 mg/kg	15 mg/kg q24–48h	6 mg/kg	Dose after HD	Dose for GFR <10
Ganciclovir (prodrug = valganciclovir)	90–100	1–2%	3.6/30	q12h	q24–48h	q48–96h	Dose after HD	Dose for GFR <10

Drug	Route of elimination (%)	% Protein binding	Half-life normal/ESRD	GFR >50	GFR 10–50	GFR <10	Supplement for hemodialysis	Supplement for CAPD
Indinavir	Hepatic	60	1.8/?	—	—	—	Dose after HD	—
Lamivudine	68–71	36	5–7/15–35	150 mg q12h	100 mg qd	50 mg qd	?	?
Lopinavir/ritonavir	Hepatic	98–99	5–6/?	?	?	?	?	?
Nevirapine	<5	60%	20–45/?	?	?	?	?	?
Ribavirin	10–40	0	30–60/?	100%	100%	50%	Dose after HD	Dose for GFR<10
Rimantadine	<25	10%	13–65/prolonged	100 mg q12h	100 mg qd	100 mg qd	?	?
Ritonavir	Hepatic	98–99%	3–5/?	?	?	?	?	?
Saquinavir	Hepatic	97%	1–2/?	?	?	?	?	?
Stavudine	40	<1	1.0–1.4/5.5–8.0	100%	50%	50% q24h	Dose after HD	?
Valacyclovir (prodrug of acyclovir)	<12%	13.5–18.0	2.5/3.3	1 g q8h	1 g q12–24h	0.5 g q24h	Dose after HD	Dose for GFR <10
Zalcitabine	75	<4	0.75 mg q12h	0.75 mg q8h	0.75 mg q12h	0.75 mg q24h	Dose after HD	?
Zidovudine	8–25	10–30	1.1–1.4/1.4–3.0	200 mg q8h	200 mg q8h	100 mg q12h	100 mg after HD	Dose for GFR <10
Cardiovascular drugs								
Adenosine	<5	0	<10 sec/unchanged	100%	100%	100%	None	None
Amiodarone	<5	96	14–120 d/unchanged	100%	100%	100%	None	None
Digoxin	76–85	20–30	36–44/80–120	100% q24h	25–75% q36h	10–25% q48h	None	None

(continued)

TABLE 29.1. (continued)

Drug	Excreted unchanged (%)	Protein bound (%)	$t_{1/2}$ Normal/renal failure (h)	Dose or frequency adjustment for GFR (ml/min)			Supplemental dose for	
				GFR >50	GFR 10-50	GFR <10	HD	Peritoneal dialysis
Dobutamine	<10	?	2 min/?	100%	100%	100%	?	?
Flecainide	25	52	12/19-26	100%	100%	50-75%	None	None
Lidocaine	10	60-66	2.2/3.0	100%	100%	100%	None	None
Mexiletine	10	70-75	8/13-16	100%	100%	50-75%	None	None
Propafenone	<1	>95	12/?	100%	100%	100%	None	None
Quinidine	20	70-95	6/4-14	100%	100%	75%	100-200 mg	None
Sotalol	60	<1	?	100%	30%	15-30%	80 mg	None
Tocainide	40	10-20	14/22-27	100%	100%	50%	200 mg	None
Angiotensin-converting enzyme inhibitors								
Benazepril	20	95	22/30	100%	75-100%	50%	25-30%	None
Captopril	30-40	25-30	1.9/21-32	100% q8-12h	75% q12-18h	50% q24h	25-30%	None
Enalapril	43	50-60	24/34-60	100% q8-12h	75-100%	50%	20-25%	None
Fosinopril	<1	95	11-12/12-20	100%	100%	75%	None	None
Lisinopril	80-90	0-10	12.6/40-50	100%	50-75%	25-50%	20%	None
Quinapril	30	97	1-2/6-15	100%	75-100%	50%	25%	None
Ramipril	10-21	55-70	5.8/15.0	100%	50-75%	25-50%	20%	None

				100%			
Angiotensin receptor blockers							
Candesartan	33	99	9/?	100%	Start 2 mg, titrate to BP (16 mg)	?	?
Eprosartan	35–50	99	5–7/?	100%	100%	100%	?
Irbesartan	20	90	12–20/?	100%	Start 75 mg, titrate to BP	?	?
Losartan	10	30	3/4	100%	100%	100%	None
Olmesartan	7	99	13/?	100%	?	?	?
Telmisartan	7	98	24/?	100%	100%	?	?
Valsartan	13.2	85–99	6.1/?	100%	100%	?	?
Beta blockers							
Atenolol	>90	3	6.7/15–35	100% q24h	50% q48h	30–50% q96h	25–50 mg
Carvedilol	<2	95	5–8/unchanged	100%	100%	100%	None
Labetalol	<5	50	3–9/unchanged	100%	100%	100%	None
Metoprolol	5	8	3.5/2.5–4.5	100%	100%	100%	50 mg
Pindolol	40	50	2.5–4.0/3–4	100%	100%	100%	None
Propranolol	<5	93	2–6/1–6	100%	100%	100%	None
Calcium channel blockers							
Amlodipine	<10	>95	35–50/50	100%	100%	100%	None
Diltiazem	<10	98	2–8/3.5	100%	100%	100%	None

(continued)

TABLE 29.1. (continued)

Drug	Excreted unchanged (%)	Protein bound (%)	$t_{1/2}$ Normal/renal failure (h)	Dose or frequency adjustment for GFR (ml/min)			Supplemental dose for	
				GFR >50	GFR 10-50	GFR <10	HD	Peritoneal dialysis
Nicardipine	<1	98-99	5/5-7	100%	100%	100%	None	None
Nifedipine	<10	97	5.5/5-7	100%	100%	100%	None	None
Verapamil	<10	83-93	3-7/2.4-4.0	100%	100%	100%	None	None
Centrally acting agents								
Clonidine	45	20-40	6-23/38-42	100%	100%	100%	None	None
Methyldopa	25-40	<15	1.5-6.0/6-16	q8h	q8-12h	q12-24h	250 mg	None
Vasodilators								
Hydralazine	5-10	87	2.0-4.5/7-16	q8h	q8h	q8-16h	None	None
Minoxidil	15-20	0	2.8-4.2/ unchanged	100%	100%	100%	None	None
Terazosin	20-30	90-94	9-12/8-12	100%	100%	100%	?	?
Antiulcer/proton pump inhibitors								
Cimetidine	50-70	20	1.5-2.0/5	100%	50%	25%	None	None
Esomeprazole	<1	97	1.0-1.5/ unchanged	100%	100%	100%	?	None
Famotidine	65-80	15-22	2.5-4.0/12-19	50%	25%	10%	None	None
Lansoprazole	None	>98	1.3-2.9/ unchanged	100%	100%	100%	?	?

Drug								
Omeprazole	<1	95	0.5–1.0/ unchanged	100%	100%	100%	?	?
Ranitidine	80	15	1.5–3.0/6–9	75%	50%	25%	50%	None
Anticonvulsants, antidepressants, antiparkinsonians, antipsychotics								
Amitriptyline	Hepatic	96	24–40/unchanged	100%	100%	100%	None	?
Carbamazepine	2–3	75	—	100%	100%	100%	None	None
Carbidopa	30	?	2/?	100%	100%	100%	?	?
Clonazepam	Hepatic	47	18–50/?	?	?	?	?	?
Citalopram	12	80	35/?	100%	100%	?	None	?
Fluoxetine	Hepatic	94.5	24–72/ unchanged	100%	100%	100%	?	?
Gabapentin	90	Unbound	5–7/132	400 mg t.i.d.	300 mg q12–24h	300 mg every other day	300 mg load, then 200–300 mg after HD	300 mg every other day
Haloperidol	Hepatic	90–92	10–19/?	100%	100%	100%	None	None
Lamotrigine	10	55	25–36/43–58	100%	100%	100%	50%	?
Levetiracetam	65	<10	7/25	500–1,000 mg b.i.d.	250–750 mg b.i.d.	250–500 mg b.i.d.	500–1,000 mg qd, then 250–500 mg after HD	?
Levodopa	None	5–8	0.8–1.6/?	100%	100%	100%	?	?
Lithium	Renal	None	14–28/40	100%	50–75%	25–50%	Dose after HD	None
Nefazodone	Hepatic	99	2–4/unchanged	100%	100%	100%	?	?
Phenobarbital	Hepatic/ renal	40–60	60–150/117–160	q8–12h	q8–12h	q12–16h	Dose after HD	50%

(continued)

TABLE 29.1. (continued)

Drug	Excreted unchanged (%)	Protein bound (%)	$t_{1/2}$ Normal/renal failure (h)	Dose or frequency adjustment for GFR (ml/min) GFR >50	GFR 10-50	GFR <10	Supplemental dose for HD	Peritoneal dialysis
Paroxetine	2%	95	15-20/?	Initial dose, 12.5 mg qd, titrate up to max 50 mg qd	?	?	?	?
Phenytoin	2	90	24/unchanged	100%	100%	100%	None	None
Sertraline	Hepatic	97	24/?	?	?	?	?	?
Topiramate	70-80	9-17	19-23/48-60	100%	50%	25%	?	?
Valproic acid	3-7	90	5-16/unchanged	100%	100%	100%	None	None
Venlafaxine	Hepatic	27	4/6-8	75%	50%	50%	None	?
Antidiabetics								
Chlorpropamide	47	91-99	24-48/50-200	50%	Avoid	Avoid	?	?
Glipizide	4.5-7.0	97	3-7/?	100%	100%	100%	?	?
Glyburide	50	99	1.4-2.9/?	?	Avoid	Avoid	None	None

Drug								
Metformin	90–100	Negligible	1–5/prolonged	50%	25%	Avoid	?	?
Pioglitazone	Hepatic	97	9/unchanged	100%	100%	100%	100%	?
Rosiglitazone	Hepatic	99	3–4/unchanged	100%	100%	100%	100%	?
Antihyperlipidemics								
Atorvastatin	<2	>98	14/?	?	?	?	?	?
Gemfibrozil	None	97–99	7.6/	100%	100%	100%	100%	None
Lovastatin	None	>95	1.1–1.7/ unchanged	100%	100%	100%	100%	?
Niacin	None	?	0.5–1.0/?	100%	50%	25%	?	?
Pravastatin	<10	40–60	0.8–3.2/ unchanged	100%	100%	100%	100%	?
Simvastatin	<0.5	>95	?/ unchanged	100%	100%	100%	100%	?

?, no data; b.i.d., twice a day; BP, blood pressure; GFR, glomerular filtration rate; HD, hemodialysis; hepatic, predominantly eliminated by hepatic metabolism; max, maximum; t.i.d., three times a day.

[a] Active metabolite (normeperidine) lowers seizure threshold, accumulates in end-stage renal disease, and is poorly dialyzed.
[b] End-stage renal disease patients have increased sensitivity to morphine's effects.
[c] Aminoglycosides: See below for alternative once-daily dose.

Creatinine clearance (ml/min)	>80	60–80	40–60	30–40	20–30	10–20	<10
Antibiotic dose	Dose q24h (mg/kg)				Dose q48h (mg/kg)		
Amikacin/kanamycin	15.0	12.0	7.5	4.0	7.5	4.0	3.0
Gentamicin/tobramycin	5.1	4.0	3.5	2.5	4.0	3.0	2.0

[d]Measure serum levels. Risk for nephrotoxicity and ototoxicity. Peritoneal dialysis pharmacokinetics variable.

[e]Imipenem lowers seizure threshold in end-stage renal disease. Cilastatin decreases potential nephrotoxicity of metabolite.

[f]Quinolone malabsorption occurs in the presence of magnesium, calcium, aluminum, and iron-containing compounds.

[g]Tetracycline drugs: Malabsorption occurs with magnesium, calcium, aluminum, and iron-containing compounds.

[h]See http://www.aidsinfo.nih.gov for updates.

Adapted from Aronoff GR, Berns JS, Brier ME, et al., eds. *Drug prescribing in renal failure: dosing guidelines for adults*, 4th ed. Philadelphia: American College of Physicians, 1999; Brater DC. Drug dosing in renal failure. In: Brady HR, Wilcox CS, eds. *Therapy in nephrology and hypertension: companion to Brenner and Rector's the kidney*, 2nd ed. Philadelphia: WB Saunders, 2003:939–954; Gilbert D, Moellering R, et al. *The Sanford guide to antimicrobial therapy*. Hyde Park, VT: Jeb C. Sanford, 2003; Kuczynska J. *Drugs in renal failure: analgesics (part 2) rofecoxib and celecoxib*. South West Medicines Information and Training: UK Medicines Information of National Health System, 2003; Sandow N. *RxList: the internet drug list*. RxList LLC, 2003. Available at http://www.rxlist.com/.

binding data and plasma drug levels are available. The ability of a drug to transit the dialyzer by convective clearance during continuous ultrafiltration is expressed as the *sieving coefficient* (S = drug concentration in ultrafiltrate/ drug concentration in plasma). Because most unbound drugs are freely cleared by continuous hemofiltration, S can be approximated by the free fraction (1 – fractional protein binding), and drug clearance becomes S × ultrafiltration rate. Drug replacement then is calculated as drug clearance × drug concentration.

VII. Peritoneal Dialysis of Drugs. Like other solutes, most drugs may be transported bidirectionally across the peritoneal membrane during continuous ambulatory peritoneal dialysis. Intraperitoneally administered drugs enter the circulation rapidly. For example, antibiotics can achieve equivalent plasma levels after intravenous or intraperitoneal dosing. Although peritoneal surface area is large, most dwell volumes are only approximately 2 L. Even if drug clearance were to approximate peritoneal creatinine clearance, it would only be 6–8 ml/min. More importantly, because peritoneal volumes are much smaller than the V_D for most drugs, only a small fraction of drug is present in the peritoneal cavity at any given time, limiting its contribution to drug clearance. Importantly, the data on the peritoneal elimination of many drugs are inconsistent, increasing the need for drug level monitoring.

VIII. Details of Drug Dosing in Renal Failure. Table 29.1 provides details of commonly used or important drugs that require dose adjustments in patients with renal insufficiency and those receiving dialysis. When specific recommendations are unavailable, data on the usual importance of renal drug elimination, half-life, V_D, and protein binding allow us to estimate dose adjustments.

IX. Suggested Readings

Aronoff GR, Berns JS, Brier ME, et al., eds. *Drug prescribing in renal failure: dosing guidelines for adults*, 4th ed. Philadelphia: American College of Physicians, 1999.

Ateshkadi A. Principles of drug therapy in renal failure. In: Greenberg A, Cheung A, Coffmann T, Folk R, eds. *Primer on kidney diseases*, 2nd ed. San Diego: Academic Press, 1998:298–306.

Brater DC. Drug dosing in renal failure. In: Brady HR, Wilcox CS, eds. *Therapy in nephrology and hypertension: companion to Brenner and Rector's the kidney*, 2nd ed. Philadelphia: WB Saunders, 2003:939–954.

Bugge JF. Pharmacokinetics and drug dosing adjustments during continuous venovenous hemofiltration or hemodiafiltration in critically ill patients. *Acta Anaesthesiol Scand* 2001;45:929–934.

Cohen LM, Germain MJ, Tessier EG. Neuropsychiatric complications and psychopharmacology of endstage renal disease. In: Brady HR, Wilcox CS, eds. *Therapy in nephrology and hypertension: companion to Brenner and Rector's the kidney*, 2nd ed. Philadelphia: WB Saunders, 2003:731–745.

Gilbert D, Moellering R, et al. *The Sanford guide to antimicrobial therapy*. Hyde Park, VT: Jeb C. Sanford, 2003.

Keller E, Reetze P, Schollmeyer P. Drug therapy in patients undergoing continuous ambulatory peritoneal dialysis. Clinical pharmacokinetic considerations. *Clin Pharmacokinet* 1990;18:104–117.

Kuczynska J. *Drugs in renal failure: analgesics (part 2) rofecoxib and celecoxib*. South West Medicines Information and Training: UK Medicines Information of National Health System, 2003.

Sandow N. RxList: the internet drug list. RxList LLC, 2003. Available at http://www.rxlist.com/.

VII

Renal Failure: Diagnosis and Management

Acute Renal Failure

Julie Raggio and Jason G. Umans

Acute renal failure (ARF) is a sudden decrease in glomerular filtration rate (GFR), resulting in retention of nitrogenous wastes, such as blood urea nitrogen (BUN) or creatinine (Cr), or in anuria.

Changes in serum Cr concentration (S_{Cr}) usually lag behind changes in GFR during the onset or recovery of ARF (see Chapter 4). A low S_{Cr} may also reflect loss of muscle or massive volume expansion that dilutes body stores of Cr.

Although Cr is cleared primarily via GFR, a portion is cleared by proximal tubular secretion. Several drugs, including cimetidine and trimethoprim, block this secretion, thereby increasing S_{Cr} without changing GFR (or BUN). This can lead to the misdiagnosis of ARF. Likewise, changes in BUN may reflect increased production (protein loading, gastrointestinal bleeding, catabolism due to corticosteroids or inflammation) or decreased production (malnutrition or liver failure).

The first step is to distinguish ARF from chronic renal failure (CRF) or from an acute decrement in GFR superimposed on long-standing, stable CRF. Unequivocal evidence of chronicity includes history or prior laboratory data, bilaterally small (<10 cm length) and echogenic kidneys on renal ultrasound, radiographic evidence of renal osteodystrophy, or broad (width >3× the size of a polymorphonuclear white blood cell) casts seen on careful urinalysis, which denote tubular dilatation in the setting of nephron loss. Additional evidence includes normocytic anemia, long-standing nocturia, and history of a disease that leads to renal failure (e.g., diabetes mellitus with long-standing proteinuria or autosomal-dominant polycystic kidney disease).

I. **Classification of Acute Renal Failure.** The primary causes of ARF can be classified as prerenal (renal hypoperfusion), intrinsic (damage to kidney parenchyma), or postrenal (obstruction). Oliguria is defined as a daily urine output of <500 ml and anuria as <100 ml.

A. **Prerenal Acute Renal Failure.** Prerenal ARF (PR ARF) occurs when actual or functional hypovolemia results in insufficient blood flow to the kidneys. Definitive diagnosis depends on improving GFR with volume repletion. Specific etiologies are discussed in Table 30.1.

Decreased renal perfusion leads to prostaglandin-dependent afferent arteriolar dilatation and angiotensin (Ang)-dependent efferent arteriolar constriction. Thus nonsteroidal antiinflammatory drugs, Ang-converting enzyme inhibitors, and Ang receptor blockers

TABLE 30.1.   Etiologies of prerenal acute renal failure

Intravascular volume depletion (effective)
    Cirrhosis
    Excessive use of diuretics
    Gastrointestinal fluid losses
    Hemorrhage
    Inadequate fluid replacement
    Nephrotic syndrome
    Renal fluid losses
    Third-spacing of fluid
Reduced cardiac output
    Cardiogenic shock
    Congestive heart failure
    Massive pulmonary embolism
    Pericardial tamponade
Systemic vasodilation
    Anaphylaxis
    Sepsis
    Vasodilator drugs
Renal vasoconstriction
    Acute hypercalcemia
    Drugs that block renal responses to volume depletion
    Early sepsis
    Hepatorenal syndrome
    Infused vasopressor drugs

can exacerbate ARF. Renal hypoperfusion is apparent from a reduced urinary Na and urea nitrogen concentration and a concentrated urine with a high specific gravity, urine osmolality, or urine Cr concentration. Increased urea reabsorption, out of proportion to the decrement in GFR, is detected by a rise in the serum BUN to Cr ratio. If hypovolemia is not corrected, PR ARF may progress to acute tubular necrosis (ATN). Common clues in the presentation of PR ARF are summarized in Table 30.2.

Hepatorenal Syndrome

Hepatorenal syndrome (HRS) is a severe and volume-unresponsive form of PR ARF, leading to a progressive renal failure in the setting of advanced liver disease (usually cirrhosis) in the absence of other identifiable causes. Oliguria results from intense renal vasoconstriction and systemic vasodilatation. The urine Na is usually <10 mEq/L, and fractional excretion of sodium (FE_{Na}) is <1%, even after a fluid challenge. HRS may be precipitated by infection or gastrointestinal bleeding. Patients with spontaneous bacterial peritonitis may have a lower incidence of HRS if treated with intravenous albumin in addition to antibiotics. Mortality remains >90%.

Management of Prerenal Acute Renal Failure

Volume resuscitation is essential in the management of PR ARF. Crystalloids (e.g., normal saline) are first-line replacement fluids, with colloids or blood as alterna-

TABLE 30.2. Clinical presentation of prerenal acute renal failure

History and symptoms	History of fluid loss (vomiting, diarrhea, burns)	Use of nonsteroidal antiinflammatory drugs, angiotensin-converting enzyme inhibitors, angiotensin receptor blockers, or calcineurin inhibitors, especially in setting of effective volume depletion	Negative fluid balance; output greater than input	Preexisting congestive heart failure or cirrhosis	Thirst
Signs	Orthostatic hypotension or tachycardia	Dry axillae	Flat neck veins in supine position	Dry skin and mucous membranes	Loss of tissue turgor

(continued)

TABLE 30.2.   (continued)

Labora-tory tests	Serum blood urea nitrogen to Cr ratio >20:1 (also seen with increased protein catabolism)	Urine specific gravity >1.03	Urine osmolality >500 mOsm/kg H_2O	U_{Na} <20 mEq/L	FE_{Na} <1%; $FE_{Na} = (U_{Na} \times S_{Cr})/(S_{Na} \times U_{Cr}) \times 100$	FE_{Un} <35%; $FE_{Un} = (U_{Un} \times S_{Cr})/(S_{Un} \times U_{Cr}) \times 100$	Urine sediment bland; may have hyaline or granular casts	Renal ultrasound; normal renal size and echogenicity

Cr, creatinine; FE_{Na}, fractional excretion of sodium; FE_{Un}, fractional excretion of urea nitrogen; S_{Cr}, serum creatine; S_{Na}, serum sodium; S_{Un}, serum urea nitrogen; U_{Cr}, urine creatinine; U_{Na}, urinary sodium concentration; U_{Un}, urine urea nitrogen.

TABLE 30.3. Some toxic causes of acute tubular necrosis

Exogenous
    Antibiotics (e.g., aminoglycosides, amphotericin B, pentamidine)
    Radiographic contrast
    Chemotherapeutic agents (e.g., cisplatin)
    Immunosuppressive agents (e.g., cyclosporin)
    Organic solvents (e.g., ethylene glycol)
    Heavy metals (e.g., mercury, lead, arsenic, bismuth)
Endogenous
    Myoglobin (from rhabdomyolysis)
    Hemoglobin

tives. It is difficult to restore effective renal perfusion in patients with redistribution of volume from the intravascular space (e.g., capillary leak, low serum albumin, congestive heart failure) without precipitating symptomatic volume overload or pulmonary edema. In these cases, packed red cell infusion and invasive monitoring should be considered.

B. Intrinsic Acute Renal Failure. Primary glomerular disease [glomerulonephritis (GN) or vasculitis] or tubular damage [ATN or acute interstitial nephritis (AIN)] can lead to intrinsic renal failure.

Acute Tubular Necrosis

Decreased renal perfusion leading to ischemia accounts for ~50% of ATN, whereas nephrotoxins, such as aminoglycosides and radiocontrast agents, account for 30% (Table 30.3). Renal dysfunction from ATN appears within hours to days and lasts from 1 week to 1 year. Because it results from irreversible cellular injury, neither hemodynamic normalization nor removal of the toxic insult restores normal function. However, restoration of normal renal perfusion should be a goal in all cases of ATN because autoregulation is impaired in the injured kidney, rendering it more susceptible to recurrent injury from even mild hypotension.

ATN is characterized by impaired tubular transport, intratubular obstruction, backleak of ultrafiltrate, and decreased renal cortical perfusion, resulting in decreased GFR, progressive azotemia, and impaired fluid and electrolyte handling. Laboratory abnormalities may include hyperkalemia, anion gap metabolic acidosis, hyponatremia, hyperphosphatemia, hypermagnesemia, hypocalcemia, and hyperuricemia. A diagnostic urine sediment may reveal free tubular epithelial cells with tubular epithelial cell casts. Many coarsely granular pigmented or muddy brown casts are suggestive of ATN. A urine Na >40 mEq/L and an FE_{Na} >1% in the setting of oliguria suggest ATN. However, FE_{Na} <1% may be observed early in nonoliguric ATN secondary to radiocontrast agents, rhabdomyolysis, or severe renal hypoperfusion due to hepatic failure, sepsis, burn injury, or congestive heart failure (Table 30.4).

TABLE 30.4. Clinical presentation of acute tubular necrosis

History and symptoms	Recent hypotension, shock, especially in the setting of anesthesia or sepsis	Recent nephrotoxin exposure				
Laboratory tests	Serum blood urea nitrogen to Cr ratio ~8–10:1	Urine specific gravity 1.010–10.012	Urine osmolality <350 mOsm/kg H_2O	Urine Na >40 mEq/L	FE_{Na} >2%; FE_{Na} = $(U_{Na} \times S_{Cr})/(S_{Na} \times U_{Cr}) \times 100$	FE_{Un} >35%; FE_{Un} = $(U_{Un} \times S_{Cr})/(S_{Un} \times U_{Cr}) \times 100$	Urine sediment with renal tubular cells, tubular cell casts, pigmented granular casts

Cr, creatinine; FE_{Na}, fractional excretion of sodium; FE_{Un}, fractional excretion of urea nitrogen; S_{Cr}, serum creatine; S_{Na}, serum sodium; S_{Un}, serum urea nitrogen; U_{Na}, urinary sodium concentration; U_{Cr}, urine creatinine; U_{Un}, urine urea nitrogen.

Aminoglycoside-Induced Acute Tubular Necrosis

Aminoglycoside-induced ATN is usually nonoliguric and not evident until 7–10 days of treatment. Advanced age, preexisting renal insufficiency, volume depletion, higher dosage, and exposure to other nephrotoxins increase the risk. All aminoglycosides are nephrotoxic. Once-daily administration may decrease the risk of aminoglycoside nephrotoxicity. Monitoring peak and trough levels is prudent but does not eliminate the risk.

Radiocontrast-Induced Acute Tubular Necrosis (Contrast Nephropathy)

Radiocontrast-induced ATN occurs in up to 50% of high-risk patients who have volume depletion, preexisting renal insufficiency, or diabetes mellitus. The BUN and S_{Cr} rise 24–48 hours after contrast administration, peak at 3–5 days, and may return to normal in 5–7 days. A low FE_{Na} and a high urine specific gravity may be seen soon after contrast injury, but there is loss of urinary concentration in established ATN. After repleting any volume deficit, 0.9% saline should be infused to maintain urine output at 1–2 ml/min before and for 12 hours after contrast exposure. Metaanalyses suggest that N-acetylcysteine also may decrease the risk of contrast nephropathy. Nonionic contrast agents are preferred in patients with preexisting renal insufficiency. Dopamine or fenoldopam is of no benefit in preventing contrast nephropathy. Diuretics increase the risk of nephrotoxicity.

Amphotericin B–Induced Acute Tubular Necrosis

The risk of nephrotoxicity increases with the dose and duration of treatment. Patients with chronic renal insufficiency and those receiving diuretics are at an increased risk. Distal nephron damage is manifested as polyuria secondary to nephrogenic diabetes insipidus, hypokalemia, hypomagnesemia, and renal tubular acidosis. Lipid complexed formulations are less nephrotoxic.

Rhabdomyolysis-Induced Acute Tubular Necrosis

Rhabdomyolysis sufficient to cause ATN can be caused by

- Muscle damage from trauma, pressure, crush, burns, or ischemia
- Increased muscle metabolism (e.g., seizures, exercise, heat stroke, myopathy)
- Metabolic disorders (e.g., ketoacidosis, hypokalemia, hypophosphatemia)
- Toxins (e.g., alcohol, carbon monoxide, statin drugs)
- Severe infections
- Drugs (e.g., statins)

The clinical features include muscle pain, dark brown urine, urine dipstick positive for blood (heme) in the absence of both apparent free hemoglobin and urinary red blood cells, hyperkalemia, hyperphosphatemia, hyperuricemia, and early hypocalcemia with hypercalcemia developing later. Elevated levels of serum creatine kinase, myoglobin, and urine myoglobin support the diagnosis.

ATN can be prevented by aggressive volume replacement with isotonic saline from 200 to 1,500 cc/hr. This must be initiated without delay. Once urine output is evident, forced alkaline diuresis may prevent cast formation. The goal of therapy is to increase urine output to >100 cc/hr, with a pH >6.5. This therapy should be terminated if the patient is anuric. Alkalemia may cause a fall in ionized calcium. Conversely, hypocalcemia should not be corrected unless the patient is symptomatic, because hypercalcemia frequently develops during the recovery phase.

Multiple Myeloma

Multiple myeloma may cause ARF even before diagnosis of the underlying condition. The ARF is accompanied by anemia, hypercalcemia, and elevated serum globulins (see Chapter 11). Hypercalcemia can cause volume depletion and intrarenal vasoconstriction, leading to PR ARF, whereas ATN, cast nephropathy, primary amyloidosis, and light chain deposition disease may cause intrinsic ARF. Monoclonal immunoglobulin light chains are not detected by standard dipstick tests, whereas sulfosalicylic acid detects all urinary proteins. Sulfosalicylic acid, urine and serum electrophoresis, and immunofixation are indicated if multiple myeloma is suspected.

Glomerulonephritis, Vasculitis, Acute Renovascular Disease, or Interstitial Nephritis

GN or vasculitis should be suspected as a cause of ARF in the setting of a multisystem illness with proteinuria and an active urine sediment (see Chapter 8). There may be a history of autoimmune disease, recent infection, or hepatitis. Signs and symptoms of GN or vasculitis may include fever, skin rash, arthralgias, hemoptysis, hypertension, and volume overload. Laboratory assays may reveal an elevated erythrocyte sedimentation rate; hypocomplementemia; and autoantibodies, including anti–double-stranded DNA or antineutrophil cytoplasmic antibodies. Careful urinalysis is key. Final diagnosis often depends on renal biopsy or angiography.

AIN is often precipitated by drugs and accompanied by eosinophilia, eosinophiluria, fever, and rash. Tubular function abnormalities may exceed the decrement in GFR. Pyuria or white blood cell casts in the absence of urinary tract infection or GN are suggestive.

Acute renovascular causes of ischemic ATN include thrombosis, dissection of aortic aneurysms, or renal arteries that often complicate trauma or a vascular intervention. Cholesterol renal atheroembolic disease usually follows an intravascular procedure. It is often associated with other signs of systemic emboli in the skin or nail beds, with fever, elevated erythrocyte sedimentation rate, hypocomplementemia, and eosinophilia. Renal vein thrombosis can complicate severe nephrotic syndrome or genetic thrombophilias. It may present as decreased renal function with flank pain and hematuria. Thrombotic microangiopathy should be suspected when ARF is accompanied by thrombocytopenia, intravascular hemolysis, fever, and neurologic abnormalities.

Pregnancy-Related Acute Renal Failure

ATN can complicate septic abortion, severe preeclampsia, placental abruption, peripartum hemorrhage, amniotic fluid embolism, or prolonged intrauterine fetal demise. Severe ATN in pregnancy may progress to irreversible cortical necrosis. Other rare disorders include ATN in the setting of acute fatty liver of pregnancy and a thrombotic microangiopathy that characterizes idiopathic postpartum ARF.

C. **Postrenal (Obstructive) Acute Renal Failure.** Obstruction of urine flow at any point from the tubules to the urethral outlet may result in postrenal ARF. Even partial obstruction with preserved urine output may decrease GFR. It is crucial to diagnose functional obstruction because bladder catheterization, urethral dilation and stenting, or percutaneous nephrostomy may restore and preserve renal function. Obstructive symptoms or the use of anticholinergic medications should raise suspicion. To cause clinically apparent ARF, obstruction must be bilateral or affect a single functioning kidney (Table 30.5). Urine chemistries early in the course of obstructive uropathy may resemble those in PR ARF due to solute reabsorption from relatively stagnant tubular fluid. Unequivocal diagnosis may depend on a furosemide renogram (see Chapter 3), retrograde pyelography, or response to urinary drainage.

Crystal-Induced Acute Renal Failure

Obstructive ARF may result from intratubular deposition of uric acid crystals during chemotherapy for malignancies with high cell turnover such as leukemia, aggressive lymphomas, or sarcomas. The collecting system is not dilatated. Therefore, imaging strategies are fruitless. Aggressive hydration, alkaline diuresis, and allopurinol may prevent renal failure. Allopurinol should be started several days before chemotherapy and maintained during induction. The benefits of alkaline diuresis may be limited because it may precipitate calcium phosphate. Recombinant urate oxidase may be preferable. Crystal-induced intratubular obstruction also may complicate therapy with high-dose acyclovir or indinavir.

II. **Making the Diagnosis of Acute Renal Failure.** The focus in diagnosing ARF should be on the time course of renal failure, its relationship to possible inciting factors, and an assessment of volume status and relevant comorbidities. Changes in S_{Cr} lag behind changes in GFR. Urinalysis requires a fresh urine specimen. It is often more sensitive when the sediment is stained with drops of methylene blue. Bladder catheterization is required when urine output is uncertain or obstruction is possible. The kidneys of most

TABLE 30.5. Clinical presentation of obstructive uropathy

History and symptoms	Elderly man (with presumed prostatism).	Previous urinary tract obstruction	Bilateral nephrolithiasis	Symptoms of bladder outflow obstruction (e.g., dysuria, nocturia, frequency, hesitation)	Symptoms of autonomic neuropathy or use of anticholinergic medications	Predisposition to papillary necrosis (e.g., diabetes mellitus, sickle cell disease, analgesic abuse).
Signs	Complete anuria or wide fluctuations in urine output. However, urine output may seem normal.	Distended bladder on physical examination	Urine specific gravity >1.02 acutely but lower with chronic obstruction	Large post-voiding residual urine volume on bladder catheterization or renal ultrasound		
Laboratory tests	Blood urea nitrogen to creatinine ratio may be normal or elevated.	Urine osmolality >400 mOsm/kg H_2O acutely but ~300 chronically	Urine Na <20 mEq/L acutely, >40 mEq/L chronically	FE_{Na} <1% acutely but >1% chronically	Urine sediment bland	Renal ultrasound shows dilatated collecting system above the level of obstruction, but may be falsely negative early or with advanced renal failure.

Additional column: Pelvic or retroperitoneal disease or surgery (History and symptoms).

FE_{Na}, fractional excretion of sodium.

ARF patients should be imaged by ultrasound. Subsequent evaluation often includes calculation of urinary diagnostic indices, then other laboratory tests or therapeutic trials focused on specific diagnoses.

Urinalysis should always include dipstick measures of urinary concentration, blood, protein, and pH. Suspected proteinuria should be confirmed by a quantitative assay indexed to urine Cr. The urine sediment may provide unequivocal diagnosis of ATN or GN. Hospital laboratories often fail to identify cellular casts, perhaps because they disintegrate before examination. Urinary eosinophils are best detected using Hansel's stain. Their presence is consistent with, but not diagnostic of, AIN.

Estimates of GFR by 24-hour Cr clearance or by formulae (see Chapter 3) usually underestimate the severity of ARF because Cr is not in a steady state after an abrupt decrease in GFR.

The FE_{Na} can often distinguish ATN from PR ARF but may fail to distinguish PR from obstructive ARF. It may be falsely elevated after administration of diuretics, when the fractional excretion of urea may be preferable.

III. Management. The clinical course of ARF can be divided into three phases:

- Initial phase: The period between the exposure to an insult and a fall in renal function when renal damage potentially can be reversed.
- Maintenance phase: May last from days to weeks or, occasionally, up to 2 months, during which renal damage cannot be reversed. Patients may be anuric, oliguric, or nonoliguric.
- Recovery phase: Marked by a return of serum BUN and Cr toward normal. Patients may enter a polyuric phase that can cause fluid and electrolyte abnormalities. Recovery of renal function may be incomplete.

Reversible causes of renal dysfunction must be sought and treated expeditiously. It is essential to maintain hemodynamics, as the ATN kidney is particularly susceptible to recurrent injury. High doses of diuretics (up to 400 mg of furosemide intravenously or infusion of 10–15 mg/hr) may increase urine output in oliguric ATN. Conversion of oliguric to nonoliguric ATN does not alter prognosis but identifies a less severely injured subgroup and can sometimes avoid the severe volume overload that limits nutrition and precipitates the need for dialysis. High doses of loop diuretics are ototoxic (see Chapter 24).

After intravascular volume is normalized, fluids should be matched to urine output plus insensible losses. Daily intake of sodium generally should be limited to <2 g (86 mEq) and potassium to <1.5 g (40 mEq). Hyponatremia may be avoided by restricting free water. Hyperkalemia should be treated with glucose and insulin, sodium bicarbonate (if the serum bicarbonate is low), sodium polystyrene sulfonate resin, intravenous calcium gluconate for cardiac instability, and dialysis (see Chapter 16). Serum pH should be maintained >7.20. Hyperphosphatemia should be controlled with phosphate binders, whereas hypocalcemia should be treated only if the patient is symptomatic (see Chapter 18).

ARF is a hypercatabolic state, but nutritional support has not been shown to be beneficial. Enteral nutrition is preferred to parenteral support but should not include more than 1.5 g of protein/kg/day. Drug doses should be adjusted (see Chapter 29). Magnesium- and phosphorous-containing medications should be avoided. Indications for dialysis are given in Chapter 33. Hemodialysis, continuous renal replacement therapy, and peritoneal dialysis are effective in treating metabolic abnormalities and fluid overload. Intermittent or continuous renal replacement therapy results may not change mortality.

IV. Prognosis. The prognosis of PR or postrenal ARF is relatively good if the precipitating insult is corrected. Intrinsic causes of ARF have poorer prognosis. The mortality from ATN is 38% among hospitalized patients and 79% among patients in the intensive care unit. Mortality increases with age, comorbidities, multiorgan failure, sepsis, and oliguria.

V. Suggested Readings

Bellomo R, Kellum JA, Ronco C. Defining acute renal failure: physiological principles. *Intensive Care Med* 2004;30:33–37.

Brady HR, Wilcox CS, eds. *Therapy in nephrology and hypertension: a companion to Brenner and Rector's the kidney*, 2nd ed. Philadelphia: WB Saunders, 2003:3–91.

Carvounis CP, Niser S, Guro-Razuman S. Significance of the fractional excretion of urea in the differential diagnosis of acute renal failure. *Kidney Int* 2002;62:2223–2229.

Esson ML, Schrier RW. Diagnosis and treatment of acute tubular necrosis. *Ann Intern Med* 2002;137:744–752.

Gines P, Guerara M, Arroyo V, Rodes J. Hepatorenal syndrome. *Lancet* 2003;362:1819–1827.

McGee S, Abernethy WB 3rd, Simel DL. The rational clinical examination: is this patient hypovolemic? *JAMA* 1999; 281:1022–1029.

Molitoris BA, Finn WF, eds. *Acute renal failure: a companion to Brenner and Rector's the kidney*. Philadelphia: WB Saunders, 2001.

Chronic Renal Failure

Francisco Llach

Chronic renal failure (CRF) is irreversible loss of renal function. End-stage renal disease (ESRD) is advanced CRF requiring dialysis or kidney transplantation.

I. **Pathophysiology.** Loss of nephron mass results in structural and functional hypertrophy of the remaining nephrons. The single nephron plasma flow and intraglomerular pressure increase as a result of preferential vasodilation of the afferent arterioles. Proximal reabsorption of NaCl, fluid, and phosphate and collecting duct secretion of K^+ and H^+ are enhanced. These adaptations initially restore homeostasis, but glomerular hyperfiltration contributes to ongoing glomerular injury, autodestruction glomerular sclerosis, and further loss of renal function.

Growth factors such as transforming growth factor-β, platelet-derived growth factor, osteopontin, angiotensin II, and endothelin contribute to interstitial fibrosis. The reduction in glomerular filtration rate (GFR) correlates with the degree of interstitial and tubular fibrosis.

II. **Clinical Predictors of Accelerated Progression to End-Stage Renal Disease.** The clinical predictors of accelerated progression to end-stage renal disease are detailed in Table 31.1.

III. **Incidence and Prevalence of Chronic Kidney Disease.** Etiologies of chronic kidney disease (CKD) are listed in Table 31.2. The National Kidney Foundation (Kidney Disease Outcomes Quality Initiative)–recommended staging of CKD is outlined in Table 31.3.

IV. **Stages of Chronic Kidney Disease and Cardiovascular Disease.** Patients with CKD are at increased risk for coronary artery disease, cerebrovascular disease, peripheral vascular disease, and congestive heart failure (CHF) (Fig. 31.1). Both traditional and nontraditional cardiovascular risk factors contribute. All patients with CKD should be considered in the highest risk group for cardiovascular disease, regardless of presence of traditional risk factors. Cardiovascular disease accounts for 40–50% of all deaths in the stage 5 CKD population, and cardiovascular mortality rates in CKD patients are approximately 15 times higher than in the general population. Forty percent of patients starting dialysis already have evidence of coronary artery disease, and only 15% are considered to have normal left ventricular structure and function by echocardiography.

V. **Uremic Syndrome.** Uremia results from retention of end products of protein metabolism. Administration of urea causes only mild symptoms. Other potential uremic toxins

TABLE 31.1.   Factors contributing to the progression of chronic renal failure

Degree of systemic and intraglomerular hypertension
Severity of proteinuria
Glomerular hypertrophy with increase of vessel wall stress
Hyperlipidemia (increased low-density lipoprotein cholesterol, low-density lipoprotein)
Impaired prostaglandin generation with the use of nonsteroidal anti-inflammatory drugs
High-protein diet
Persistent metabolic acidosis and increased ammonia production
Extent of tubulointerstitial disease

TABLE 31.2.   Etiology of end-stage renal disease

Condition	Fraction of total patients (%)
Diabetes mellitus	39
Hypertension and large-vessel disease	28
Glomerulonephritis, primary or secondary	13
Hereditary cystic and congenital renal disease	4
Interstitial nephritis and pyelonephritis	4
Neoplasm/tumor	2
Miscellaneous	3
Missing	3

TABLE 31.3.   Progression and prevalence of chronic kidney disease by stage of disease

Stage	Glomerular filtration rate (ml/min/1.73 m^2)	Number of individuals (% of population)
1	Normal with persistent albuminuria	5.9 million (3.3)
2	60–89 with persistent albuminuria	5.3 million (3.0)
3	30–59	7.6 million (4.3)
4	15–29	400,000 (0.2)
5	<15 or renal replacement therapy	300,000 (0.2)

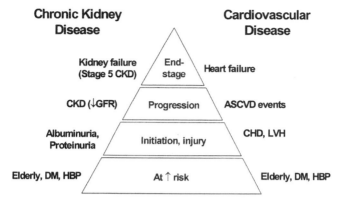

FIG. 31.1. Stages of kidney and cardiovascular disease. ASCVD, atherosclerotic cardiovascular disease; CHD, coronary heart disease; CKD, chronic kidney disease; DM, diabetes mellitus; GFR, glomerular filtration rate; HBP, high blood pressure; LVH, left ventricular hypertrophy.

include guanidine, guanidinosuccinic acid, β_2-microglobulin, hippurate, homocysteine, parathyroid hormone (PTH), phenols, phosphates, polyamines, asymmetric dimethyl arginine, and purines. Symptoms are common when the creatinine clearance falls below 15 ml/min, but diabetics become symptomatic earlier.

VI. **Metabolic and Electrolyte Abnormalities in Chronic Renal Failure**

A. **Carbohydrate Intolerance.** Insulin is degraded by the liver and kidneys. However, the decrease in insulin clearance is generally offset by peripheral insulin resistance. Hyperparathyroidism inhibits insulin secretion and worsens glucose intolerance. There is generally a decrease in requirements for insulin and oral hypoglycemic agents in diabetic patients as they develop renal failure.

B. **Hyperlipidemia.** Decreased plasma levels of high-density lipoprotein cholesterol and increased plasma levels of triglycerides and lipoprotein(a) antigen are common in CRF. These adverse lipid changes are usually mitigated by a decreased level of low-density lipoprotein cholesterol due to a decrease in lipoprotein lipase activity. The dyslipidemia can be ascribed primarily to hyperparathyroidism and insulin resistance.

C. **Fluid and Electrolytes.** There is an impaired ability to excrete because of defective tubular function and a reduction in the GFR resulting in a subtle or overt expansion of the plasma and extracellular fluid volumes, salt-sensitive hypertension, and edema. Hyponatremia can result from failure to excrete free water when intakes exceed 1.5 L/day. Hypertension is common unless Na^+ intake is restricted to 100 mEq/day.

Some patients with tubulointerstitial disease or primary diseases of the medulla cannot conserve NaCl and develop orthostatic hypotension and prerenal azotemia. These patients with salt-losing nephropathy require stepwise increases in NaCl and fluid intake.

K^+ elimination in CRF is initially maintained by enhanced K^+ secretion by surviving nephrons and by colonic K^+ secretion dictated by aldosterone stimulated by hyperkalemia and metabolic acidosis. However, as the GFR decreases, K^+ elimination is curtailed. Cellular K^+ uptake is impaired by insulin resistance, β_2-adrenergic resistance, decreased Na^+/K^+-ATPase activity, and metabolic acidosis. Therefore, hyperkalemia is frequent in CRF.

D. **Acid–Base Abnormalities.** Metabolic acidosis in CRF occurs primarily because of a defect in ammoniagenesis that limits distal tubular H^+ trapping as NH_4^+ and, hence, decreases renal bicarbonate regeneration. Additionally, there may be proximal HCO_3^- wasting or reduced distal H^+ secretion. Chronic metabolic acidosis should be corrected because it is accompanied by skeletal demineralization. As the GFR falls below 10 ml/min, there is a progressive retention of organic acids that raises the anion gap with a reciprocal fall in serum $[HCO_3^-]$.

E. **Calcium and Phosphate Abnormalities and Renal Osteodystrophy.** Phosphate retention and metabolic acidosis begin when the GFR is less than 25 ml/min. Acidosis increases bone resorption and serum calcium and phosphate concentrations. Hyperphosphatemia, per se, increases PTH secretion, reduces ionized serum calcium, and inhibits the renal hydroxylation of $25(OH)D_3$ to its active metabolite, $1,25(OH)_2D_3$ (calcitriol), thereby decreasing intestinal absorption of Ca. The resulting hypocalcemia increases PTH further.

Hyperphosphatemia (>6–6.5 mg/dl) is an independent factor in the increased morbidity and mortality of stage 5 CKD patients from cardiovascular events. Furthermore, hyperphosphatemia, an increase in the calcium–phosphorus product (>55 mg^2/dl^2), and an increase in the total calcium load (dietary + dialysate) predict coronary artery calcifications ($>50\%$ of stage 5 CKD patients) as evaluated by electron beam computed tomography.

Renal osteodystrophy is classified in Table 31.4. Adynamic bone disease (low bone turnover) now occurs in 30–40% of stage 5 CKD patients because of overtreatment with large doses of calcium-containing phosphorus binders and the overuse of nonselective vitamin D compounds, which cause hypercalcemia and oversuppression of PTH. Adynamic bone disease has also been observed in elderly diabetic patients and in those receiving peritoneal dialysis using a high dialysate $[Ca^{2+}]$ (3.5 mEq/L). Proximal muscle weakness, bone pain, and bone fractures occur late in the course of CKD and reflect severe high bone turnover (secondary hyperpara-

TABLE 31.4. Different forms of renal osteodystrophy

Type of bone disease	Prevalence (%)
High-turnover bone disease	
Osteitis fibrosa cystica	50–70
Mixed uremic osteodystrophy	10
Low-turnover bone disease	
Adynamic bone disease	30–40
Osteomalacia	<5

thyroidism). This can be prevented with early therapy to control hyperphosphatemia with non–calcium-containing phosphorus binders and new selective vitamin D analogs such as paricalcitol.

VII. Cardiovascular Abnormalities of End-Stage Renal Disease

A. Hypertension. Hypertension occurs in 85–95% of patients with ESRD. It is ascribed primarily to excessive salt and water retention, but inappropriate secretion of renin and angiotensin and increased sympathetic tone contribute. Blood vessels generate excessive quantities of the vasoconstrictor endothelin and diminished quantities of the vasodilator nitric oxide. Treatment of hypertension slows the progression of renal failure in those with moderate or heavy proteinuria.

B. Cardiomyopathy and Pericarditis. The prevalence of left ventricular hypertrophy, coronary artery disease, and CHF is increased two- to fivefold in ESRD. Approximately one-half of all hemodialysis patients have significant ischemic heart disease. Dyslipidemia, hypertension, hyperhomocystinemia, diabetes mellitus, and insulin resistance contribute to atherosclerosis.

Diastolic dysfunction commonly causes heart failure and hypertension in ESRD. Other causes of cardiac dysfunction include hyperparathyroidism, amyloidosis, and iron overload. Anemia aggravates left ventricular hypertrophy.

Pericarditis can present with a sharp pericardial chest pain that changes with breathing or posture and is accompanied by a rub. Pericardial fluid is usually hemorrhagic, and tamponade can occur. Some patients have milder uremic pericarditis that responds to extra dialysis.

VIII. Neuromuscular Abnormalities. Central nervous system (CNS) dysfunction is characterized by decreased attention span, agitation, confusion, insomnia, and impaired memory. Patients may develop depression, hallucinations, delusions, hiccups, cramps, asterixis, myoclonus, fasciculation, and seizures.

Peripheral neuropathy is usually symmetric and preferentially affects the lower extremities. Sensory involvement precedes motor dysfunction. Restless legs syndrome and burning feet are early phases of uremic peripheral neuropathy. Postural hypotension can be a manifestation of autonomic dysfunction.

IX. **Hematologic Abnormalities**

   A. **Anemia.** The hematocrit falls as the serum creatinine increases >2–3 mg/dl (see Chapter 36).

   B. **Uremic Bleeding Diathesis.** Uremic bleeding diathesis causes frequent bruising, ecchymoses, and bleeding from mucous membranes and, occasionally, subdural hematomas. There is a defect in platelet function that impairs platelet activation and adhesion to the endothelium. This has been ascribed to abnormalities of the von Willebrand factor, which facilitates the interaction between platelets and endothelium through its binding to platelet glycoprotein (IIb–IIIa) receptors. Anemia exacerbates uremic bleeding. Erythrocytes enhance platelet function by increasing the interaction of platelets with the vessel wall.

X. **Gastrointestinal Abnormalities.** Gastrointestinal complaints include anorexia and early morning nausea and vomiting. As renal failure progresses, patients may develop uremic fetor, stomatitis, esophagitis, gastritis, duodenitis, and peptic ulcer disease. Gastrin is degraded by the liver and the kidney and has a prolonged half-life in CRF. Gastroparesis and gastrointestinal bleeding are increased by vascular ectasia and peptic ulcer disease.

XI. **Dermatologic Abnormalities.** Uremic pruritus is related to calcium and phosphorus deposition (secondary hyperparathyroidism), hypercalcemia, peripheral neuropathy, dry skin, and anemia. The most important cause is inadequate dialysis therapy. A yellow discoloration is related to the retention of urochrome pigments and urea.

XII. **Evaluation of Chronic Renal Failure.** The history should document the presence of uremic symptoms and possible etiology from diabetes mellitus, hypertension, CHF, multiple myeloma, or prolonged intake of nonsteroidal antiinflammatory drugs. A family history suggests the diagnosis of polycystic kidney disease or hereditary nephritis. A reduced kidney size by ultrasound imaging suggests CRF, although patients with diabetic nephropathy, amyloid, or multiple myeloma often have large kidneys. The degree of renal insufficiency may be determined by measuring blood urea nitrogen, serum creatinine, and creatinine clearance or by nuclear medicine methods (see Chapter 3). Volume depletion and obstructive nephropathy should be identified and treated promptly.

XIII. **Prevention of Progression of Renal Disease.** Prevention of the progression of renal disease is discussed in Chapter 32.

XIV. **Management of Complications of Chronic Renal Failure**

   A. **Fluid and Electrolyte Disorders.** Dietary NaCl restriction is required to control hypertension and prevent edema. The goal should be a daily Na^+ intake of <100 mEq. More severe restriction to 80 mEq is needed for severe hypertension or diuretic resistance. Frequently, loop diuretics are also required (see Chapter 24). Hyponatremia is treated by fluid restriction (1–1.5 L/day). Hyperkalemia is a life-threatening complication. Exogenous sources of potassium (foods with high K^+ content, such as citrus fruits, chocolate, dried fruits, and salt substitutes) and medications that can cause hyperkalemia (angiotensin-converting enzyme inhibitors, angiotensin receptor blockers, nonsteroidal antiinflammatory drugs, K^+-sparing diuretics, beta blockers, and heparin) should be discontinued. Patients with hyperkalemia and electrocardiographic changes should be treated promptly with intravenous calcium gluconate or calcium chloride (10 ml of 10% solutions) followed by an infusion of 25 ml of 50% dextrose solutions with insulin. A β_2-adrenergic agonist (nebulized albuterol) is a useful adjunct to lower serum potassium. Bicarbonate administration lowers serum potassium more gradually over 6–24 hours (see Chapter 16). Oral alkali supplementation with sodium bicarbonate or citrate (650 mg or 8 mEq/tablet) should be instituted if the serum bicarbonate concentration falls below 15–17 mEq/L. Sodium citrate should be avoided in patients taking aluminum-containing antacids, as it enhances intestinal aluminum absorption.

B. **Hyperphosphatemia and Secondary Hyperparathyroidism.** Dietary phosphorus intake in moderate or severe CRF must be reduced to <10 mg/kg/day. Adequate control of hyperphosphatemia (phosphorus <5.5–6 mg/dl) requires phosphorus binders. Calcium-containing phosphorus binders such as calcium carbonate (Oscal, Tums) or calcium acetate (Phoslo) have been related to coronary artery calcifications. Thus, non–calcium-containing phosphorus binders such as sevelamer hydrochloride (RenaGel) are now preferred. This has been shown in randomized studies to decrease the severity of coronary artery calcification. Another new binder, lanthanum carbonate, is effective and safe.

Vitamin D (calcitriol) is usually required to replace decreased renal production of calcitriol. It must be withheld until the serum phosphate concentration has been controlled to <6 mg/dl because it may cause diffuse soft tissue calcification. The usual starting dose is 0.25 µg daily, which is increased in 2- to 4-week intervals to normalize the serum calcium concentration.

Vitamin D compounds can cause hypercalcemia and hyperphosphatemia, which may increase coronary calcification. Paricalcitol (Zemplar 19-nor-1α, 25-dihydroxyvitamin D_2) is an analog that inhibits PTH synthesis and causes these adverse effects less commonly. It is effective therapy for secondary hyperparathyroidism of stage 5 CKD patients. The initial dose (in µg per dialysis) can be calculated by dividing the PTH level by 100.

Parathyroidectomy is indicated for secondary hyperparathyroidism (PTH >800 pg/ml), with symptoms of bone disease (myopathy or bone pain), persistent hyperphosphatemia, and/or soft tissue calcification that are refractory to appropriate paricalcitol therapy.

C. Anemia. Anemia is discussed in Chapter 36.

D. Hyperlipidemia. The goal for management of hyperlipidemia should be to maintain the low-density lipoprotein cholesterol <100 mg/dl. Patients should be started on a step I American Heart Association diet that provides <30% of total calories from fat and <300 mg cholesterol daily. If goals are not achieved, drug therapy with hydroxy-3-methylglutaryl coenzyme A reductase inhibitors is usually indicated. In patients who are refractory to monotherapy, nicotinic acid may be added. Nicotinic acid specifically reduces the elevated levels of lipoprotein(a) antigen in CRF.

XV. Suggested Readings

Coresh J, Astor BC, Greene T, et al. Prevalence of chronic kidney disease and decreased kidney function in the adult US population: third national health and nutrition examination survey. *Am J Kidney Dis* 2003;41:1–12.

Ganesh SK, Stack AG, Levin NW, et al. Association of elevated serum PO(4), Ca × PO(4) product, and parathyroid hormone with cardiac mortality risk in chronic hemodialysis patients. *J Am Soc Nephrol* 2001;12(10):2131–2138.

Kopple JD, Levey AS, Greene T, et al., for the Modification of Diet in Renal Disease Study Group. Effect of dietary protein restriction on nutritional status in the Modification of Diet in Renal Disease Study. *Kidney Int* 1997;52:778–791.

Llach F, Yudd M. Paricalcitol in dialysis patients with calcitriol-resistant secondary hyperparathyroidism. *Am J Kidney Dis* 2001;38[Suppl 5]:S45–S50.

National Kidney Foundation. K/DOQI clinical practice guidelines. *Am J Kidney Dis* October 2003;42[Suppl 3]:S52–S102.

Prevention of Progression of Chronic Kidney Disease and Its Cardiovascular Complications

Awad A. El-Magbri and Shakil Aslam

Some interventions can slow the otherwise relentless progression of chronic kidney disease (CKD) to end-stage renal disease (ESRD). In addition the progressive decline in glomerular filtration rate (GFR) is associated with several complications, including a many-fold increased risk for cardiovascular disease (CVD).

I. **Mechanisms of Progression of Chronic Kidney Disease.** The response to renal injury follows common pathways of progression. Hyperfiltration in remaining glomeruli initially maintains the GFR but leads to intraglomerular hypertension and glomerular hypertrophy that worsen proteinuria and eventually cause glomerulosclerosis. This is apparent as worsening proteinuria and a progressive decline in GFR. The high-molecular-weight proteinuria accompanying many glomerular diseases may contribute directly to the progression of CKD, whereas minimal-change disease with extensive albuminuria rarely progresses to ESRD. Some of the filtered protein is reabsorbed by the proximal tubular cells, where it induces proinflammatory cytokines, including nuclear factor-κB; RANTES (regulated on activation, normally T cell expressed and secreted); monocyte chemoattractant protein-1; complement components; transforming growth factor-β; and endothelin. Angiotensin II, acting on type I receptors, is implicated in activation of these cytokines, which leads to an influx of inflammatory cells in the renal parenchyma, causing tubulointerstitial injury and, eventually, fibrosis. The degree of tubulointerstitial injury on biopsy predicts the progression of CKD. Reduction in proteinuria in experimental models ameliorates these changes.

II. **Risk Factors for Progression of Chronic Kidney Disease.** Proteinuria and its response to therapy are strong predictors of CKD progression. In the African American Study of Kidney Disease and Hypertension, the patients with a urinary protein to creatinine ratio >0.22 exhibited a twofold higher rate of decline in GFR. Proteinuria >3 g/day portends a poor renal prognosis. Patients who have increased excretion of α_1-microglobulin, β_2-microglobulin, immunoglobulin (Ig) G, and IgM are also at higher risk of progression.

Hypertension predicts a faster decline in proteinuric renal diseases.

Ethnicity is important in the progression of CKD. Black patients with diabetes have a two- to threefold higher risk for development of ESRD compared with whites. Modifiable factors, such as lack of access to medical care, socioeconomic status, and lifestyle, explain less than one-half of the increased risk for ESRD in blacks, indicating a genetic predisposition to CKD.

Dyslipidemia was predictive of the development of ESRD in the Multiple Risk Factor Intervention Trial. However, clinical trials have yet to show that lipid-lowering therapy delays the progression of CKD. The National Cholesterol Education Program Guidelines should be followed in patients with CKD. Low levels of serum high-density lipoprotein and transferrin were predictors of CKD progression in the Modification of Diet in Renal Disease trial.

Smoking is associated with CKD progression. Smoking cessation slows the decline in GFR in type I diabetic patients.

III. **Prevention of Progression of Chronic Kidney Disease.** CKD is a multisystem disease with predictable complications as GFR declines. The treatment of its major complications improves morbidity and mortality. A multidisciplinary approach involving the primary care physician, a dietitian, and a nephrologist should be adopted.

A. **Treatment of Hypertension and Choice of Agent.** Hypertension can be a cause or a complication of CKD. It is an important contributor to progression of CKD. Treatment of hypertension is the cornerstone of therapy to delay progression of CKD. The target blood pressure (BP) goal and the choice of antihypertensive agent are controversial. The approach should be tailored to the patient's underlying renal disease and other comorbid conditions, including cerebrovascular and cardiovascular disease. Only patients with >1 g/day of proteinuria benefit from more aggressive control of hypertension. The VII Joint National Commission on the Detection, Evaluation and Treatment of Hypertension recommends a BP target of <130/80 mm Hg in patients with CKD and diabetes. This usually requires two to three antihypertensive drugs.

Several randomized trials have shown that angiotensin-converting enzyme inhibitors (ACEIs) and angiotensin receptor blockers (ARBs) are superior to other agents in delaying progression of renal disease in diabetes (e.g., the Collaborative Study Group, IDNT, IRMA, and RENAAL) and in other proteinuric (>1 g/day) nephropathies (e.g., AIPRI and REIN) (see Chapter 26, Table 26.3). This renoprotective effect appears to be somewhat independent of BP lowering, but this remains controversial. However, the UKPDS trial failed to show superiority of an ACEI over a beta blocker in patients with diabetes (see Chapter 26, Table 26.2). ACEIs and ARBs reduce proteinuria by 35–

60%, which correlates with an improved outcome. In proteinuric patients unable to tolerate ACEIs or ARBs, a non-dihydropyridine calcium channel blocker (CCB) (e.g., verapamil and diltiazem) is preferred. They reduce proteinuria and enhance the antiproteinuric effects of ACEIs and ARBs (see Chapter 28). In contrast, dihydropyridine CCB proteinuria may activate the sympathetic nervous system. Thus, CCBs should not be used as first-line agents, but they remain useful as third- or fourth-line agents to achieve a low BP goal.

Combination therapy with an ACEI and an ARB has been found to be beneficial. The CALM trial (n = 199) documented additional benefit of combination therapy for diabetic nephropathy, although BP in the combination group was lower. The COOPERATE trial (n = 263) documented improved outcome in nondiabetic proteinuric CKD with similar BP control (see Chapter 27, Table 27.3). Management of ACEI and ARB therapy in these patients is detailed in Chapter 27 and outlined in Figure 32.1.

B. **Dietary Protein Restriction.** The Modification of Diet in Renal Disease study did not detect a benefit for GFR decline among groups of patients with CKD randomized to a protein-restricted diet. However, a meta-analysis of 13 randomized studies (n = 1,919) found that dietary protein restriction decreases progression, but by only 0.53 ml/min/year. This effect was greater in patients with diabetes. Protein restriction should not

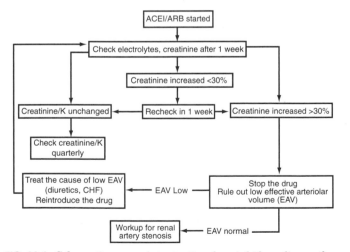

FIG. 32.1. Schematic approach to starting chronic kidney disease therapy with angiotensin-converting enzyme inhibitors (ACEIs) or angiotensin receptor blockers (ARBs). CHF, congestive heart failure.

exceed 0.6 g/kg/day in moderate or advanced CKD plus an amount equivalent to any urinary protein losses, and ingested protein should be of high quality. More severe restriction can cause malnutrition. The steady-state protein intake can be assessed from the 24-hour excretion of urea (see Chapter 3). Protein restriction requires the assistance of a skilled nutritionist.

In addition to the above measures, glycemic control in patients with diabetes reduces proteinuria and should be strongly advised. Patients with CKD should be counseled to cease smoking. Use of nonsteroidal antiinflammatory drugs, aminoglycosides, and radiocontrast agents should be discouraged in patients with CKD. Future interventions may include use of aldosterone antagonists and antifibrotic agents such as Pirfenidone.

IV. **Prevention of Cardiovascular Disease in Chronic Kidney Disease.** CVD includes coronary heart disease, cerebrovascular disease, peripheral vascular disease, and congestive heart failure. Approximately 40% of patients initiating dialysis have evidence of coronary artery disease, and 85% have left ventricular hypertrophy or depressed left ventricular function. The Framingham Heart study shows a strong relationship between increased creatinine (1.4–3.0 mg/dl) and CVD or all-cause mortality. Patients with all grades of CKD are more likely to die from CVD than to progress to ESRD.

The mortality from CVD in patients with ESRD is approximately 9% per year. This is approximately 30 times the risk in the general population. The cardiac mortality of dialysis patients younger than 45 years is approximately 100 times greater than that in the general population. Patients with CKD have a higher incidence of traditional CVD risk factors, including hypertension, diabetes, and dyslipidemias. Diabetes and smoking are strongly associated with CVD. These traditional factors account for only a small fraction of CVD. Other nontraditional CVD risk factors in this patient population include oxidative stress, endothelial dysfunction, nitric oxide deficiency, hyperhomocystinemia, vascular calcification, a high level of lipoprotein(a), hyperfibrinogenemia, and chronic inflammation.

The Secondary Meneution with Antioxidants of Cardiovascular Disease in End-Stage Renal Disease (SPACE) study randomized dialysis patients who had recovered from a myocardial infarction to vitamin E (800 IU daily) or placebo for 18 months. Those receiving the antioxidant had a significantly reduced rate of new cardiovascular events or myocardial infarction. Other controlled trials are awaited to evaluate the significance of these nontraditional CVD risk factors. Current guidelines are that patients with CKD should be considered at the highest risk for CVD. They should be evaluated for dyslipidemias at presentation, after a change in clinical status, and annually. Drug therapy is recommended for patients with low-density lipoprotein ≥100 mg/dl. Hepatic 3-methylglutaryl coenzyme A reductase inhibitors are indicated if dietary manipulations fail

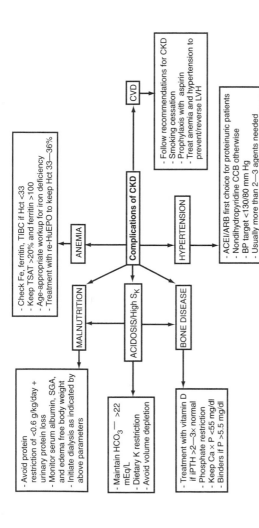

FIG. 32.2. Summary of complications of chronic kidney disease (CKD) and their therapy. ACEI, angiotensin-converting enzyme inhibitor; ARB, angiotensin receptor blocker; BP, blood pressure; Ca, calcium; CCB, calcium channel blocker; CVD, cardiovascular disease; Fe, iron; Hct, hematocrit; iPTH, immunoreactive parathyroid hormone; K, potassium; LVH, left ventricular hypertrophy; P, phosphate; re-HuEPO, recombinant human erythropoietin; SGA, Subjective Global Assessment; S_K, serum potassium; TIBC, total iron-binding capacity; TSAT, Transferrin Saturation.

after 3 months. Fibrates are recommended for patients with triglycerides ≥500 mg/dl without a correctable underlying cause and in patients with triglycerides ≥200 mg/dl and low-density lipoprotein cholesterol ≥130 mg/dl who are not able to tolerate statins. Slow-release nicotinic acid can reduce elevated levels of low-density lipoprotein. Modification of traditional risk factors, including smoking, diabetes, hypertension, and obesity, should also be pursued aggressively. The American Diabetes Association recommends use of low-dose aspirin in diabetic patients with CKD.

V. Preparation for Renal Replacement Therapy. Delayed referral to a nephrologist is associated with poorer outcomes, more hospitalizations, and higher costs. Such patients are less likely to have received erythropoietin and to have a functioning vascular access or to have a serum albumin or hematocrit at target levels. Patients with GFR <25 should be evaluated for receiving a preemptive renal transplantation or should be listed for a cadaveric kidney if there are no contraindications. Patients should also be counseled about the choice between peritoneal dialysis and hemodialysis. Both modalities are equally effective in treating ESRD. An early referral also allows a timely initiation of dialysis once GFR is below 10 ml/min/1.73 m^2 or if patients exhibit signs of malnutrition or uremia. A summary of CKD complications and their management is provided in Figure 32.2 and is detailed further in Chapter 31.

VI. Suggested Readings

Coresh J, Astor BC, Greene T, et al. Prevalence of chronic kidney disease and decreased kidney function in the adult US population: Third Health and Nutrition Examination Survey. *Am J Kidney Dis* 2003;41:1–12.

Jafar TH, Schmid CH, Landa M, et al. Angiotensin-converting enzyme inhibitors and progression of nondiabetic renal disease. A meta-analysis of patient-level data. *Ann Intern Med* 2001;135(2):73–87.

Klahr S, Levey AS, Beck GJ, et al. The effects of dietary protein restriction and blood-pressure control on the progression of chronic renal disease. Modification of Diet in Renal Disease Study Group. *N Engl J Med* 1994; 330:877–884.

National Kidney Foundation. Clinical practice guidelines, K/DOQI. http://www.kidney.org/professionals/kdoqi/guidelines.cfm (accessed 5/04).

Hemodialysis and Continuous Therapies

Edward A. Ross and Janet M. Caruso

Hemodialysis is defined as a primarily diffusion-based therapy in which solute from the patient's blood crosses a semipermeable membrane (the dialyzer) into the dialysate. Removal of excess fluid is accomplished by ultrafiltration, in which hydrostatic pressure causes the bulk flow of plasma water through the membrane. With advances in vascular access, anticoagulation, and the production of reliable and efficient dialyzers, hemodialysis has become the predominant method of treatment for acute and chronic renal failure.

I. **Indications for Hemodialysis.** Most patients with acute renal insufficiency are successfully managed without dialysis (see Chapter 30). Factors to be considered before initiating hemodialysis in patients with chronic renal failure should include comorbid conditions and patient preference. Timing of therapy is dictated by serum chemistries and symptoms. Hemodialysis is usually started when creatinine clearance decreases to <10 (<15 for diabetic patients) ml/min, which typically corresponds to a serum creatinine of 8–10 mg/dl. However, more important than the absolute laboratory values is the presence of uremic symptoms. Most uremic patients who are not terminal from another progressive illness or who are not so mentally incompetent as to present a danger to themselves or others are offered dialysis therapy (Table 33.1). Practice guidelines have been developed by the National Kidney Foundation for chronic kidney disease (CKD) patients to assist in the management of complications of CKD, choice of renal replacement therapy modality, creation of vascular access, administration of erythropoietin, and timing of the initiation of dialysis. These Kidney Disease Outcomes Quality Initiative Clinical Practice Guidelines have had a profound impact on the treatment of CKD patients. Dialytic therapies can also be used to correct certain emergent electrolyte problems, including hyperkalemia, hypercalcemia, hyperphosphatemia, hyperuricemia (such as that seen in the tumor lysis syndrome), as well as to treat some toxin or drug overdoses.

II. **Vascular Access.** Provision of dialysis requires reliable repeated access to the patient's circulation that can provide blood flow of approximately 200–450 ml/min. Ideally, the access should be created well before the need for chronic dialysis, typically when the creatinine clearance falls below approximately 20–25 ml/min, depending on the tempo of the renal deterioration.

**TABLE 33.1.   Indications and contraindications
for hemodialysis**

Indications
   Relative
      Symptomatic azotemia, including encephalopathy
      Dialyzable toxins (drug poisoning)
   Absolute
      Uremic pericarditis
      Hyperkalemia, severe (see Chapter 16)
      Diuretic unresponsive fluid overload (pulmonary edema)
      Intractable acidosis
Contraindications
   Relative
      Hypotension unresponsive to pressors
      Terminal illness
      Organic brain syndrome

A. **Acute Vascular Access.** Internal jugular or femoral catheters have become the preferred method to obtain temporary vascular access for emergent dialysis and are useful until a more permanent access is ready. Although previously common, subclavian vein catheterization is now avoided for temporary access in all patients with chronic renal failure due to the risk of central venous stenosis, which may later cause problems establishing permanent dialysis access in the involved arm. Modern catheters with dual lumens can provide excellent bidirectional blood flow rates and can often be used in the internal jugular location for 2–3 weeks. Highly flexible silicone-based cuffed catheters, which are tunneled subcutaneously, may be used for much longer periods and have improved flow and infection rates. Femoral vein catheters, in comparison, are typically used for only 48–72 hours. They are not suitable for ambulatory patients, and long-term use carries a significant risk of infection. Possible catheter complications include bleeding, infection, thrombosis or stenosis of the vessel, pneumothorax, and air embolus. Dialysis catheters should not be used as routine intravenous lines, because breaks in sterile technique greatly increase the risk of infection and catheter thrombosis. Catheters obstructed by clot can often be successfully cleared using thrombolytic agents (streptokinase, urokinase, tissue plasminogen activator).

In the presence of systemic bacteremia, temporary dialysis catheters should be removed, the appropriate cultures taken, including the catheter tip, and systemic antibiotics administered. The empiric antibiotic of choice has traditionally been vancomycin; however, initial therapy with another agent, such as a cephalosporin (with gram-positive organism coverage), may be appropriate in an attempt to avoid development of vancomycin-resistant antibiotic strains until culture results are available. Effective blood levels of vancomycin may be maintained for up to 1 week with a single dose; however, close monitoring of blood levels is recommended, especially when high-flux dialysis is used. Dosing of antibiotics often requires much more frequent administration, which can be problematic for outpatients.

B. Chronic Vascular Access

Arteriovenous Fistula

The arteriovenous (AV) fistula is the preferred vascular access for chronic hemodialysis and may last for years. When progression to end-stage renal failure is imminent, an effort should be made to spare the nondominant arm from venipuncture and arterial puncture. Fistulae are created by the surgical anastomosis of an artery and vein, most commonly the radial artery to the cephalic vein. Typically, a new primary fistula should be allowed to mature for 2–4 months, during which time the vein enlarges ("arterializes"), and is then used for cannulation by two needles (to and from the dialyzer). Examination of the functioning AV fistula reveals a palpable pulsation ("thrill") and a bruit by auscultation. In most instances, aggressive pursuit of an AV fistula is superior to chronic use of the other types of vascular access described below, which are often used as a "bridge" to development of a mature AV fistula.

Arteriovenous Grafts

When the patient's own vessels are inadequate to create an AV fistula, polytetrafluoroethylene grafts (i.e., Gore-Tex®) are typically used to form a conduit from artery to vein. Antibiotic prophylaxis to safeguard synthetic grafts should precede procedures for which bacteremia is anticipated. AV grafts should be placed at least 2–4 weeks before the anticipated need for hemodialysis.

Tunneled Catheters

Tunneled cuffed catheters are often used as a bridge to development of a mature AV fistula if a mature fistula is not in place at the time of initiation of chronic hemodialysis. Most often, they are configured as dual-lumen devices (with a single exit site, tunnel and venotomy), which then split into separate catheters once inside the large central vein. Due to the risk of catheter-related complications, it is preferable to develop permanent vascular access with an AV fistula. Tunneled devices are often placed in patients with acute renal failure if dialysis is still needed after 3 weeks of using a temporary catheter.

Assessment of Vascular Access

To optimize dialysis delivery, it is important to ensure that the access blood flow meets that of the desired extracorporeal pump rate. Inadequate blood supply would cause recirculation of a portion of the extracorporeal circuit and decrease dialysis effectiveness. In the past, it was recommended that recirculation studies be performed at regular intervals, and, if recirculation was >10–15%, radiologic imaging was advised. Now, however, newer technologies allow direct measurement of intra-access blood flow, which is a superior monitoring method. Fistulograms are particularly helpful in studying an access, and, in the presence of stenosis, angioplasty and stenting may correct the abnormality. In addition, imaging helps the surgeon to define the anatomy if revision is necessary.

Complications of chronic vascular access include

- Stenosis leading to inadequate blood flow
- Thrombosis requiring surgical intervention in 24–48 hours
- Infection, skin erosion, or both
- Failure to develop adequate venous outflow
- Ischemic limb caused by vascular steal
- Venous hypertension syndrome
- High-output cardiac failure
- Pseudoaneurysms

III. **Hemodialysis: Procedure.** The equipment used for hemo-dialysis prepares the dialysate, regulates dialysate and blood flow past a semipermeable membrane, and monitors functions involving the dialysate and extracorporeal blood circuit. Heparin is typically used for systemic anticoagula-tion. Blood and dialysate are perfused on opposite sides of the semipermeable membrane in a countercurrent direc-tion for maximal efficiency of solute removal. Dialysate composition, the characteristics and size of the membrane in the dialyzer, and blood and solute flow rates all affect solute removal.

A. **Dialysate Composition.** Sodium, potassium, magne-sium, and calcium concentrations are prescribed as the clinical situation dictates. The electrolyte composition of the dialysate is chosen with great care because ion fluxes (potassium in particular) can induce arrhyth-mias. Low calcium baths may be used in the acute and chronic therapy of hypercalcemia. Bicarbonate is used as the base buffer in modern dialysates, and its concen-tration can be changed as needed. The standard glucose concentration of dialysate is 200 mg/dl.

B. **Dialyzers.** Dialyzers are manufactured in hollow-fiber configurations composed of thousands of small-diameter fibers through which blood flows. Commonly used mem-branes have included cuprophane, cellulose acetate, and several high-porosity synthetic copolymer membranes (polyacrylonitrile, polymethyl-methacrylate, and polysul-fone). The nonsynthetic cellulosic membranes have become relatively uncommon because they are bioincom-patible in that they can activate the alternate complement pathway and lead to leukoagglutination and cytokine release. In comparison, the synthetic polymer membranes are being used more frequently because they exhibit bet-ter biocompatibility, improved ultrafiltration characteristics, and increased solute clearance, especially in the middle molecule (molecular mass, 300–2,000 dalton) range; they are also less thrombogenic, allowing no heparin dialysis when indicated. There are reports that outcomes in acute renal failure are improved by use of biocompatible synthetic dialyzers. These membranes are also used in high-flux dialysis and hemofiltration. A disadvantage of the synthetic membranes is their high cost. Reprocessing or reuse of these dialyzers is commonly performed for chronic outpatient dialysis.

Allergic reactions, which may be due to the membrane plastic compounds or disinfectants, are manifested by pruritus and respiratory distress on initiation of dialysis. Reactions may be prevented by rinsing the dialyzer; however, once they occur, cessation of dialysis, treatment with antihistamines, and expectant management of respiratory difficulty are required.

  C. High-Flux Dialysis. High-flux dialysis has gained rapid acceptance and is accomplished using very permeable membranes that are also biocompatible. High blood and dialysate flow rates are used to further increase the efficiency of dialysis. These strategies may improve the clearance of larger metabolites and sometimes can permit shortening of the treatment time. Urea kinetic modeling is used to determine the adequacy of dialysis (see the next section).

IV. Aims of Dialytic Therapy. Incomplete understanding of the pathogenesis of uremic symptoms makes it difficult to define an optimum dialysis prescription. Although a predialysis blood urea nitrogen concentration of <80 mg/dl was once an aim of therapy, correlation of toxic manifestations of uremia with blood urea nitrogen is often poor. The National Cooperative Dialysis Study has shown low morbidity in chronic stable dialysis patients when time-averaged concentration urea levels reach 50 mg/dl. Time-averaged urea concentration is calculated from pre- and postdialysis blood urea nitrogen, dialysis time, and interdialytic time. More comprehensive mathematical approaches were then developed, and dialysis prescriptions are now guided by these methods of urea kinetic modeling. Key concepts in one model include the protein catabolic rate (a measure of the dietary protein intake), residual renal function, and the dimensionless parameter, Kt/V urea. The latter term expresses the fractional urea clearance, where K is dialyzer urea clearance, t is dialysis treatment time, and V is body urea distribution volume. This ratio determines the magnitude of decline of blood urea nitrogen during a dialysis, and it serves as a measure of the dose of dialysis related to urea removal. In practice, this parameter should be at least 1.2 to minimize uremic symptoms and is calculated using a complex set of equations. Alternatively, the more simplistic urea reduction ratio (i.e., target of a 65% reduction in blood urea nitrogen levels) has gained favor and provides much insight into dialysis adequacy. New technology for continuous monitoring of urea losses into dialysate may overcome the pitfalls of basing adequacy determination on just blood levels. Even though a switch to high-flux dialysis can be shown to provide significantly higher clearances, it still does not yield the dramatic increases needed to approach that of native kidney function. This is the most likely explanation for the failure of high-flux methodology to improve patient outcomes over that from standard-flux treatments in the most recent multicenter international trial.

V. Complications of Hemodialysis

A. Hypotension. Hypotension, which is the most frequent complication during hemodialysis, has been related to prior use of acetate buffer dialysate, low sodium dialysate (130–135 mEq/L), atherosclerotic heart disease, autonomic neuropathy, and excessive fluid weight gain. Prevention of symptomatic hypotension can be achieved by accurate determinations of dry weight, precise ultrafiltration with newer-technology dialysis machines, biocompatible dialysis membranes, prevention of temperature fluxes, careful choice of the dialysate sodium and calcium concentrations, reduction of antihypertensive medications immediately before dialysis, and, if necessary, use of sympathomimetic agents.

B. Muscle Cramps. Muscle cramps occur commonly during rapid, high-volume ultrafiltration, due to plasma volume contraction and rapid sodium fluxes. Preventive measures include fluid restriction to gain no more than 2 kg between treatments, use of a transiently high sodium concentration in the dialysate (sodium modeling), stretching exercises, possibly carnitine supplementation, and, if clinically disabling, small doses of quinine sulfate, such as 325 mg orally before dialysis).

C. Dialysis Disequilibrium Syndrome. The dialysis disequilibrium syndrome is believed to result primarily from less rapid clearance of urea and other osmoles from the brain than from the blood, which results in an osmotic gradient between these compartments. This osmotic gradient leads to a net movement of water into the brain that results in cerebral edema. The syndrome is uncommon and is usually seen with the first dialytic treatments in severely azotemic patients. Other predisposing factors include severe metabolic acidosis, older age, pediatric patients, and the presence of other central nervous system disease, such as a preexisting seizure disorder. Symptoms, which can occur during or after the procedure, include headache, lethargy, nausea, muscular twitching, and malaise, with rare progression to mental status changes, seizures, and even cardiorespiratory arrest. After recognition of high-risk patients, the use of smaller surface area dialyzers and lower blood flow rates will lessen osmotic shifts. Intradialysis mannitol infusion (25–50 g) may lessen the frequency and severity of symptoms but carries a risk of pulmonary edema.

D. Hypoxemia. Hypoxemia during dialysis is important in patients with compromised cardiopulmonary function. Research implicates membrane incompatibility, acid–base changes induced by the dialysate base buffer, and hypoventilation. Predisposed patients should be given supplemental oxygen and dialyzed with synthetic copolymer membranes using bicarbonate dialysate.

E. Arrhythmias. Hypoxemia, hypotension, removal of antiarrhythmic agents during dialysis, and rapid changes in serum bicarbonate, calcium, magnesium, and potassium (especially in patients taking digoxin) all contribute to arrhythmias in predisposed patients. Continuous electrocardiogram monitoring during dialysis is necessary in high-risk patients.

F. Bleeding. Although uremia causes platelet dysfunction (i.e., assessed by measuring the bleeding time), anticoagulation is still usually needed to prevent clotting of the extracorporeal circuit. Heparin is typically used, and the dose can be adjusted according to the clotting time. Dialysis may be attempted without heparin if indicated, using special protocols involving biocompatible membranes and saline rinses. Cryoprecipitate, 1-deamino-8-arginine vasopressin (0.3 µg/kg body weight), and conjugated estrogen may prove successful when uremic bleeding is unresponsive to adequate dialysis.

G. Transfusion-Related Diseases. The incidence of hepatitis B infection has decreased dramatically since the screening of donor blood and implementation of isolation techniques. Hepatitis B vaccine induces seroconversion in 40–70% of hemodialysis patients. The incidence of non-A, non-B (hepatitis C) infection is also declining as blood donors are screened for hepatitis C virus antibodies. Other possible infections include human immunodeficiency virus and cytomegalovirus. Generally, fewer blood transfusions are required with the introduction of erythropoietin therapy, and this decreases the risk of bloodborne disorders.

H. Metabolic Bone Disease. The causes of metabolic bone disease include secondary hyperparathyroidism, oversuppression of parathyroid hormone (adynamic bone disease), aluminum deposition (from aluminum-containing antacids used as phosphate binders), and a unique form of amyloid deposition (β_2-microglobulin). Clinical features common to dialysis bone disease include bone pain, arthralgias, fractures, bone cysts, and carpal tunnel syndrome (for management, see Chapter 31).

I. Acquired Renal Cystic Disease. Multiple renal cysts develop in the kidneys in up to 80% of dialysis patients treated >3 years. Screening of hemodialysis patients by ultrasonography or computed tomography after 3 years on dialysis is recommended to detect malignant changes.

J. Pericarditis. Two distinct patterns of pericarditis are encountered in patients with renal failure. Pericarditis can occur in uremic nondialyzed patients and in those already receiving dialysis therapy. Uremic pericarditis usually responds to intensive daily dialysis, and a correlation between resolution of pericarditis and improvement in the uremia has been shown. Conversely, pericarditis that occurs in patients already on hemodialysis may be related to occult inadequate dialysis or concurrent illnesses, such as systemic lupus erythematosus or viral pericarditis. Treatment is intensive dialysis without heparin anticoagulation. The patient should be monitored clinically and by echocardiography for features suggestive of pericardial tamponade. A pericardiocentesis tray should be kept at the bedside. Patients need to be intensively monitored to detect hemodynamic instability, changes in pericardial friction rub, and pulsus paradoxus. If pericardial tamponade develops, percutaneous pericardiocentesis, placement of a pericardial window, or pericardiectomy may be necessary.

K. **Anemia and Recombinant Human Erythropoietin.** The causes of anemia in dialysis patients include decreased red blood cell production and survival and blood loss in the extracorporeal circuit. Recombinant human erythropoietin is used routinely to correct the anemia. The recommended starting dose in hemodialysis patients is typically 50 U/kg body weight intravenously or subcutaneously three times weekly. The dose is adjusted to keep the hematocrit between 30% and 36%, with 33–36% being the range associated with the best cardiovascular outcomes. In addition to correction of anemia, recombinant human erythropoietin improves patient well-being, exercise tolerance, and cognitive function. Potential side effects include hypertension, seizures, thrombosis, iron deficiency, hyperkalemia, and flu-like symptoms. Resistance to recombinant human erythropoietin occurs in the presence of iron deficiency, aluminum toxicity, severe secondary hyperparathyroidism, infection, or other inflammatory diseases.

L. **Dialytic Therapies in the Intensive Care Unit.** Critically ill, hemodynamically unstable intensive care unit (ICU) patients are typically the most challenging to treat with conventional dialytic modalities. The intermittent volume and solute fluxes may cause significant morbidity, which includes worsening of hypotension and arrhythmias. Although there are only limited convincing data that mortality can be improved, many investigators have proposed benefits from various forms of continuous renal replacement therapy. Continuous renal replacement therapy may be indicated for the treatment of acute renal failure with hemodynamic instability, cardiogenic shock with pulmonary edema and inadequate urine output, and diuretic-unresponsive congestive heart failure, and for patients who need aggressive parenteral nutrition. Because acute peritoneal dialysis often cannot yield adequate solute removal or is precluded by abdominal surgery, peritoneal leaks, or peritonitis, a variety of blood clearance modalities were devised. Continuous arterio venous hemofiltration or hemodialysis has largely been replaced by pumped venovenous systems [continuous venovenous hemofiltration (CVVH), continuous venovenous hemodialysis (CVVHD), continuous venovenous hemodiafiltration (CVVHDF)], avoiding arterial puncture and providing regulated extracorporeal blood flow.

These modalities have the disadvantage of the risks of continuous blood pumps (ICU setting only, poor emergent treatment for hyperkalemia and acidosis, access site infection, strict fluid monitoring) but may offer the luxury of microprocessor-controlled fluid delivery and removal rates, user-friendly interfaces, and automated troubleshooting. CVVHD is similar conceptually to traditional hemodialysis but enhances patient stability by the slow fluid and solute fluxes accomplished at low blood and dialysate flow rates. CVVH instead relies on convective solute clearance (rather than diffusion), by using hydraulic pressure to drive ultrafiltration of bulk fluid across a high-porosity hemofilter membrane. This approach necessitates generation of very large volumes of ultrafiltrate (i.e., up to 3 L/hr), which has a composition similar to that of plasma water. The quantity of solute removed (the renal replacement "dose") is thus a function of the amount of ultrafiltrate generated. These losses must be accurately replaced by a balanced electrolyte solution in amounts determined by desired fluid and electrolyte losses or gains. Solute removal may be further enhanced by combining these two modalities into hemodiafiltration (CVVHDF). There are a variety of dialysate and replacement fluid options available commercially or prepared locally. The base buffer can be either bicarbonate or citrate. The latter can also serve as a regional anticoagulant, but its use necessitates the careful monitoring and replacement of calcium as indicated. There currently is no clear outcomes study favoring either CVVH or CVVHD. At high pump speeds, the daily solute and fluid clearance rates can match or even exceed those of daily conventional hemodialysis, which is particularly appropriate for very catabolic patients (i.e., those with sepsis or burns) who require high-dose or high-volume parenteral nutrition. Venovenous access is typically obtained by placement of a dual-lumen dialysis catheter in the femoral or internal jugular position. To prevent thrombosis in the extracorporeal circuit, anticoagulation is usually required and can be accomplished with either heparin or regional anticoagulation with citrate. These machines may also be used for fluid removal alone (slow continuous ultrafiltration) for "renal support," as in select patients with severe congestive heart failure and inadequate urine volume. There is a growing appreciation that there are other special circumstances for which this modality may be particularly helpful, such as in neonates with congenital enzyme deficiencies and in hypo- and hyperthermia.

There has long been controversy in the choice of the appropriate dialysis modality for management of acute renal failure; options include routine care with three-times-per-week hemodialysis, daily intermittent hemodialysis (which provides a higher total dialysis dose, improved volume control, and, possibly, improved mortality in the ICU setting), CVVH, CVVHD, CVVHDF, or slow, low-efficiency hemodialysis via prolonged treatments with conventional machines. With a paucity of outcomes data clearly favoring one modality, the choice is sometimes determined by local machine resources (expense and availability of new equipment), nursing care availability (requires training large numbers of ICU staff), cost (equipment, custom sterile fluids, nursing), anticoagulation technique (none, heparin, or citrate), or even schedules for other patient procedures (slow, continuous modalities are not usually portable outside of the ICU). The hypothesis that harmful mediators of sepsis can be cleared with any current nonresearch technology or dose is unproven.

VI. **Dialytic Techniques in Drug Overdose.** Hemodialysis and a related technique, hemoperfusion, are occasionally helpful in the management of overdose or toxins. Charcoal hemoperfusion uses coated or uncoated charcoal particles to adsorb toxins or drugs. Complications are due to its bioincompatibility and include thrombocytopenia.

In acute poisonings, hemodialysis has the advantage of correcting any concurrent acid–base and electrolyte disturbances. Table 33.2 gives a brief listing of medications removed

TABLE 33.2.   Common drugs and toxins removed by hemodialysis or hemoperfusion, or both

Acetaminophen
Alcohols (ethanol, methanol, isopropyl alcohol, ethylene glycol)
Amphetamines
Antiarrhythmics (procainamide and *N*-acetyl-procainamide, sotalol)
Antihypertensives (angiotensin-converting enzyme inhibitors, beta blockers)
Antimicrobials (many)
Antineoplastics (busulphan, cyclophosphamide, 5-fluorouracil)
Arsenic
Aspirin
Barbiturates
Carbamazepine
Lithium
Mannitol
Monoamine oxidase inhibitors
Theophylline
Valproic acid

by hemodialysis or hemoperfusion. Antidepressants and benzodiazepines are poorly removed by dialytic techniques. Dialysis for poisoning should be considered only when supportive measures are ineffective or there is impending irreversible organ toxicity.

VII. **Other Considerations in Care of Dialysis Patients.** The following are important practical aspects in the care of hemodialysis patients that must be emphasized.

- Fluid intake should be limited to 1–1.5 L/day to avoid fluid overload because these patients are usually oligoanuric. For dietary therapy, refer to Chapter 37.
- Phosphate binders, such as calcium carbonate, calcium acetate, sevelamer HCl, and aluminum hydroxide, should be administered with meals.
- Many drugs, such as antibiotics and antiarrhythmics, are removed by hemodialysis. Therefore, alteration of dosage, supplemental doses, and monitoring of blood levels are frequently required. This may be especially problematic in patients undergoing hemofiltration or frequent dialysis. In these situations, coordination of medication dosing with the renal team is important.
- These patients are often on intravenous medications such as recombinant human erythropoietin and vitamin D as outpatients. These usually should be continued when the patients are admitted to the hospital. Coordination with the renal team is essential.
- Magnesium-containing antacids and laxatives or phosphorus-based (Fleet®) enemas should be avoided to prevent hypermagnesemia and hyperphosphatemia, respectively.
- If blood transfusions are required, they should be administered during hemodialysis to avoid fluid overload and hyperkalemia.
- Because these patients are immunosuppressed and frequently hypothermic, there should be a low threshold for an intensive workup if they present with features suggestive of infection.
- Specific dialysis treatment goals, such as optimum fluid removal and target pulmonary capillary wedge pressure, should be discussed with the nephrologist.
- If invasive procedures are planned, the nephrologist should be informed in advance to modify the dialysis schedule, alter heparin dosage, and correct bleeding time abnormalities.
- Protection of the vascular access arm is crucial. This includes avoidance of blood pressure determination, venipuncture, and arterial puncture in this extremity. If access is still in the planning stage, protection of the nondominant arm is indicated. Protection involves informing the patient and hanging a sign above the hospital bed.

VIII. **Suggested Readings**

Couch P, Stumpf JL. Management of uremic bleeding. *Clin Pharm* 1990;9:673–681.

Daugirdas JT, Ing TS, Blake PG, eds. *Handbook of dialysis*, 3rd ed. New York: Lippincott Williams & Wilkins, 2000.

Eknoyan G, Beck GJ, Cheung AK, et al. Hemodialysis (HEMO) Study Group. Effect of dialysis dose and membrane flux in maintenance hemodialysis. *N Engl J Med* 2002;347:2010–2019.

Forni LG, Hilton PJ. Continuous hemofiltration in the treatment of acute renal failure. *N Engl J Med* 1997;336:1303–1309.

Hakim RM, Wingard RL, Parker RA. Effect of the dialysis membrane in the treatment of patients with acute renal failure. *N Engl J Med* 1994;331:1338–1342.

Levin NW, Lazarus JM, Nissenson AR. National cooperative rHu erythropoietin study in patients with chronic renal failure—an interim report. The National Cooperative rHu Erythropoietin Study Group. *Am J Kidney Dis* 1993; 22[2 Suppl 1]:3–12.

National Kidney Foundation, Kidney Disease Outcomes Quality Initiative. *Clinical practice guidelines*. Available at: http://www.kidney.org/professionals/kdoqi. Accessed 2003.

Nissenson AR, Fine RN, Gentile DE, eds. *Clinical dialysis*. New York: McGraw-Hill Professional, 1996.

Ronco C, Bellomo R, Homel P, et al. Effects of different doses in continuous veno-venous haemofiltration on outcomes of acute renal failure: a prospective randomized trial. *Lancet* 2000;356(9223):26–30.

Ronco C, Bellomo R, Kellum JA. Continuous renal replacement therapy: opinions and evidence. *Adv Ren Replace Ther* 2002;9:229–244.

Winchester JF. Dialysis and hemoperfusion in poisoning. *Adv Ren Replace Ther* 2002;9:26–30.

Wood JE, Mahnensmith RL. Pericarditis associated with renal failure: evolution and management. *Semin Dial* 2001;14:61–66.

34

Peritoneal Dialysis

Joyce M. Gonin

I. **Overview.** Currently, 14% of the 300,000 patients on renal replacement therapy in the United States receive peritoneal dialysis (PD). Continuous ambulatory PD (CAPD) involves manual exchanges of 2–3 L of fresh dialysis fluid approximately four times daily. A total daily fluid exchange of 8–12 L includes approximately 2 L of ultrafiltrate. Continuous cyclic PD (CCPD) involves exchanges of dialysis fluid by a machine during the night. It can be combined with a daytime dwell of fluid. CCPD is more convenient but more costly than CAPD. The dialysis fluid contains hypertonic dextrose solution (1.5%, 2.5%, and 4.25%) to achieve fluid ultrafiltration, with added Ca^{2+}, Mg^{2+}, Na^+, Cl^-, and lactate to correct acidosis or replace deficiencies. CAPD entails four exchanges of 1.5–3.0 L of warmed peritoneal dialysate infused into the abdomen through a peritoneal catheter to dwell for 4–5 hours. The overnight exchange is approximately 8 hours. With CCPD, the exchange fluid is derived from two to three 5- to 6-L bags delivered at preselected volumes and dwell times. Patients treated with CAPD or CCPD must connect and disconnect themselves from the dialysis tubing using aseptic technique. They flush one limb of a Y-shaped tubing set with spent dialysate to wash out any bacterial contamination (the "flush before fill" technique) before infusing the new dialysis fluid.

II. **Principles of Solute and Fluid Removal**

    A. **Solute Removal.** As residual renal function declines, the frequency and volumes of dialysis must increase. Exchanges are timed when solutes such as urea have almost equilibrated between plasma and dialysate. Consequently, higher molecular weight solutes (*middle molecules*) are removed less effectively, but their slow, continuous, convective transport by PD is more effective than the abrupt, but relatively short, periods of transport provided by conventional hemodialysis. Only expensive, high-flux hemodialysis filters can surpass the efficiency of CAPD for removing middle molecules.

        The adequacy of PD is assessed by measurement of Kt/V. This dimensionless number is derived from the calculated dialysis removal of urea (K), the time (t), and the volume of distribution of urea (V, or whole body water) corrected for any residual renal function. A goal for weekly Kt/V is 2.2. The peritoneal equilibration test quantifies the solute transport of the peritoneal membrane from the 4-hour accumulation of urea and creatinine and the disappearance of dextrose from the dialysate. Low transporters require longer dwell times to achieve

TABLE 34.1.   Advantages and disadvantages of peritoneal dialysis

Advantages	Disadvantages
Ease of performance	Low efficiency
High safety margin	Requires a dialysis catheter
Portability	Potential pulmonary compromise
Fewer dialysis-related symptoms	Potential protein loss and malnutrition
Better control of parathyroid hormone levels	Potential for infection
More liberal diet	Hypertriglyceridemia
No routine anticoagulation	
Fewer medications	
Better control of hypertension	

solute clearance, whereas high transporters may fail to ultrafilter fluid because of loss of osmotic pressure with the absorption of dextrose. They require shorter dwell times.

  B. **Fluid Removal.** Dextrose in concentrations of 1.5%, 2.5%, and 4.25% (equivalent to 347, 400, and 486 mOsm/kg H_2O) produces an ultrafiltrate of 300–1,000 ml per exchange. This is adjusted for fluid and blood pressure control.

III. **Indications for Peritoneal Dialysis.** The indications for PD are based on lifestyle requirements and suitability (Table 34.1). Relative indications include patients with cardiovascular or hemodynamic instability, those with problematic vascular accesses, those living far from a dialysis center, and those at high risk from the anticoagulation needed for hemodialysis. Contraindications to CAPD are listed in Table 34.2.

IV. **Technical Aspects of Peritoneal Dialysis**
  A. **Catheters.** These are flexible 30-cm tubules with distal perforations. They are often spiral to keep the tip in the pelvis and to prevent the pain caused by dialysis fluid streaming onto the rectal wall. The catheter is anchored with Dacron cuffs. Approximately 15 cm of catheter is tunneled through the abdominal wall laterally below the belt line. Catheters should not be used for 4 weeks after placement to permit them to seal.
  B. **Composition of Standard Dialysate Solution.** Dialysate (Table 34.3) is provided in premixed, flexible, plastic bags of 250–750 ml for children and 1–3 L for adults. Most adults tolerate 2-L volumes. Special low calcium and magnesium formulations are available. Icodextrin, a glucose polymer, can be used in place of dextrose. It is removed far more slowly from the dialysate and prolongs ultrafiltration in high transporters. Icodextrin is used only once daily during the long (8- to 16-hour) dwell.

TABLE 34.2. Contraindications of peritoneal dialysis

Absolute
    Peritoneal fibrosis (50%)
    Pleuroperitoneal leak (hydrothorax)
Major
    Colostomy or nephrostomy
    Severe hypercatabolic state (e.g., burns)
    Fresh aortic prosthesis
    Recent thoracic or abdominal surgery
    Extensive abdominal adhesions
    Inguinal or abdominal hernia
    Blindness
    Quadriplegia
    Mental retardation
    Poor motivation and compliance
    Crippling arthritis
Minor
    Polycystic kidney disease
    Diverticulosis
    Obesity
    Peripheral vascular disease
    Hyperlipidemia
    Lack of a telephone for communication

C. **Management of the Diabetic Patient Receiving Peritoneal Dialysis.** Dextrose complicates the control of diabetes. Regular insulin can be added to the dialysis solution in a dose that is decided empirically and increased in proportion to the dextrose concentration. A usual starting dose is 5–7 U per exchange. Because peritoneal fibrosis has been associated with intraperitoneal insulin, subcutaneous insulin is preferred.

V. **Complications of Peritoneal Dialysis.** *Mechanical complications* include pain with exchanges, dialysate leakage (usually early after catheter placement), poor outflow drainage (omental wrapping and trapping of the catheter), scrotal edema (which usually indicates a patent processus vaginalis and the need for hernia repair), hernias, catheter cuff extrusion, and lower back pain. Intestinal perforation is rare. *Car-*

TABLE 34.3. Peritoneal dialysate composition

Dialysate component	Concentration
Dextrose monohydrate	1.5%, 2.5%, 4.25%
Sodium	132 mEq/L
Calcium	2.5 mEq/L
Magnesium	1.5 mEq/L
Chloride	102 mEq/L
Lactate	35 mEq/L

TABLE 34.4.   Signs, symptoms, and diagnosis of peritonitis

Cloudy dialysis fluid.
A peritoneal dialysis white blood cell count >100/ml with >50% poly-
  morphonuclear leukocytes.
Gastrointestinal symptoms (e.g., abdominal pain, cramps, constipa-
  tion, diarrhea) occur in 75%.
Gram's stain of peritoneal fluid that demonstrates organisms.

diovascular complications include fluid overload and hyper-
and hypotension. *Pulmonary complications* include atelectasis, hydrothorax, and hypoxemia. *Infectious and inflammatory
complications* include bacterial, fungal, and sclerosing peritonitis; catheter tunnel infections; catheter exit-site infections;
and pancreatitis. *Metabolic complications* include hypertriglyceridemia and hyperglycemia.

A. **Peritonitis.** Peritonitis occurring more than approximately once every 2 years should prompt a reevaluation
of the exchange procedure and retraining. Peritonitis is
usually caused by a single organism introduced by touch
contamination. Multiple organisms should prompt consideration of bowel perforation. Signs and symptoms of
peritonitis are shown in Table 34.4.

Etiology

Infections with gram-positive organisms, such as *Staphylococcus epidermidis*, *Staphylococcus aureus*, and
Streptococcus species, are common. Gram-negative organisms causing peritonitis include Enterobacteriaceae,
Proteus species, *Escherichia coli*, Klebsiella species,
Enterobacter cloacae, Acinetobacter species, and Xanthomonas (Pseudomonas) species. *Candida albicans*, *Nocardia asteroides*, Aspergillus species, Fusarium species,
Mycobacterium tuberculosis, and nontuberculous myco-
bacteria occur rarely.

Treatment

Because of the emergence of resistant enterococcus and
staphylococci, vancomycin is reserved for the following situations: methicillin-resistant *S. aureus*, β-lactam–resistant
organisms, serious peritonitis in patients allergic to other
antibiotics, and *Clostridium difficile* enterocolitis unresponsive to metronidazole. Commonly selected antibiotic
regimens are outlined in Table 34.5 and at the Web site of
the International Society for Peritoneal Dialysis at http://
www.ispd.org.

Three steps of management are usually performed as
an outpatient over 2 weeks:

1. Abdominal lavage with three rapid in-and-out flushes of
   dialysate fluid.
2. Empirical antibiotic coverage (intraperitoneal third-
   generation cephalosporin plus an aminoglycoside or ceftazi-
   dime) until dialysate cultures and sensitivities allow specific

TABLE 34.5. Common therapeutic regimens for peritonitis

Organism	Regimen
Gram-positive bacteria	Third-generation cephalosporin IP or vancomycin IP
Gram-negative bacteria	Aminoglycoside alone or third-generation cephalosporin
Mixed organisms suggest bowel perforation	Third-generation cephalosporin IP or vancomycin (or ampicillin) + aminoglycoside + metronidazole (or clindamycin)
No organism present on Gram's stain	Third-generation cephalosporin IP or vancomycin + aminoglycoside
Fungal forms	Amphotericin IP or intravenous, fluconazole IP

IP, intraperitoneal.

antibiotic selection. Rifampin is added in cases of *S. aureus* peritonitis.

3. Catheter removal if fungal infection occurs or if symptoms or dialysate cell counts fail to improve rapidly.

Indications for hospitalization for peritonitis include the following:

- Infection that has not responded to routine therapy after 2–3 days.
- Unusually painful and severe peritonitis or the isolation of organisms such as *Pseudomonas* (*Xanthomonas*), fungi, and *S. aureus* that are difficult to treat
- Suspicion of bowel perforation.
- Failure to respond to initial antibiotic therapy.
- Fecal or mycobacterial peritonitis.

VI. Suggested Readings

Gokal R, Mallick NP. Peritoneal dialysis. *Lancet* 1999;353:823–828.

Jassal SV, Oreopoulos DG. Techniques in peritoneal dialysis. In: Brady HR, Wilcox CS, eds. *Therapy in nephrology and hypertension*, 2nd ed. Philadelphia: WB Saunders, 2003:839–849.

Oreopoulos DG. The optimization of continuous ambulatory peritoneal dialysis. *Kidney Int* 1999;55:1131–1149.

Ronco C. Peritoneal dialysis: the state of the art in Europe. *Am J Kidney Dis* 1999;33:1–3.

United States Renal Data System. *USRDS 1998 Annual Data Report*. Bethesda, MD: The National Institutes of Health, National Institute of Diabetes and Digestive and Kidney Diseases, 1998.

Winchester JF, Rakowski TA. End-stage renal disease and its management in the elderly. *Clin Geriatr Med* 1998;14:255–265.

Renal Transplantation

Joyce M. Gonin

Renal transplantation is the preferred modality for end-stage renal disease replacement therapy. In the United States, 15,000 kidney transplants were performed in 2002. It is the least expensive method of replacement therapy. Life expectancy is higher in transplant recipients than in dialysis patients. Living related donors are most immunologically compatible. However, living unrelated transplants are becoming more prevalent and have superior graft survival compared to cadaveric transplants. Current 1-year graft survival rates are 94% for living donor transplants and 88% for cadaveric transplants. The half-life for long-term survival is 8.6 years for cadaveric transplants and 12.1 years for living related transplants but increases to 23.6 years in human leukocyte antigen (HLA)-identical sibling transplants.

I. **Immune Response.** The process of organ rejection resembles the normal response to a foreign antigen (infection) and the abnormal response to self-antigens (autoimmunity). The class I histocompatibility antigen molecules are named *HLA-A*, *-B*, and *-C*, whereas class II molecules are designated *HLA-DP*, *-DQ*, and *-DR*. HLA-A, -B, and -DR are the most important. Tissue typing involves measuring two A, two B and two DR. A *0-antigen mismatch* transplant carries survival benefits.

Class I molecules are expressed constitutively on the plasma membranes of most cells and react with $CD8^+$ (cytotoxic) T cells. Class II molecules are expressed constitutively on B lymphocytes, macrophages, and monocytes and react with $CD4^+$ (helper) T cells. A complex interaction among the histocompatibility antigens, T and B cells, macrophages, monocytes, endothelial cells, and cytokines determines whether rejection occurs. Immunosuppressive drugs manipulate this system.

II. **Recipient Evaluation.** Cardiac evaluation is especially important because of the high incidence of cardiovascular disease in patients with end-stage renal disease. Cardiovascular disease remains the leading cause of morbidity and mortality in renal transplant recipients and is a major limitation for graft survival. Diabetics have a high incidence of angiographically significant coronary disease in asymptomatic individuals.

In general, patients who have had a malignancy should be disease free for at least 2 years before consideration for transplantation. Immunosuppressive drugs predispose toward the development of skin cancer and lymphoproliferative disorders. Some centers have transplanted patients infected with the human immunodeficiency virus if they are stable with an undetectable viral load and a CD4 count >200.

III. Donor Evaluation

A. **Cadaveric Donor.** Acceptable candidates for renal transplantation should be entered into the United Network for Organ Sharing cadaveric waiting list, provided the glomerular filtration rate is <20 ml/min, or may obtain a transplant from a properly evaluated living donor. The United Network for Organ Sharing point system accounts for time on the waiting list, number of B or DR antigen mismatches, and age. Pediatric patients receive preference. Kidneys generally are offered locally, but a 0-antigen mismatch mandates shipping an organ anywhere in the United States. A donor must be brain dead and free of human immunodeficiency virus or any other systemic disease. However, some centers transplant organs from hepatitis B and C–positive donors into recipients who are hepatitis B or C positive. With the increased need for organs, donor kidneys have been taken from older subjects, those with hypertension or diabetes, and non–heart-beating subjects.

B. **Living Donor.** Potential living related donors should be screened similarly to cadaveric donors. Patients with familial renal disease require an especially careful evaluation. Relative contraindications have included age >65 years, advanced medical illness, severe hypertension, diabetes mellitus, preexisting renal disease, and active infection. Kidney donors have no apparent decline in function of the remaining kidney over 25 years, but there is a slight increase in hypertension and a modest proteinuria.

IV. Immunosuppressive Drugs. Maintenance immunosuppression is necessary to prevent allograft rejection except for an identical twin transplant. Even with 0-antigen mismatches, some degree of immunosuppression is provided, often for life. The strategy of immunosuppression generally involves three distinct phases: (a) *Induction* is the use of high doses of immunosuppressive drugs to initiate acceptance of the allograft; (b) *maintenance* is the continued use of drugs at tapered doses, ultimately allowing long-term immunosuppression with a minimum of side effects; and (c) *antirejection therapy* is higher doses of drugs to treat an episode of rejection. Immunosuppression typically entails a triple-drug regimen of corticosteroids, an antiproliferative drug [azathioprine, mycophenolate, or sirolimus (SRL)], and cyclosporine (CsA) or tacrolimus. Monoclonal or polyclonal antibodies can be used as induction therapy (especially in high-risk patients) and for treatment of rejection.

A. **Corticosteroids.** Corticosteroids are used in all phases of immunosuppressive therapy. They have nonspecific antiinflammatory properties and also block the elaboration of interleukin (IL)-1 and IL-6 and tumor necrosis factor by activated macrophages. Prednisone is usually started at 0.5–2.0 mg/kg/day and tapered to 10 mg/day within 1–3 months. Some patients can be managed on 5 mg/day or an alternate-day regimen.

Complications of corticosteroid therapy include impaired glucose metabolism, hyperlipidemia, weight gain, osteoporosis and osteonecrosis, cataracts, myopathy, easy bruisability, acne, hypertension, mood lability, psychosis, and sleep disturbances. Wound healing may be delayed or impaired.

B. **Azathioprine.** Azathioprine is an imidazole derivative of 6-mercaptopurine that is bioactivated in the liver to 6-mercaptopurine. It depletes purines that are required by rapidly dividing cells to synthesize DNA. Side effects associated with azathioprine include pancytopenia (more commonly, leukopenia), megaloblastic erythropoiesis, hepatocellular injury, cholestatic jaundice, pancreatitis, pneumonitis, and alopecia. The dose of azathioprine should be lowered in the presence of hepatic injury, and it should not be prescribed with allopurinol, which inhibits xanthine oxidase, which is critical in the degradation of azathioprine.

C. **Mycophenolate Mofetil.** Mycophenolate mofetil has replaced azathioprine in most transplant programs. It inhibits inosine monophosphate dehydrogenase, which is the rate-limiting enzyme in the *de novo* synthesis of purines in lymphocytes. Mycophenolate mofetil is more effective than azathioprine at reducing the incidence of early rejections. The adverse effects of mycophenolate mofetil include bone marrow suppression and gastrointestinal side effects, including abdominal pain, nausea, and diarrhea. The average dose is 2 g/day.

D. **Cyclosporine.** CsA inhibits the production of IL-2 and other cytokines critical to T-cell activation and proliferation. It is eliminated by biliary excretion. Monitoring of CsA trough levels is required because of variability in its absorption and enterohepatic recirculation.

The usual starting dose is 8–10 mg/kg/day. Some centers avoid using CsA until renal function has clearly improved and substitute a polyclonal or monoclonal antibody (sequential immunosuppression). Approximately 6 months after transplantation, the dose of CsA is gradually tapered to a maintenance dose of 3–6 mg/kg/day (given in two divided doses). Ultimately, trough levels should dictate dosing. CsA measured by high-performance liquid chromatography provides lower levels than by radioimmunoassay. Levels of 200–250 ng/ml are usually adequate in the first 6 months, after which levels of 150–200 ng/ml may be sufficient.

The major complication of CsA is nephrotoxicity. An acute, reversible decline in renal function due to renal vasoconstriction is the most common finding. Less commonly, CsA may cause hemolytic-uremic syndrome. Both usually respond to dose reduction or discontinuation of

CsA. Chronic CsA nephrotoxicity is caused by irreversible small vessel obliteration, leading to glomerular ischemia and sclerosis, tubular atrophy, and interstitial fibrosis.

Other adverse effects of CsA include hyperkalemia, hypomagnesemia, and hyperuricemia with gout. Salt-sensitive hypertension is common. Neurotoxicity is dose related and manifests as tremor or paresthesias. Hirsutism and gingival hyperplasia are problematic.

Drugs that increase CsA levels through inhibition of hepatic P_{450} activity may result in nephrotoxicity, whereas those that induce P_{450} activity lower CsA levels, with the risk of rejection. Cholestyramine interferes with the intestinal absorption of CsA (Table 35.1).

E. Tacrolimus. Tacrolimus is a macrolide antibiotic resembling CsA that inhibits the activation of DNA-binding proteins that activate the promoter sequence of the IL-2 gene. Nephrotoxicity is its major side effect, but neurotoxicity, perhaps more severe than with CsA, is also a problem. A serious side effect is drug-induced diabetes mellitus, which may become irreversible. Benefits over CsA include an absence of hirsutism and gingival hyperplasia. A trial comparing tacrolimus with CsA reported a reduction in rejection episodes but no difference in graft survival. Tacrolimus is often preferred in retransplants, children, and African Americans who are at high risk for rejection. Plasma levels of 10–12 ng/ml in the first 6 months posttransplant and 8–10 ng/ml thereafter are typical. Drug interactions are the same as for CsA (Table 35.1).

F. Sirolimus. SRL is a macrolide antibiotic that blocks signal transduction through IL-2 and inhibits cell cycle progression. SRL plasma levels should be 6–12 ng/ml. Dose-related adverse effects include anemia, thrombocytopenia, leukopenia, and exacerbation of CsA-induced hypercholesterolemia and steroid-induced hypertriglyceridemia. Diarrhea, hepatotoxicity, pneumonitis, ototoxicity, and dermatologic effects occur less frequently.

G. Polyclonal and Monoclonal Antibodies. Equine antithymocyte globulin and rabbit antithymocyte globulin (Thymoglobulin) are polyclonal antibodies raised against thymocytes that are used for induction and for treatment

TABLE 35.1. Drugs that affect the level of cyclosporine A

Increase	Decrease
Ciprofloxacin	Carbamazepine
Diltiazem	Isoniazid (INH)
Erythromycin	Phenobarbital
Fluconazole	Rifampin
Metoclopramide	
Nicardipine	
Verapamil	

of steroid-resistant rejection. Therapy is complicated by a serum sickness syndrome in up to 15% of patients and by thrombocytopenia and anemia.

The highly effective monoclonal antibody OKT3 is directed against the CD3 antigen complex expressed on mature human T cells. It prevents lymphocytes from recognizing and responding to alloantigens. An initial lymphocyte activation causes fever, chills, capillary leak, pulmonary edema, and, occasionally, aseptic meningitis. Aggressive volume control is important to mitigate capillary leakage.

Delayed complications of antibodies include susceptibility to viral infections [herpes, cytomegalovirus (CMV), and Epstein-Barr virus] and posttransplant lymphoproliferative disease. The humanized monoclonal antibody daclizumab and the chimeric monoclonal antibody basiliximab appear to be better tolerated. These are directed against the high-affinity IL-2 receptor, thereby preventing the clonal expansion of primed T cells.

V. **Surgical Procedure.** The renal allograft generally is placed retroperitoneally in the right iliac fossa. The ureter is implanted into the bladder by creating a submucosal tunnel to prevent reflux. Immunosuppressive drugs delay wound healing and increase infection.

VI. **Early Postoperative Course.** A bladder catheter is usually placed for 3–5 days. Fluid intake and output must be measured scrupulously. Medications must be adjusted for the degree of renal dysfunction. Dietary intake of potassium, phosphorus, and magnesium should be restricted. Delayed graft function occurs in 10–50% of cadaveric transplants, and some require initial dialysis. Excessive ultrafiltration and associated hypotension can prolong allograft dysfunction.

VII. **Allograft Dysfunction**

A. **Etiology.** Immunologic rejection, surgical complications, and nephrotoxicity from CsA or tacrolimus are the unique problems.

B. **Prerenal Disease.** Prerenal azotemia occurs from excessive fluid losses from diuretics or an osmotic diuresis during the correction of uremia. Assessment requires daily weights, fluid intake, and output and orthostatic changes. A high plasma bicarbonate (contraction alkalosis) and a low fractional excretion of sodium may be seen. An elevated blood urea nitrogen–to–creatinine ratio is inconsistent because corticosteroids can elevate the blood urea nitrogen independently.

C. **Parenchymal Disease**
Acute Tubular Necrosis
The most common cause of parenchymal renal disease and delayed graft function in the transplant recipient is acute, ischemic tubular necrosis (ATN). The causes of ATN include a prolonged time from harvesting to engraftment, intraoperative hypotension, and adverse effects of the preservative solution, nephrotoxic drugs, and radiographic contrast agents. ATN may require dial-

ysis and mandates dose adjustments of all medications. If function does not return in 1 week, a renal biopsy should be considered to diagnose associated acute rejection.

Rejection

Immunologic rejection can be hyperacute, accelerated, acute, or chronic. *Hyperacute* rejection occurs minutes to hours after the transplant procedure. It is caused by pre-existing antibodies directed against the donor blood ABO or histocompatibility leukocyte antigens on the transplant endothelium. This causes complement activation, inflammatory cell infiltration, thrombosis, cortical necrosis, and graft loss requiring nephrectomy.

Accelerated rejection resembles hyperacute rejection but occurs over 2–4 days. It is mediated by previously primed cellular (T cell) or humoral (antibody) mechanisms. There is either primary nonfunction or rapid deterioration. The graft is usually lost.

Acute rejection usually occurs in 20–40% of recipients within the first 3 months. Later episodes suggest noncompliance. Acute rejection results from a cellular and humoral immune response. Mononuclear cells infiltrate the interstitium and invade the tubular basement membrane and vessels. There is a rise in the serum creatinine, but the classic signs of fever and graft tenderness are less pronounced with CsA. Low levels of CsA or tacrolimus may promote acute rejection. Certain individuals are at increased risk of rejection (Table 35.2).

Chronic rejection is better termed *chronic allograft nephropathy* (CAN), because immunologic and nonimmunologic insults may contribute. It may occur within a few weeks. It is the major cause of graft loss. The newer immunosuppressive protocols have had little impact on CAN. The number of acute rejection episodes and the presence of delayed graft function predict subsequent CAN. Other factors include donor and recipient age and immunologic matching. CAN is characterized by glomerulosclerosis, thickening and reduplication of the glomerular basement membrane, tubular atrophy, interstitial fibrosis, and small vessel obliteration. There is progressive azotemia, proteinuria, and hypertension. No strategy prevents CAN, but recommendations include prevention of acute rejection, control of hypertension, and perhaps the use of angiotensin-converting enzyme (ACE) inhibitors.

TABLE 35.2. Characteristics of recipients at higher risk for rejection

High panel-reactive antibodies (>50%)
African American race
Younger age
Second or subsequent transplant
Presence of delayed graft function

Other Intrarenal Processes

Renal dysfunction can be a complication of antibiotics or the use of ACE inhibitors in patients with transplant renal artery stenosis and may occur in patients taking nonsteroidal antiinflammatory agents. It may also complicate bacterial infection of the single functioning allograft or recurrence of the native kidney disease. Diabetic nephropathy recurs in all patients eventually, although most diabetics lose their allografts to other causes before recurrence becomes clinically important. Immunoglobulin A nephropathy recurs in 10–50% of transplant patients. Focal segmental glomerulosclerosis recurs in 30–50% of patients; other complications include membranous glomerulopathy, membranoproliferative glomerulonephritis, hemolytic uremic syndrome, and, rarely, lupus nephritis.

D. Postrenal Disease. Blood (hematoma), urine (urinoma), or lymph (lymphocele) can cause obstruction that can be detected by ultrasound. An aspirate can aid diagnosis. Lymph has a high protein content and a creatinine equal to that of serum, whereas urine has a high creatinine. Blood clots in the bladder require irrigation with a bladder catheter. Bladder outlet obstruction from prostatic hypertrophy, neoplasms, and neurogenic bladder (especially in diabetics) can cause postrenal obstruction.

E. Vascular Disease. Acute arterial or venous thrombosis occurs usually within the first 2 weeks and leads to graft loss. Risk factors include surgical problems and hypotension, whereas acute rejection is the most common cause later.

Renal artery stenosis usually occurs up to 2 years after the transplant in 12% of recipients. It presents with hypertension and graft dysfunction exacerbated by ACE inhibition. An allograft bruit is a nonspecific finding (see Chapter 22).

F. Diagnosis of Allograft Dysfunction. A thorough evaluation should include history of offending drugs (nonsteroidal antiinflammatory drugs, diuretics, ACE inhibitors), timing of CsA or tacrolimus doses, symptoms of rejection or infection, orthostatic blood pressure readings, and manual evaluation of the allograft. Laboratory data should include electrolytes, blood urea nitrogen, serum creatinine, urine analysis and possibly culture, a complete blood count, and a trough CsA or tacrolimus level. If proteinuria is present, it should be quantitated with a 24-hour urine collection.

Patency of the urinary catheter should be ascertained. Unless contraindicated, a fluid challenge should be prescribed. The CsA or tacrolimus dose should be adjusted according to blood levels, and the serum creatinine and drug levels should be repeated in 2 days. An ultrasound can detect hydronephrosis or fluid collections, and a duplex Doppler velocimetry can detect blood flow, which can be confirmed by a renal nuclear scan or an angiogram. If obstruction is detected, a retro grade or antegrade pyelogram (after a percutaneous nephrostomy drainage) can localize the obstruction. Bladder outlet obstruction may be relieved by a Foley catheter. A fluid collection associated with hydronephrosis should be aspirated. A similar creatinine in the fluid and urine suggests urine leak, whereas a similar protein in the fluid and serum suggests a lymphocele. An allograft biopsy may be required to diagnose rejection.

G. **Management of Allograft Dysfunction.** Prerenal azotemia is managed with volume repletion, discontinuation of diuretics, and optimization of cardiac function. ATN may require dialysis when primary nonfunction is presumed due to ATN; a biopsy is appropriate at 7–10 days to exclude concurrent rejection. Avoidance of nephrotoxins and adjustment of medication dosing are imperative. Pyelonephritis is treated with antibiotics (see Chapter 20).

Patients with acute rejection can be given high-dose (pulse) corticosteroids or intravenous methylprednisolone (0.5 g every day for 3–4 days) or oral prednisone (100–200 mg every day for 3–5 days). Antithymocyte globulin or OKT3 is given for steroid-resistant or severe vascular rejection.

For chronic rejection, baseline immunosuppressive drugs should be optimized and hypertension controlled aggressively. Protein restriction (0.6–0.8 g/kg/day + urine protein losses) may be beneficial in those with heavy proteinuria. Protein excretion may be reduced by ACE inhibition (see Chapter 32). Fluid collections are drained only if they are causing obstruction. Arterial or venous thrombosis usually leads to graft loss.

VIII. **Long-Term Complications of Transplantation**

A. **Infection.** The most common infections immediately after transplant are bacterial and involve the urinary tract, the wound, the respiratory tract, and intravenous lines. Infections can be avoided by prompt removal of bladder catheters, prophylactic intraoperative antibiotics, meticulous wound management, and avoidance of prolonged use of intravenous lines. Opportunistic infections can arise at any time, but immunosuppression is maximal 6 weeks to 3 months posttransplant. Urinary tract infection is the most common infection. Routine infections must not be overlooked.

Reactivation of herpes simplex virus is reduced by prophylactic acyclovir. Orolabial, esophageal, and genital involvement is treated with acyclovir.

CMV infection may occur in the first 6 months and may be *de novo* or reactivation of disease. Prophylaxis with acyclovir, ganciclovir, valganciclovir, and CMV immunoglobulin may attenuate the disease, which can be detected by the emergence of CMV antigen. CMV causes fever, malaise, leukopenia, chorioretinitis, pneumonitis, and gastrointestinal ulceration. CMV-seronegative recipients of CMV-seropositive donor kidneys should receive prophylactic treatment. Active disease is treated with intravenous ganciclovir and reduction of immunosuppression. Foscarnet can treat ganciclovir-resistant CMV infection but is nephrotoxic.

Pneumocystis carinii, *Listeria*, *Legionella*, *Nocardia*, *Toxoplasma*, and *Cryptococcus* are rare infections in transplant patients. Prophylaxis with trimethoprim-sulfamethoxazole has reduced the incidence of *P. carinii*.

All prospective transplant recipients should be vaccinated against hepatitis A and B, tetanus, diphtheria, and pneumococcal disease.

B. **Cardiovascular Disease.** Cardiovascular disease is the most common cause of death after renal transplantation. Special risk factors in the transplant population include prior renal disease, proteinuria, and hyperlipidemia exacerbated by corticosteroids, CsA, and SRL. Pharmacologic therapy for hyperlipidemia is similar to that in the general population, but liver function tests and creatine phosphokinase should be followed to detect myositis and rhabdomyolysis.

Diabetic patients have a high incidence of asymptomatic coronary artery disease, which has led to the proposal for a coronary angiogram in all type I diabetics older than age 45 and in young diabetics with multiple cardiac risk factors or abnormal noninvasive tests.

C. **Malignancies.** Immunosuppressive drugs predispose transplant recipients to develop squamous cell carcinoma of the skin. Patients should avoid sun exposure and wear sunscreen. Other predisposed malignancies include non-Hodgkin's lymphoma (posttransplant lymphoproliferative disorder), Kaposi's sarcoma, and carcinomas of the cervix, uterus, vulva, perineum, and hepatobiliary system. Pap smears are required annually. Malignancy in the transplant patient may require a reduction or cessation of the immunosuppression, especially for non-Hodgkin's lymphoma and Kaposi's sarcoma, in which tumor regression and even cure can occur.

D. **Hypertension.** Hypertension occurs in 50–60% of transplant recipients. It may be exacerbated by CsA, tacrolimus, and high-dose corticosteroids, but most is due to essential hypertension. Transplant renal artery stenosis should be suspected in those with worsening hypertension, a rise in the serum creatinine, and a graft bruit.

Calcium channel blockers not only reduce blood pressure but can reverse renal vasoconstriction caused by CsA. Verapamil and diltiazem can increase CsA levels, whereas nifedipine and amlodipine do not alter CsA levels. They may cause lower extremity edema and gingival hyperplasia (see Chapter 27). α-Adrenergic blockers can improve lipid parameters and regress prostatic hypertrophy (see Chapter 25). ACE inhibitors moderate posttransplant erythrocytosis but may exacerbate hyperkalemia seen with CsA.

E. Bone Disease. Osteoporosis and osteonecrosis are complications of corticosteroids. Bisphosphonates are widely used for those with osteopenia or osteoporosis. All patients should take calcium supplements and vitamin D. Transplantation promotes the healing of renal osteodystrophy and aluminum bone disease and the resolution of hyperparathyroidism.

IX. Suggested Readings

Morris PJ, ed. *Kidney transplantation*. Philadelphia: WB Saunders, 2001.

Pascual M, Theruvath T, Kawai T, et al. Strategies to improve long-term outcomes after renal transplantation. *N Engl J Med* 2002;346;580–590.

Vincenti F. Immunosuppression minimization: current and future trends in transplant immunosuppression. *J Am Soc Nephrol* 2003;14:1940–1948.

Wheeler DC, Steiger J. Evolution and etiology of cardiovascular disease in renal transplant recipients. *Transplantation* 2000;70;SS41–SS45.

Anemia of Chronic Kidney Disease

Aaron Francis Kulick and Robert J. Rubin

I. **Definition.** An anemia workup in chronic kidney disease (CKD) should be initiated when the hemoglobin/hematocrit (Hgb/Hct) level declines to Hgb <11 g/dl (Hct is <33%) in premenopausal females and prepubertal patients and Hgb <12 g/dl (Hct is <37%) in adult males and post-menopausal females.

II. **Evaluation.** Anemia of CKD occurs because the diseased kidneys are unable to produce adequate erythropoietin. It is characterized by a normocytic, normochromic anemia with a low corrected absolute reticulocyte count. Typically, the anemia of CKD develops when the glomerular filtration rate declines to <30 ml/min and the serum creatinine to >2 mg/dl. The minimum workup of anemia in the patient with CKD should include Hgb/Hct, red blood cell indices, reticulocyte count, stool guaiac for evaluation of occult gastrointestinal blood loss, and iron studies. Iron deficiency may be present in one-third of such patients. Serum erythropoietin levels are often variable and seldom helpful in the workup of anemia of CKD. An algorithm is presented in Figure 36.1.

    A. **Target Hemoglobin/Hematocrit.** Significant anemia increases the likelihood of left ventricular hypertrophy, decreases quality of life, and reduces survival in patients on hemodialysis. Conversely, targeting Hct levels as high as 42% may be associated with coronary events and, possibly, increased mortality. National Kidney Foundation–Kidney Disease Outcomes Quality Initiative guidelines recommend that Hgb be targeted between 11 and 12 g/dl and Hct between 33 and 36%.

    B. **Target Iron Levels.** The percent transferrin saturation (TSAT) reflects iron available for erythropoiesis. Serum ferritin reflects overall iron stores. Iron deficiency normally has a TSAT <16% and a serum ferritin <12 ng/ml. However, in the patient with CKD, a TSAT >20% and ferritin >100 ng/ml can occur despite iron deficiency. CKD patients who are unable to achieve the target Hgb/Hct or who require comparatively large doses of erythropoietic drugs may require a trial of intravenous (IV) iron therapy. Supplemental iron should be withheld if TSAT is >50% or ferritin is >800 ng/ml because the risk of iron overload is increased.

    C. **Distinguishing between Functional Iron Deficiency and Anemia of Chronic Disease.** Anemia of chronic disease (AOCD) results in an inflammatory block of iron

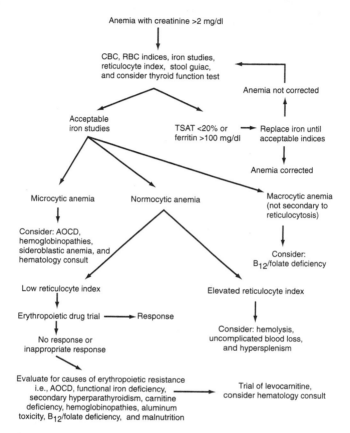

FIG. 36.1. Approach to the patient with anemia of chronic kidney disease. AOCD, anemia of chronic disease; CBC, complete blood cell count; RBC, red blood cell; TSAT, transferrin saturation.

utilization for erythropoiesis. AOCD can complicate an active inflammatory disorder. Like iron deficiency, it is manifested by a normal to low TSAT and a ferritin >100 ng/ml. Serum ferritin generally decreases after erythropoietic therapy in functional iron deficiency, whereas it increases in AOCD. If the diagnosis is unclear and the ferritin is <800 ng/ml, the Hgb/Hct may be monitored after a trial of IV iron.

III. Monitoring of Iron Levels. After initiation of erythropoietic therapy, the TSAT and serum ferritin should be checked every month in patients not receiving IV iron and at least once every 3 months in patients receiving IV iron until the target Hgb/Hct is reached.

IV. Treatment Guidelines

A. Oral Iron.
In non–end-stage renal disease CKD patients, oral iron supplementation should be given either 1 hour before meals or 2 hours postprandial, as food tends to reduce gastrointestinal absorption. At least 200 mg of elemental iron should be given daily in two to three doses (Table 36.1). In dialysis patients, oral iron therapy is not recommended, as ongoing iron losses tend to be higher (approximately 25–100 mg weekly).

B. Intravenous Iron.
The usual dose of IV iron is 1 g of iron dextran, ferric gluconate (Ferrlecit), or iron sucrose (iron saccharate, Venofer) divided into 10 doses of 100 mg given with each dialysis session. Delayed adverse reactions of arthralgias and myalgias are dose related above 100 mg. There is a small incidence of anaphylactoid reactions, which are more common in patients with a history of multiple drug allergies. Thus, a small test dose (25 mg) of IV iron is given 15–60 minutes before the first dose of any iron preparation. Iron sucrose may be given to patients with a prior history of an allergic reaction to iron dextran.

C. Epoetin Alfa (Epogen, Procrit).
Epoetin alfa (Epogen/Procrit) is a 165–amino acid recombinant glycoprotein (30.4 kd). Patients with anemia related to CKD respond to epoetin with improved energy level, work capacity, sexual function, appetite, sleep habits, exercise capacity, and well being. Although it is generally more effective when given subcutaneously, most patients on hemodialysis receive epoetin intravenously. The starting dose of IV epoetin is 120–180 IU/kg/wk with dialysis. In predialysis patients with CKD and peritoneal dialysis patients, epoetin should be given as a weekly subcutaneous injection, initially at 80–120 IU/kg/wk. The Hct/Hgb should be measured 3–4 weeks after initiation of treatment and 2 weeks after a dosage adjustment and should be monitored every 4 weeks. The most common side effects are headache, hypertension, arthralgias, and diarrhea.

Resistance to Epoetin

When high levels of epoetin are required to maintain adequate Hgb/Hct, or when this is not achieved despite

TABLE 36.1.   Oral iron preparations

Oral iron preparation	Trade names	Generic available	Approximate % elemental iron
Ferrous gluconate	Fergon	Yes	10
Ferrous sulfate	Feosol	Yes	20
Ferrous fumarate	Femiron, Ferretts	No	30
Polysaccharide-iron complex	Niferex, Nu-Iron	Yes	100

TABLE 36.2. Conversion dose equivalence for epoetin alfa and darbepoetin alfa

Epoetin alfa (U/wk)	Darbepoetin alfa (μg/wk)
<2,500	6.25
2,500–4,999	12.5
5,000–10,999	25
11,000–17,999	40
18,000–33,999	60
34,000–89,999	100
≥90,000	200

adequate dosing, patients should be evaluated for anemia of other causes—notably, iron deficiency. A trial of IV iron supplementation may be warranted if TSAT is <50% and ferritin is <800 ng/ml. In the iron-replete patient, infection/inflammation (AOCD), chronic blood loss, secondary hyperparathyroidism, aluminum toxicity, hemoglobinopathies, folate or B_{12} deficiency, and malnutrition should all be ruled out. If no reversible causes are identified, anemia may be treated with a trial of levocarnitine for 6 months.

D. Darbepoetin Alfa (Aranesp)
Darbepoetin alfa (Aranesp) is a recombinant erythropoiesis-stimulating glycoprotein with a half-life that is threefold longer intravenously and twofold longer subcutaneously than that of epoetin. The recommended starting dose is 0.45 μg/kg subcutaneously weekly or double the dose every other week (Table 36.2). The side effect profile is similar to that of epoetin.

V. Suggested Readings

Mikhail AI, Macdougau IC. Iron and erythropoietin—related therapies. In: Brady HR, Wilcox CS, eds. *Therapy in nephrology and hypertension*, 2nd ed. Philadelphia: WB Saunders, 2003:681–688.

National Kidney Foundation–Kidney Disease Outcomes Quality. Initiative guidelines for the treatment of anemia of chronic renal failure: http://www.kidney.org/professionals/kdoqi/guidelines_updates/doqi_uptoc.html.

Pemuzzi G, Schieppati A, Minetti L. Anemia and coagulopathy. In: Brady HR, Wilcox CS, eds. *Therapy in nephrology and hypertension*, 2nd ed. Philadelphia: WB Saunders, 2003:689–700.

Nutrition in Renal Failure

Thomas G. Baumgartner and Edward A. Ross

Patients with kidney disease have nutritional requirements that vary with the degree of renal insufficiency. Diet is modified to reduce uremic symptoms from the accumulation of toxic metabolites, to address acid–base imbalances, to facilitate electrolyte and water homeostasis, and to prevent renal osteodystrophy. Patients with advanced chronic renal failure ultimately may develop protein-calorie malnutrition and require dietary supplementation. Depression, low socioeconomic status, and multiple medications are associated with malnutrition. Other causes of malnutrition in the renal patient include concurrent illnesses, depletion of water-soluble vitamins removed with dialytic procedures, inadequate dialysis, and consequences of uremia (fatigue, muscle cramps, anorexia, nausea, vomiting, stomatitis, altered sense of taste, altered mental status, insulin resistance, increased catabolic hormones, decreased anabolic hormones, gastroparesis, and malabsorption).

I. General Nutritional Concepts

A. Protein-Calorie Malnutrition.
Patients with advanced renal insufficiency are at risk for malnutrition because uremic symptoms (anorexia, nausea, vomiting, and altered taste) are superimposed on the restricted diet, malabsorption, and urinary protein losses. This often results in hypoalbuminemia, abnormal profiles of blood amino acid levels, decreased protein and fat stores, and deranged white blood cell function. The institution of an appropriate diet or initiation of dialysis therapy may not, however, correct these deficits. It is frequently necessary to enlist the aid of a clinical nutritionist to assist in an aggressive program of enteral or parenteral nutrition. This includes the careful monitoring of nutritional parameters, such as serum prealbumin, albumin, and anthropometric measurements of fat and muscle bulk (respectively, triceps skinfold thickness and midarm muscle circumference). Performance of the Subjective Global Assessment has also become an important tool used to quantify and periodically monitor the nutritional status of hemodialysis and peritoneal dialysis patients. This tool has been modified for use in renal failure and is still undergoing revisions and validation in subsets of patients. Currently, brief training is recommended for rating the four items (weight change over the preceding 6 months, dietary intake and gastrointestinal symptoms, visual assessment of subcutaneous tissue for fat and muscle wasting, and muscle mass) on a seven-point scale. Impairment of gastric motility can lead to mal-

nutrition in both diabetic and nondiabetic patients. Radionuclide studies can be used to assess gastric emptying and to test the therapeutic response of promotility agents (i.e., metoclopramide, erythromycin, bethanechol).

B. **Caloric Requirements.** Patients with uncomplicated renal insufficiency have normal basal energy expenditure and caloric requirements. A diet containing 30–35 Kcal/kg body weight is usually prescribed. Patients who are catabolic or have proteinuria have greater requirements; without additional carbohydrate intake, these patients deplete their fat and protein stores. Portable indirect calorimeters are now available to ascertain actual energy expenditure, respiratory quotients (PCO_2/PO_2), and oxygen consumption (VO_2). This technology points the clinician in the right direction with regard to caloric mix.

C. **Macronutrients**

Protein

Stable patients with renal disease have normal minimum daily protein requirements. Protein restriction delays the need for dialysis by preventing the uremic symptoms caused by nitrogenous wastes. The quantity of protein necessary to avoid malnutrition depends on the food's biologic value (ratio of essential to nonessential amino acids). Fish, eggs, and milk are of higher biologic value than poultry or beef, especially when compared with grains. Approximately 75% of the protein in renal diets should be of the high-biologic-value type.

The amount of protein prescribed is based on the patient's renal function, proteinuria, type of dialysis, and body weight. As described below, the protein recommendation ranges from 0.6–1.5 g/kg/day. For edematous patients, the calculation should be based on the usual or estimated dry weight. For obese patients, calculate the adjusted body weight from the ideal body weight plus 25% of the excess weight. Generally, the diet limitations are reasonably tolerated if they contain ≥40 g of protein per day, with 75% being of high biologic value. Patients are usually in negative protein balance if their intake is restricted to <0.6 g protein/kg/day, unless they are provided with essential amino acid supplementation. α-Ketoanalogs (ketoacids) are experimental supplements that contain no nitrogen yet undergo liver transamination into the corresponding amino acid.

Intensive and repeated dietary counseling is helpful to improve compliance for protein restriction. A very useful monitor of dietary nitrogen intake (in grams) in a patient with stable renal function is to measure the 24-hour urine urea nitrogen (urine urea nitrogen × V), where V is the urine volume:

$$IN = (\text{urine urea nitrogen} \times V) + NUN$$

where IN is the daily nitrogen intake and NUN is nonurea nitrogen (i.e., creatine, creatinine, uric acid, ammonia) excretion (in grams) and is estimated to be

$$NUN = 0.031 \times body\ weight\ (kg)$$

Because protein contains approximately 16% alpha nitrogen, IN is then converted to protein intake (in grams) as follows:

$$protein\ intake = 6.25 \times IN$$

As an example, consider a lean, nonedematous 70-kg man whose 24-hour urine reveals 5 g of urea N:

$$IN = 5\ g + (0.031 \times 70\ kg) = 7.17\ g\ nitrogen$$

Estimated protein intake (in g/day) = $6.25 \times 7.17 = 44.8$, which is then compared with dietary protein prescription. In patients with significant proteinuria, the amount of protein lost in the urine also has to be taken into account, and the dietary protein prescription should be adjusted for this. Because stool contains approximately 1 g of nitrogen per 300 ml, great losses may occur in patients with diarrhea.

Carbohydrates

Carbohydrates are a major source of calories in renal patients with multiple dietary restrictions and, thereby, are protein sparing. Sugars also permit the complete oxidation of fatty acids, which avoids ketone production. Grains, vegetables, and fruits are common sources of carbohydrate and have the added benefits of dietary fiber. Excessive carbohydrate can also lead to hypertriglyceridemia and hyperglycemia, which can increase morbidity (immunocompromise, steatosis, and hypercapnia).

The most common cause of hypophosphatemia in institutionalized patients is the iatrogenic introduction of excessive dextrose, especially in the setting of dialytic removal of phosphate. This so-called refeeding syndrome is, therefore, frequently reported in renal failure patients and is particularly important in the intensive care unit. Glucose loading is a major reason for a phosphate shift from the intravascular compartment, which may deplete erythrocytes of 2,3-diphosphoglycerate, tighten hemoglobin:oxygen affinity, and shift the oxygen dissociation curve to the left.

Although glucose (dextrose) or glucose polymers are the most common carbohydrate sources, many other carbohydrate products are available, including parenteral glycerol and fructose, that have different insulin action. In the setting of insulin insensitivity or resistance, high doses of exogenous insulin have been associated with profound antinatiuretic activity and microalbuminuria.

Lipids

Hyperlipidemia occurs in >50% of chronic renal failure patients and is of great concern because of the high mortality due to atherosclerotic cardiovascular disease. Causes of the hypercholesterolemia and hypertriglyceridemia are multifactorial and include proteinuria in the nephrotic range, depressed lipoprotein lipase activity, decreased metabolism of remnant lipoproteins, and impaired cholesterol transport. Initiation of dialysis does not correct these disorders. Indeed, hypertriglyceridemia often worsens during peritoneal dialysis owing to the absorption of large quantities of dextrose from the dialysate. The vast majority of patients require pharmacologic therapy to achieve the increasingly stringent cholesterol target levels.

Dietary lipid guidelines and goals for renal patients are the same as those for nonuremic individuals. These include performing routine lipoprotein analyses, restricting fats to 30% of total calories (to include protein, carbohydrate, and lipid), substituting polyunsaturated fats for saturated fats, creating a balance between omega-3 and omega-6 lipids, and reducing cholesterol intake to <200 mg/day. Under particular circumstances (i.e., elevated PCO_2, hyperinsulinemia), it may be appropriate to increase the percentage of total calories from fat, with some investigators suggesting as much as 83% fat in parenterally fed patients.

Reducing low-density-lipoprotein cholesterol levels is especially important in patients with cardiovascular risk factors because of the now well-established increased mortality risk with poorly controlled lipid levels. However, it may be difficult to design a diet that provides adequate calories with concurrent fat and protein restrictions. Fruits (limited by their potassium content), sugars, and syrups are often useful.

Essential fatty acid requirements (for prevention) are estimated to be approximately 1–4% of total energy requirements and should be in the form of linoleic acid (omega-6) or linolenic acid (omega-3).

D. Micronutrients. Virtually all anabolic and catabolic processes in humans are intimately related to micronutrients. Electrolytes are responsible for seemingly limitless metabolic reactions, play key roles in structure, and maintain acid–base balance. Acid–base considerations must be assessed before any electrolytes can be provided to patients. If a patient is alkalemic, acid salts (chloride, phosphate, and sulfate) should be used, whereas an acidemic patient requires the use of bicarbonate precursors, such as acetate, citrate, gluconate, or lactate. Each salt must be carefully selected with pathophysiologic insight. Trace elements also facilitate complex metabolic reactions and, not unlike vitamins, play key roles in antioxidant activities.

Electrolytes

SODIUM AND CHLORIDE. Most patients with advancing renal insufficiency develop salt retention. This can be a management problem in patients with nephrotic syndrome or oliguric renal failure. The dietary prescription is commonly expressed in either milliequivalents of NaCl or grams of sodium (100 mEq NaCl contains 2.3 g of sodium and 3.5 g of chloride).

Renal disease also may impair the patient's ability to conserve salt, which may lead to a superimposed prerenal azotemia. Many patients with acute renal failure have an initial oliguric phase, when salt must be restricted, and then a polyuric phase, in which salt must be supplemented.

POTASSIUM. The degree of dietary potassium restriction depends on the amount of both renal and nonrenal losses. Because 40 g of oral protein may contain 1 g (25 mEq) of potassium, a high-protein diet would preclude severe potassium restriction. Particularly good sources are oranges and orange juice, other citrus products, bananas, potatoes, tomatoes, melons, spinach, and legumes. In fact, many fruits (such as peaches or nectarines) and vegetables are very rich sources of potassium and, at the same time, low in sodium. Some salt substitutes also contain potassium, and these products can contribute a significant amount to the diet. In most patients, a diet limited to 1 mEq of potassium/kg body weight/day prevents hyperkalemia. Additional potassium may need to be prescribed because of peritoneal dialysate or gastrointestinal losses (nasogastric losses or diarrhea). The impact of acid–base must also be appreciated with respect to potassium. For every 0.1 U acute decline in pH, serum potassium rises approximately 0.5 mEq/L.

PHOSPHORUS AND CALCIUM. Hyperphosphatemia and secondary hyperparathyroidism develop with advancing renal insufficiency, unless dietary phosphate is restricted concurrent with the use of oral phosphate binders. Patients on diets relatively high in protein have an obligatory source of phosphorus and may require higher doses of binders. Calcium carbonate and calcium acetate are the preferred binders for the approximately 200 mg (7 mmol) of phosphate that is excreted in the stool daily. However, these must be administered directly with the meals; a delay can lead to significant calcium absorption and cause hypercalcemia. The interpretation of calcium levels (i.e., total or ionized concentrations) and management of calcium administration are covered in more detail in Chapter 18. Evolving national guidelines are limiting the total daily calcium intake and are thereby leading to the greater use of non–calcium-based phosphate binders. Unless carefully specified in the physician orders, the proper timing of phosphate binders can be problematic in hospitalized patients because of variable meal schedules. Aluminum-containing antacids and sucralfate (Carafate®) are also used for phosphate chelation but are restricted in light of the hyperaluminumemia that occurs in acute and chronic renal failure. Sevelamer hydrochloride (Renagel®) is a nonabsorbed, calcium-free, and aluminum-free polymer that can be used in hyperphosphatemia. It may become especially useful in hyperphosphatemic patients who have coexisting hypercalcemia, as it avoids the administration of aluminum hydroxide and its associated potential long-term toxic effects. It has the secondary benefit of binding dietary cholesterol and can lead to significant decreases in low-density-lipoprotein cholesterol levels. Hypophosphatemia is rare in patients with renal failure, unless it is accompanied by poor nutritional intake. It must be remembered, however, that conventional hemodialysis removes approximately 8 mmol of phosphorus per 4- to 5-hour run, and 10 mmol of phosphorus is removed with daily peritoneal dialytic procedures. It is important to monitor patients for the occurrence of hypophosphatemia because it is becoming a more frequent finding with aggressive daily hemodialysis (especially with dialyzer membranes with relatively high phosphate clearance) and high-volume continuous renal replacement protocols (such as continuous venovenous hemodialysis). Repletion may often be accomplished by the enteral route but, at times, requires intravenous therapy, especially because diarrhea is associated with oral phosphate replacement.

MAGNESIUM. Because renal insufficiency decreases magnesium excretion, magnesium-containing laxatives and antacids should be avoided. Approximately 30–40% of oral magnesium is absorbed in the ileal/jejunal parenchyma. High-dose intermittent or continuous hemodialysis or hemofiltration therapies, as well as peritoneal dialysis, may be associated with hypomagnesemia and require repletion.

Trace Elements

IRON. Iron deficiency has become quite common in renal patients because of increased use during erythropoietin therapy. Repetitive, albeit small, blood losses during hemodialysis also contribute to the iron deficit. Oral repletion is difficult in renal patients because of poor dietary intake of iron and decreased absorption when administered with phosphate-binding antacids. Even when oral iron is administered in high doses (65–150 mg of elemental iron) between meals, it has only 10–20% bioavailability. Parenteral repletion is often necessary because yearly requirements may exceed 2 g. The scheduled (i.e., weekly or monthly maintenance dosing) supplementation of parenteral iron is controversial and carries with it the theoretical risk of tissue and vascular damage mediated by toxic free radicals generated from transiently increased free iron levels. Similarly, raising the target levels for iron repletion (ferritin of 100 ng/ml and transferrin saturation of 20%) may enhance responsiveness to erythropoietin or darbepoetin alfa but carries the risk of iron toxicity. It has been suggested that intensive care unit patients not receive iron supplementation because of the concern that it would facilitate the growth of certain microorganisms.

ZINC. Zinc may become deficient in patients with advanced renal insufficiency because of decreased intake and absorption. This can be one of many causes of dysgeusia, alopecia, or impotence, and these may at least partially respond to zinc supplementation. Excess zinc supplementation may not be desirable for several reasons. Zinc can antagonize copper absorption and result in sideroblastic anemia. Parenteral zinc supplementation can exacerbate the mild acute-phase reaction in intensive care unit patients, as evidenced by a significantly higher febrile response.

Vitamins

Vitamin nutrition is complex in renal patients because some of these nutrients are deficient, whereas others can accumulate to the point of toxicity. The fat-soluble vitamins (A, E, and K) do not require supplementation, and excess vitamin A or vitamin K can be toxic in dialysis patients. Vitamin D deficiency is of great concern and is discussed elsewhere (see Chapter 18). The water-soluble vitamins, however, can become deficient because of losses into dialysate and decreased availability from the restricted diet, anorexia, or abnormal metabolism. For most water-soluble vitamins, supplementation should be 100% of the dietary reference intake (DRI). Vitamin C is not supplemented beyond the normal recommended daily requirement because its metabolite (oxalate) accumulates and contributes to secondary oxalosis in dialysis patients. An association between high levels of homocysteine and vascular morbidity (stroke, coronary artery disease, peripheral vascular disease) has recently emerged. Homocysteine levels rise with advancing renal failure and persist after initiation of dialysis. Studies have shown that, although supplemental vitamin B_6, vitamin B_{12}, and folate can lower homocysteine levels in healthy patients, these agents have a very attenuated effect in the end-stage renal disease population. It is unclear whether this resistance can be overcome with higher vitamin doses, and results from the use of two to five times the DRI of vitamin B_6 and folate have been disappointing. It has also been suggested that hyperhomocysteinemia may arise from the shrinking of endogenous nitrogen pools as a result of decreased protein intake or stress-induced losses. It has been proposed that increased total homocysteine may result from the attempt of the malnourished or stressed body to preserve methionine homeostasis.

Because of the unique vitamin requirements of renal patients, routine over-the-counter multivitamin preparations are best avoided in preference for those formulated specifically for this population. Typical contents include folic acid, 1 mg; pyridoxine, 10 mg; thiamine, 1.4–1.6 mg; riboflavin, 1.6–2.0 mg; pantothenic acid, 5–10 mg; and ascorbic acid, 60 mg.

CARNITINE. Carnitine is an important intermediate in fatty acid metabolism, and its deficiency has been associated with diverse and poorly characterized organ dysfunctional syndromes, including cardiomyopathy, infections, muscle weakness, and anemia refractory to erythropoietin. Benefits of carnitine repletion are often subjective and have not been shown to correlate well with plasma carnitine levels, as these may not reliably reflect tissue concentrations. If carnitine deficiency is suspected, it can be repleted at a dose of 3–20 mg/kg intravenously after dialysis or approximately 330 mg orally three times per day.

II. Specific Recommendations

A. Acute Renal Failure Patients Managed without Dialysis

Macronutrients

The goal is to provide adequate nutrition without exceeding the patient's excretory capacity and inducing uremic symptoms. Caloric requirements typically increase with the stress of the acute illness to approximately 40–45 Kcal/kg/day, reflecting a rise in the metabolic rate by >20%. These extra calories are provided by a high-carbohydrate diet, because protein must be limited to 0.6–0.8 g (high biologic value) per kg/day. Patients who cannot tolerate oral feeding need parenteral nutrition with essential and nonessential amino acids, dextrose, and lipids. Patients older than 60 years of age often require fewer calories (i.e., 30 Kcal/kg/day).

Micronutrients

Oliguric patients at risk of volume overload need sodium to be restricted to 1–2 g/day and fluid intake decreased to 1.0–1.5 L/day. Depending on the degree of hyperkalemia, potassium may need to be limited to 50 mEq/day or less. Phosphate binders and a phosphorus intake of 0.6–1.0 g (20–33 mmol) per day are necessary to prevent hyperphosphatemia. These restrictions must be liberalized in the setting of excessive nonrenal salt and water losses as well as after the onset of the diuretic phase of acute renal failure. Combination trace elements are generally supplied to renal patients. It must be remembered, however, that the kidney is the primary excretion route for all trace elements, with the exception of copper and manganese, which are primarily excreted through the biliary system.

B. Chronic Renal Failure Patients (Predialysis)

Macronutrients

Because of the risk of malnutrition from chronically restricted diets, careful monitoring with the assistance of a clinical nutritionist is necessary. Clinical studies have suggested that low-protein diets have a small benefit in slowing the decline of renal function in patients with moderate renal insufficiency. It is recommended that the daily protein intake be decreased to 0.6–0.8 g/kg with a diet containing approximately 35 Kcal/kg/day. Compliance with the diet can be assessed by periodically measuring the urine urea nitrogen appearance rate, as previously described. The nonprotein calories are provided by fats (such as poly- or monounsaturated vegetable oils) and simple carbohydrates. However, diabetic patients may benefit from the use of complex carbohydrates. Once the glomerular filtration rate has fallen below approximately 15 ml/min, a 0.6- to 0.8-g protein/kg/day diet clearly minimizes uremic symptoms and permits a brief delay in the initiation of dialysis to establish appropriate vascular or peritoneal access.

Micronutrients

The degree of salt and water restriction needs to be individualized based on the patient's residual renal function and associated electrolyte disorders (i.e., hyperkalemia, renal tubular acidosis). A daily 2- to 4-g sodium and 50- to 70-mEq potassium diet is often adequate in individuals retaining these salts. When the glomerular filtration rate declines below approximately 50 ml/min, patients benefit from a phosphate restriction of 0.8–1.2 g (25–40 mmol) per day [later decreased to 0.6–0.8 g (20–25 mmol) per day] and phosphate binders, as well as monitoring of intact parathyroid hormone levels and initiating some form of vitamin D therapy as necessary. There is a growing realization that a substantial portion of these patients are deficient in vitamin D and may respond to its repletion, even before needing the more costly 1-hydroxylated analog.

C. Patients with Nephrotic Syndrome

Macronutrients

Patients with the nephrotic syndrome present unique dietary problems because of urinary protein losses, hypoalbuminemia, edema, and hyperlipidemia. Very-high-protein diets are generally ineffective in raising the serum albumin level and may exacerbate the proteinuria. There is recent evidence that dietary protein limited to 0.8 g/kg/day (supplemented with the amount lost in the urine) provides adequate substrate for albumin synthesis and decreases proteinuria. Because of the associated lipid disorders, it is usually necessary to limit cholesterol intake to <200 mg/day with 30% of the dietary calories as fat (2 to 1 polyunsaturated to saturated fat ratio). The remainder of the 35 Kcal/kg/day preferably consists of complex carbohydrates.

Micronutrients

The degree of sodium restriction depends on the magnitude of edema and typically ranges from 2–4 g sodium/day (i.e., a 5-g or 70-mEq sodium chloride diet). Potassium and phosphorus dosing is dependent on glomerular filtration rate.

D. Patients on Hemodialysis

Macronutrients

Once hemodialysis is initiated, there are small protein and amino acid losses into the dialysate, and the dialysis prescription should be adjusted periodically to optimize clearance of nitrogenous waste products. The dietary protein should be liberalized as indicated below, with additional quantities prescribed to compensate for any residual renal losses. The Kidney/Disease Outcomes Quality Initiative guidelines recommend the assessment of dialytic patient dietary protein intake by frequent (usually monthly) measurement of the protein catabolic rate (PCR). This is accomplished by urea kinetic modeling software programs that use blood urea nitrogen levels drawn both after a dialysis session and before the next treatment, as well as the amount of urea nitrogen in a simultaneous collection of any residual urine output. A dietary protein prescription that equals or exceeds the PCR is important to avoid negative nitrogen balance. The minimum PCR should be 0.8 g protein/kg/day, but a target of 1.0–1.2 g/kg/day has been associated with improved survival. In predialysis patients, a calculated spontaneous protein intake of <0.8 g/kg/day may indicate such severe uremic symptoms that it can be used as a criterion to initiate hemodialysis independent of serum creatinine or urea clearance.

Another important parameter to follow is the serum albumin concentration. Because a low serum albumin (especially <3 g/dl) at the commencement of dialytic therapy is associated with high patient morbidity and mortality, it is hoped that these individuals will benefit from very aggressive feeding. A precise evaluation of serum albumin concentration is needed to avoid misinterpreting changes (in the range of 10%) that could be due to positional, circadian, and dilutional factors.

Various palatable dietary supplements are now commercially available for patients unable to consume standard meals because of anorexia, nausea, or vomiting.

Intradialytic parenteral nutrition with solutions of 5–50% dextrose, 10–20% amino acids, and 20% lipids is reserved for those who cannot achieve adequate oral intake. The diet generally contains 35 Kcal/kg/day, of which 35–50% of the calories are from carbohydrates and 30% are from fat (2 to 1 polyunsaturated to saturated fat ratio). Intradialytic administration of carbohydrate should not exceed hepatic oxidative rates (5–7 mg carbohydrate/kg/min in adults or 15–20 mg carbohydrate/kg/min in neonates). Rapid infusion of intravenous lipid over short intervals that are used in intradialytic feeding has been associated with free fatty acid shower, hypertriglyceridemia, and cholecystokinin stimulation (all of which normalize with longer infusion times). Cholesterol intake should be guided by periodic lipoprotein analyses. For anabolic patients gaining weight, calories must be increased with the use of fats and simple carbohydrates.

Critically ill patients in an intensive care setting are, in general, hypermetabolic and have increased caloric requirements, as well as catabolic rates. Serial measurements of the PCR best reflect their nutritional needs because protein requirements can vary widely and may exceed four times their basal values. As parenteral nutrition supplementation often necessitates the administration of large fluid volumes, continuous renal replacement modalities (such as continuous venovenous hemodialysis) are sometimes superior to intermittent hemodialysis to assure volume removal and thereby permit adequate nutrition.

Micronutrients

Sodium, potassium, and water restriction depend on the residual renal function and urine output. Anuric patients typically require a daily restriction of 1.0–1.5 L fluid, 2–3 g (85–130 mEq NaCl) sodium, and 1 mEq/kg potassium. Phosphorus is limited to 0.8–1.0 g (25–32 mmol) per day. Adherence to fluid restriction is important to avoid volume-dependent hypertension and adverse postdialytic symptoms associated with excess fluid removal (such as intradialytic hypotension or cramping).

VITAMINS. Dialysis patients should receive supplements of water-soluble vitamins because of the potential for increased removal of these vitamins, especially during high-flux dialysis. For most water-soluble vitamins, supplementation should be 100% of the DRI. The removal of fat-soluble vitamins by hemodialysis is negligible, and their supplementation is generally not recommended. Exceptions include treatment with vitamin D for renal osteodystrophy and possible supplementation of vitamin K in patients on long-term antibiotics.

E. Patients on Chronic Peritoneal Dialysis

Macronutrients

Malnutrition is a very common problem in peritoneal dialysis patients. Diminished appetite is mainly due to the dialysate, which distends the abdomen, causes intermittent discomfort, and leads to dextrose absorption. The calories from dextrose are significant and can be estimated based on a 70–80% peritoneal absorption rate and 3.4 Kcal/g. For example, 2 L of 4.25% dextrose yields a total of 85 g, of which an estimated 80% (or 68 g) can be absorbed after a long dwell time. This would provide 68 g × 3.4 Kcal/g or approximately 231 Kcal/2 L peritoneal dialysate solution. The advent of newer osmotic agents (i.e., icodextrin) for fluid removal will help avoid the adverse effects from the chronic use of high-dextrose solutions. Protein nutrition is, however, much more of a problem, because in some patients (so-called fast solute transporters), >2 g can be lost with each dialysate exchange. During episodes of peritonitis, the losses can exceed 15 g protein/day. For this reason, patients are placed on a 1.2- to 1.5-g protein/kg/day diet, which is increased during peritonitis. Balancing the types of nutrients to provide a total of 35 Kcal/kg/day is further complicated when fat intake is limited because of hyperlipidemia. Dietary fat is usually reduced to 30% of the prescribed calories, with a 2:1 polyunsaturated to saturated fat ratio. Malnutrition is so common that it has led to the development of aggressive strategies for enteral food supplementation, as well as the use of experimental dialysate solutions containing amino acids. As peritoneal dialysis adequacy targets are better defined, it has become apparent that poor nutritional intake is often due to uremic symptoms associated with an inadequate dialysis prescription. However, to achieve more rigorous solute clearance goals, the use of larger fill volumes can exacerbate early satiety, gastroesophageal reflux symptoms, and anorexia.

Micronutrients

Salt and water balance is less problematic in peritoneal dialysis than in hemodialysis because patients can compensate for their diet by adjusting the type and frequency of peritoneal dialysate exchanges. However, the chronic use of high dextrose concentrations to increase ultrafiltration may worsen the hyperlipidemia. Thus, sodium intake occasionally needs to be limited to 2–4 g/day in 1.0–1.5 L of fluid. Hyperkalemic patients should limit their potassium intake to 1 mEq/kg/day. Hypokalemia occasionally occurs because of significant peritoneal potassium losses when patients fail to meet the protein intake targets, especially with high-volume peritoneal fluid prescriptions. Cautious use of potassium supplementation with frequent monitoring of blood levels may be indicated in these situations. The high-protein prescription makes it difficult to decrease phosphorus to less than approximately 1 g/day.

F. **Kidney Transplant Patients.** Postoperative kidney transplant patients receiving glucocorticoids require close attention to assure that they are receiving increased nutrients. Even if the allograft has initial nonfunction, these patients should receive 1.5 g protein/kg/day, and the increased protein and caloric intake commonly demands more intensive dialytic therapy. Subsequent dietary guidelines depend on the degree of allograft function. Steroid-induced hyperglycemia may limit the permissible simple carbohydrate intake. Calcium intake should be monitored to achieve approximately 1 g/day. Particular attention should be focused on dietary modification for control of hyperlipidemia. In addition, potassium and magnesium intake may need to be adjusted because of the electrolyte imbalances associated with immunosuppressive therapy (i.e., cyclosporine and hyperkalemia/hypomagnesemia; mycophenolate and hypophosphatemia; tacrolimus and hypercalcemia/hyperkalemia).

III. **Summary.** Nutrition in the renal failure patient must be carefully assessed, prescribed, and monitored to minimize morbidity and mortality. Synthetic amino acids or protein must be empirically adjusted in a dose of 0.6–1.7 g protein/kg/day depending on the patient and, if used, the dialytic procedure. Energy mix can be most scientifically measured using indirect calorimetry for both the ambulatory and the hospitalized patient in the range of 30–45 Kcal/kg/day. Much remains to be learned about preferred carbohydrate sources (i.e., fructose, glycerol, or xylitol, which are associated with different insulin actions) and fat sources (i.e., polyunsaturated versus saturated ratios, omega-6 versus omega-3 ratios).

An empiric approach is similarly used for micronutrient supplementation. After acid–base assessment, the salt is selected, and electrolytes are dosed depending on tolerance.

Deficiencies of chromium (hyperglycemia), selenium (muscle pain, cardiomyopathy, low triiodothyronine), and zinc (alopecia, delayed wound healing, depression) are dosed as per symptomatology and loss quantification, whereas copper and manganese are primarily excreted through the biliary system. Iron is generally not used or needed with recombinant erythropoietin or darbepoetin therapy in the critically ill renal patient. Trace elements and vitamins can generally be dosed as per the DRI (which is the oral requirement). Fat-soluble vitamin supplementation can be deleterious (i.e., vitamins A and K are osteolytic) and is, as possible, avoided in the renal failure patient.

IV. Suggested Readings

Adequacy of dialysis and nutrition in continuous peritoneal dialysis: association with clinical outcomes. Canada-USA (CANUSA) Peritoneal Dialysis Study Group. *J Am Soc Nephrol* 1996;7:198–207.

Collins AJ, Roberts TL, St. Peter WL, et al. United States Renal Data System assessment of the impact of the National Kidney Foundation-Dialysis Outcomes Quality Initiative guidelines. *Am J Kidney Dis* 2002;39:784–795.

Hoy WE, Sargent JA, Freeman RB, et al. The influence of glucocorticoid dose on protein catabolism after renal transplantation. *Am J Med Sci* 1986;291:241–247.

Ingenbleek Y, Hardillier E, Jung L. Subclinical protein malnutrition is a determinant of hyperhomocysteinemia. *Nutrition* 2002;18:40–46.

Kalantar-Zadeh K, Kleiner M, Dunne E, et al. A modified quantitative subjective global assessment of nutrition for dialysis patients. *Nephrol Dial Transplant* 1999;14:1732–1738.

Klahr S, Levey AS, Beck GJ, et al. The effects of dietary protein restriction and blood-pressure control on the progression of chronic renal disease. *N Engl J Med* 1994;330:877–884.

Leverve X, Barnoud D. Stress metabolism and nutritional support in acute renal failure. *Kidney Int* 1998;53[Suppl 66]:S62–S66.

Levey AS, Greene T, Beck GJ, et al. Dietary protein restriction and the progression of chronic renal disease: what have all of the results of the MDRD study shown? Modification of Diet in Renal Disease Study group. *J Am Soc Nephrol* 1999;10[Suppl 11]:2426–2439.

Mitch WE. Dietary protein restriction in chronic renal failure: nutritional efficacy, compliance and progression of renal insufficiency. *J Am Soc Nephrol* 1991;2[Suppl 4]:823–831.

National Kidney Foundation Kidney/Disease Outcomes Quality Initiative (K/DOQI) guidelines 2000. Clinical practice guidelines for nutrition in chronic renal failure. National Kidney Foundation Web site: http://www.kidney.org/professionals/kdoqi/guidelines_updates/doqi_nut.html.

Nutrition Work Group: Clinical practice guidelines for nutrition in chronic renal failure. *Am J Kidney Dis* 2000;35:S36–S37.

Rocco MV, Makoff R. Appropriate vitamin therapy for dialysis patients. *Semin Dial* 1997;10:272–277.

Index

Note: Page numbers followed by *t* indicate tables; page numbers followed by *f* indicate figures.